AF687080

Clinical Scenarios in Urologic Surgery

Clinical Scenarios in Urologic Surgery

Editor: Brynn McKenzie

AMERICAN
MEDICAL PUBLISHERS
www.americanmedicalpublishers.com

AMERICAN
MEDICAL PUBLISHERS
www.americanmedicalpublishers.com

Cataloging-in-Publication Data

Clinical scenarios in urologic surgery / edited by Brynn McKenzie.
p. cm.
Includes bibliographical references and index.
ISBN 979-8-88740-011-2
1. Genitourinary organs--Surgery. 2. Urinary organs--Surgery. 3. Urinary organs--Diseases--Treatment.
4. Urology. 5. Surgery, Operative. I. McKenzie, Brynn.
RD571 .C55 2023
61746--dc23

© American Medical Publishers, 2023

American Medical Publishers,
41 Flatbush Avenue,
1st Floor, New York,
NY 11217, USA

ISBN 979-8-88740-011-2 (Hardback)

This book contains information obtained from authentic and highly regarded sources. Copyright for all individual chapters remain with the respective authors as indicated. All chapters are published with permission under the Creative Commons Attribution License or equivalent. A wide variety of references are listed. Permission and sources are indicated; for detailed attributions, please refer to the permissions page and list of contributors. Reasonable efforts have been made to publish reliable data and information, but the authors, editors and publisher cannot assume any responsibility for the validity of all materials or the consequences of their use.

Trademark Notice: Registered trademark of products or corporate names are used only for explanation and identification without intent to infringe.

Contents

Preface

This book has been an outcome of determined endeavour from a group of educationists in the field. The primary objective was to involve a broad spectrum of professionals from diverse cultural background involved in the field for developing new researches. The book not only targets students but also scholars pursuing higher research for further enhancement of the theoretical and practical applications of the subject.

Urologic surgery combines procedures for the urogenital, colon and gynecological organs in the pelvis, with the goal of treating malignancies, dysfunction, blockages and inflammatory conditions. It is frequently required for conditions, such as chronic digestive and urologic disorders, spinal cord injury, pelvic organ injuries as well as prostate infections and inflammations. Common urologic procedures include bladder surgery, testicular surgery, renal surgery, ureter surgery, urethra surgery, prostatic surgery, etc. Major urologic surgeries encompass implantation and diversion surgeries. It also includes partial and radical resections for benign and malignant diseases. The risk of urologic surgery varies according to the surgical technique, as well as the extent to which organ has been damaged. This book aims to understand the clinical perspectives of urologic surgery. It presents researches and studies performed by experts across the globe. The extensive content of this book provides the readers with a thorough understanding of the subject.

It was an honour to edit such a profound book and also a challenging task to compile and examine all the relevant data for accuracy and originality. I wish to acknowledge the efforts of the contributors for submitting such brilliant and diverse chapters in the field and for endlessly working for the completion of the book. Last, but not the least; I thank my family for being a constant source of support in all my research endeavours.

Editor

1

Effect of prostate gland weight on the surgical and oncological outcomes of extraperitoneal robot-assisted radical prostatectomy

Min Seok Kim[1], Won Sik Jang[1], Doo Yong Chung[1], Dong Hoon Koh[1], Jong Soo Lee[1], Hyeok Jun Goh[1] and Young Deuk Choi[2*]

Abstract

Background: Robot-assisted radical prostatectomy (RARP) is performed by urologists as one of the surgical procedures for treating prostate cancer. Numerous studies have been published with regard to the impact of prostate weight on performing RARP but were limited by the insufficient number of patients and use of the transperitoneal approach. This study aimed to determine the effect of prostate gland weight on the surgical and short-term oncological outcomes of RARP using the extraperitoneal approach.

Methods: In total, 1168 patients who underwent extraperitoneal RARP (EP-RARP) performed by a single surgeon at Yonsei University Severance Hospital between May 2009 and May 2016 were included in the study. The patients were divided into 4 groups according to the prostate weight measured by transrectal ultrasonography preoperatively. Intraoperative and postoperative outcomes were analyzed retrospectively. One-way analysis of variance and the chi-square test were used in the statistical analyses.

Results: Age, the Gleason score, clinical stage, and pathological stage were significantly different. Patients with a larger prostate size had a longer console time and higher estimated blood loss ($P < 0.05$). There were no significant differences between the 4 groups in length of hospital stay, duration of catheterization, blood transfusion, body mass index, prostate-specific antigen (PSA) level, history of abdominal surgery, intraoperative complications, positive surgical margin, incidence of lymphocele, and PSA recurrence after 1 year.

Conclusions: The console time and estimated blood loss were significantly increased with a larger prostate size. However, there were no significant differences in the oncologic outcome and intraoperative complications, suggesting that EP-RARP requires meticulous bleeding control in patients with a prostate weighing > 75 g, and if appropriate management is implemented for blood loss intraoperatively, EP-RARP can be performed regardless of the prostate size.

Keywords: Radical prostatectomy, Prostate weight, Robot, Prostate cancer

* Correspondence: youngd74@yuhs.ac
[2]Department of Urology, Severance Hospital, Urological Science Institute, Yonsei University College of Medicine, 50-1, Yonsei-ro, Seodaemun-gu, Seoul 03722, Republic of Korea
Full list of author information is available at the end of the article

Background

Since Blinder and Kramer first performed robot-assisted radical prostatectomy (RARP) in 2000, RARP has been performed by numerous urologists as one of the surgical procedures for treating prostate cancer (PCa) [1]. Several studies comparing the operative outcomes of RARP with those of open radical prostatectomy (ORP) have been published and showed no significant differences in oncologic and functional outcomes, and better outcomes for bleeding in RARP [2–4].

Among the several factors affecting radical prostatectomy (RP), prostate weight has been reported by many studies. According to the studies on the impact of prostate weight on the operative outcomes of ORP, the larger the prostate size, the greater the risk of blood loss and blood transfusion, and the smaller the prostate size, the greater is the incidence of a positive surgical margin [5]. In laparoscopic RP, similar to what is observed in ORP, there is proportionate increase in the amount of bleeding as the prostate enlarges in size, and the smaller the prostate size, the higher the incidence of a positive margin [6]. Numerous studies have been published on the impact of prostate weight on RARP. However, there were limitations to these studies in that the number of patients was insufficient and most surgical methods were performed using the transperitoneal approach [7–12]. Generally, the operative space is narrower in the extraperitoneal approach than in the transperitoneal approach. Thus, it may be more difficult to perform RP using the extraperitoneal approach than to perform RP using the transperitoneal approach in the case of a larger prostate size.

Consequently, we aimed to determine whether the prostate size affects perioperative or oncological outcomes when the extraperitoneal approach is used. We retrospectively analyzed 1168 patients who underwent RARP using the extraperitoneal approach performed by a single surgeon. In this paper, we evaluated the effect of prostate gland weight on the surgical and short-term oncological outcomes of RARP performed using the extraperitoneal approach.

Methods

After institutional review board approval (approval number: YUHS 4–2018-0555) was obtained, we retrospectively analyzed 1509 patients with PCa who underwent extraperitoneal RARP (EP-RARP) performed by a single surgeon in Yonsei University Severance Hospital between May 2009 and May 2016. In total, 1168 patients were included after excluding patients with inadequate medical records and suspected metastasis (clinical T4 or M1) on preoperative magnetic resonance imaging (MRI) of the prostate or whole body bone scan prior to surgery for prostate cancer. The operator was an expert surgeon who had previously performed 250 cases of RARP [13]. The patients were divided into 4 groups (group 1: < 25 g, group 2: 25–50 g, group 3: 51–75 g, and group 4: > 75 g) according to the prostate weight measured by transrectal ultrasonography preoperatively. The prostate weight was calculated using the following formula: height × length × width × π/6. The clinical stage was classified according to TNM staging, which was established by the American Joint Committee on Cancer in 2010 using preoperative pelvic magnetic resonance imaging and whole-body bone scanning [14]. Transfusion records were included in all cases intraoperatively and during hospitalization. Prostate-specific antigen (PSA) recurrence was defined as a continuous increase in the PSA level of 0.2 or more after 1 year [15].

Operative technique

All RPs were performed using the extraperitoneal approach with the da Vinci Surgical System (Intuitive Surgical, Sunnyvale, CA, USA). The operation was performed using the same procedure as previously reported [16]. Six ports (4 robot arm ports and 2 assistant ports) were used for RARP. A 1.5-cm vertical infraumbilical incision was made, exposing the anterior rectus sheath. The anterior rectus sheath was incised, and the rectus abdominis muscle was swept. Then, an extraperitoneal space was created using blunt finger dissection. A PDB balloon dilator (Tyco, Princeton, NJ, USA) was used to expand the extraperitoneal cavity. A 5-mm suction port was inserted into the left upper side of the umbilicus using the left index finger. A 12-mm camera port was inserted into the infraumbilical incision site, and an 8-mm port was placed 8 cm away from the umbilicus in both directions. A 12-mm assistant port was inserted 2 cm above the left anterior superior iliac spine, and an 8-mm port was inserted 2 cm above the right anterior superior iliac spine. The endopelvic fascia was dissected. The prostatic-vesical junction was identified, and the proximal urethra was exposed. The vas deferens and seminal vesicles were separated from Denonvilliers' fascia. The dorsal vein complex was resected without ligation, and the distal urethra was exposed. The prostate apex was separated from the apical urethra and Denonvilliers' fascia. Both vascular pedicles were resected, and the prostate was completely dissected with the prostate specimen placed inside the entrapment bag (Lap-bag, Sejong Med, Paju, Korea). Vesicourethral anastomosis was performed using Monosyn 3–0 double arm sutures (Aesculap, Center Valley, PA, USA). In a posterior direction from the bladder, a continuous suture was started 3 times on the right side and 3 times on the left side. Then, an 18-French Foley catheter was inserted into the bladder. Suturing was performed twice on both sides. After approximating the puboprostatic collar and bladder, a knot was made.

Histopathological analysis of the specimens

All prostate specimens were processed in accordance with a well-established protocol and reviewed by a pathologist [17]. The pathologist recorded the tumor location, extracapsular extension (ECE), seminal vesicle invasion (SVI), vas invasion, pathological Gleason score, pathological stage, and positive surgical margin. A positive surgical margin was defined as a cancer gland reaching the inked margin.

Statistical analysis

Statistical analysis was performed using SPSS 23 software (IBM Corp., Armonk, NY, USA). One-way analysis of variance was used for normally distributed continuous data. The chi-square test was used for categorical data. Parameters with a P-value < 0.05 were considered statistically significant.

Results

Of the 1168 patients, 157 were in group 1, 824 in group 2, 149 in group 3, and 38 in group 4. Patient characteristics are shown in Table 1. The larger the prostate, the older the patient's age ($P < 0.001$). There were no significant differences in history of abdominal surgery, body mass index, and PSA level in terms of prostate weight. The larger the prostate, the lower the Gleason score ($P < 0.05$) and higher the incidence of clinical T1 stage cancer ($P < 0.05$).

Perioperative characteristics are presented in Table 2. Length of hospital stay and duration of catheterization were not correlated with prostate weight, and the incidence of lymphocele was not significantly correlated with prostate weight. The mean console time and mean estimated blood loss were significantly increased with increasing prostate weight ($P < 0.001$). Blood transfusion, rectal injury, lymph node dissection, and nerve sparing were not associated with prostate weight. There were no other complications, except for rectal injury intraoperatively, and there were no open conversions.

Table 3 shows the pathologic outcomes. SVI and a positive surgical margin were not significantly associated with prostate weight. There was no significant difference in PSA recurrence after 1 year in terms of prostate weight. ECE significantly increased as the prostate weight decreased ($P < 0.05$), and in the pathologic stage, T2 increased as the prostate weight increased ($P < 0.001$).

Discussion

This study's results showed that EP-RARP is as feasible as transperitoneal RARP (TP-RARP) regardless of the prostate weight. In our study, the greater the prostate weight, the lower the Gleason score and lower the T stage. This result is thought to be the effect of a lead time bias, as described by Link et al. [7] Benign prostatic hyperplasia (BPH) can lead to an increased PSA level, so patients with BPH are more likely to be diagnosed at a relatively early stage; in addition, prostate biopsy is performed more often in patients with BPH than in those without BPH [18]. In our study, ECE significantly increased in patients with a lower prostate

Table 1 Patient characteristics classified according to the prostate weight

Prostate weight measured by TRUS (g)	< 25 g	25–50 g	51–75 g	> 75 g	P-value
Patients (n)	157	824	149	38	
Mean age (years)	64.1 ± 8.7	64.6 ± 7.4	65.9 ± 5.8	70.2 ± 5.4	< 0.001
Mean BMI (kg/m^2)	23.8 ± 2.9	24.2 ± 2.6	25.1 ± 8.4	25.1 ± 3.4	0.07
Mean PSA level (ng/ml)	10.1 ± 9.5	10.5 ± 8.7	10.9 ± 8.6	15.9 ± 12.6	0.08
Prior abdominal surgery	29 (18.5%)	109 (13.2%)	26 (17.4%)	6 (15.8%)	0.55
Mean prostate weight by TRUS (g)	16.8 ± 2.9	31.0 ± 6.7	53.6 ± 6.7	92.1 ± 23.9	< 0.001
Mean pathologic prostate weight (g)	22.4 ± 5.2	35.4 ± 9.4	55.7 ± 10.1	81.2 ± 24.2	< 0.001
Preoperative Gleason score					0.03
2–6	57 (36.3%)	332 (40.3%)	80 (53.7%)	16 (42.1%)	
7	62 (39.5%)	274 (33.3%)	43 (28.9%)	11 (28.9%)	
8–10	38 (24.2%)	218 (26.5%)	26 (17.4%)	11 (28.9%)	
Clinical stage					0.02
T1	35 (22.3%)	152 (18.4%)	43 (28.9%)	14 (36.8%)	
T2	77 (49.0%)	430 (52.2%)	74 (49.7%)	14 (36.8%)	
T3	45 (28.7%)	242 (29.4%)	32 (21.5%)	10 (26.3%)	

TRUS transrectal ultrasonography, *BMI* body mass index, *PSA* prostate-specific antigen

Table 2 Perioperative characteristics of patients classified according to the prostate weight

Prostate weight measured by TRUS (g)	< 25 g	25–50 g	51–75 g	> 75 g	*P*-value
Patients (n)	157	824	149	38	
Length of hospital stay (days)	5.5 ± 2.0	5.3 ± 2.0	5.1 ± 1.8	5.8 ± 2.9	0.30
Duration of catheterization (days)	11.0 ± 1.9	10.9 ± 2.0	11.1 ± 2.1	10.9 ± 1.8	0.49
Mean console time (min)	45.1 ± 14.8	47.0 ± 13.8	49.5 ± 14.1	61.7 ± 18.3	< 0.001
Mean estimated blood loss (ml)	347 ± 250	386 ± 262	456 ± 303	646 ± 423	< 0.001
Transfusion (n)	2 (1.3%)	2 (0.2%)	1 (0.7%)	1 (2.6%)	0.67
Rectal injury	1 (0.6%)	0 (0.0%)	2 (1.3%)	0 (0.0%)	0.44
Incidence of lymphocele	5 (3.2%)	31 (3.8%)	4 (2.7%)	2 (5.3%)	0.89
Lymph node dissection					0.88
No	115 (73.2%)	597 (72.5%)	114 (76.5%)	26 (68.4%)	
Yes	42 (26.8%)	227 (27.5%)	35 (23.5%)	12 (31.6%)	
Nerve sparing					0.89
None	8 (5.1%)	38 (4.6%)	5 (3.4%)	3 (7.9%)	
Unilateral	2 (11.1%)	14 (1.7%)	2 (1.3%)	0 (0.0%)	
Bilateral	147 (93.6%)	772 (93.7%)	142 (95.3%)	35 (92.1%)	

TRUS, transrectal ultrasonography

weight, and the T stage was increased more in patients with a low prostate weight than in those with a high prostate weight. Our results are consistent with those of previous studies. Briganti et al. [19] reported that PCa in smaller glands is more aggressive and therefore there are higher rates of ECE than when PCa involves larger glands. Hong et al. [20] reported that prostate size is not useful in predicting tumor recurrence, but it is associated with the progression of PCa. These explanations have not yet been clearly elucidated. However, several hypotheses have been developed, including the following. First, men with a small prostate secrete less testosterone. Low testosterone levels are associated with progressive PCa [21, 22]. Second, the benign tissues of BPH play an inhibitory role in cancer cell progression [21, 23].

Table 3 Pathologic outcomes of patients classified according to the prostate weight

Prostate weight measured by TRUS (g)	< 25 g	25–50 g	51–75 g	> 75 g	*P*-value
Patients (n)	157	824	149	38	
Extracapsular extension					0.003
Negative	87 (55.4%)	430 (52.2%)	104 (69.8%)	26 (68.4%)	
Positive	70 (44.6%)	394 (47.8%)	45 (30.2%)	12 (31.6%)	
Seminal vesicle invasion					0.88
Negative	146 (93.0%)	742 (90.0%)	143 (96.0%)	32 (84.2%)	
Positive	11 (7.0%)	82 (10.0%)	6 (4.0%)	105 (9.0%)	
Pathological Gleason score					0.01
3–6	35 (22.3%)	201 (24.4%)	62 (41.6%)	12 (31.6%)	
7	86 (54.8%)	419 (50.8%)	57 (38.3%)	17 (44.7%)	
8–10	36 (22.9%)	204 (24.8%)	30 (20.1%)	9 (23.7%)	
Pathological stage					0.01
T2	85 (54.1%)	434 (52.7%)	103 (69.1%)	25 (65.8%)	
T3	72 (45.9%)	379 (46.0%)	46 (30.9%)	12 (31.6%)	
T4	0 (0.0%)	11 (1.3%)	0 (0.0%)	1 (2.6%)	
Positive surgical margin	60 (38.2%)	351 (42.6%)	51 (34.2%)	10 (26.3%)	0.12
PSA recurrence (1 year)	16 (10.2%)	127 (15.4%)	14 (9.4%)	4 (10.5%)	0.65

TRUS transrectal ultrasonography

In our study, there was no correlation between the prostate size and a positive surgical margin in RARP. However, Allaparthi et al. [8] and Link et al. [7] reported that the lower the prostate weight, the more positive the surgical margin is. This is because a small-sized prostate has a higher cancer density than a large-sized prostate [24].

The mean console time and mean estimated blood loss were significantly increased with increasing prostate weight in our study. Boylu et al. [9] and Yasui et al. [10] reported that the greater the prostate weight, the longer the operative time, and Hirasawa et al. [11] reported that the greater the prostate weight, the more the blood loss, as it is thought that men with enlarged prostate glands usually have more vascularity and broader resection margins. However, the transfusion rate was not significantly associated with the prostate weight, so even though there is a greater amount of bleeding with a greater prostate weight, it would not be clinically meaningful. Surgeons feel technically challenged when operating on an enlarged prostate because BPH affects the structure of the prostate in terms of its size and shape [25]. As mentioned previously, the large amount of bleeding and broad resection margin may have prolonged the console time.

Numerous studies have been published about the impact of the prostate weight on performing RARP, but the surgical technique most commonly used was the transperitoneal approach. Most studies reported that using the transperitoneal approach was feasible regardless of the prostate weight [7–12].

EP-RARP is associated with a lower incidence of bowel injury and postoperative hernia compared to TP-RARP, and there are no reports of symptoms of peritoneal irritation caused by gas, urinary leakage, or bleeding. However, there is a disadvantage in that the operative space is narrow and accompanied by difficulty in obtaining operative visibility [16, 26]. Because of these advantages and disadvantages, we felt that it was necessary to study the extraperitoneal approach.

According to previous studies conducted using the extraperitoneal approach, Boczko et al. [27] reported that blood loss is associated with a greater prostate weight. Allaparthi et al. [8] reported that the prostate weight is associated with a positive surgical margin. However, the study by Boczko et al. has some limitations. In particular, the statistical reliability of the data was not good, and the effect of the small prostate was not determined because the prostate weight was divided into only 2 categories [27]. The study by Allaparthi et al. was limited in terms of statistical reliability of the data because the numbers of patients with a prostate weight < 30 g and > 80 g were small [8]. In comparison, our study analyzed more patients than those of prior studies on the extraperitoneal approach and had an increased power of data analysis.

There are some limitations to our study. First, the number of patients was higher than that of prior studies, but the number of patients with a prostate weight > 70 g was relatively small compared to that in the other groups. Second, the follow-up period was relatively short (12 months), so the long-term evaluation of biochemical recurrence was not possible. Third, as all procedures were performed by a single expert surgeon, it was difficult to generalize the results. Finally, we did not perform multiple linear regression analyses of factors associated with operative outcomes. If we had performed it, we would have been able to increase the validity of the study.

Conclusions

We found that the prostate size did not significantly affect the oncologic outcomes or surgical complications in performing EP-RARP. There was also no significant difference in the length of hospital stay and duration of catheterization. In this study, the size of the prostate was correlated with the amount of estimated blood loss and console time. However, there were no statistically significant negative operative outcomes, such as transfusion, longer hospitalization, longer catheterization, operative complications, or oncologic outcomes due to increased estimated blood loss. Therefore, we concluded that we could perform EP-RARP safely regardless of the size of the prostate.

Abbreviations

BPH: benign prostatic hyperplasia; ECE: extracapsular extension; EP-RARP: extraperitoneal robot-assisted radical prostatectomy; ORP: open radical prostatectomy; PCa: prostate cancer; PSA: prostate-specific antigen; RARP: robot-assisted radical prostatectomy; RP: radical prostatectomy; SVI: seminal vesicle invasion; TP-RARP: transperitoneal robot-assisted radical prostatectomy

Acknowledgments

Not applicable.

Author details

[1]Department of Urology and Urological Science Institute, Yonsei University College of Medicine, 50-1, Yonsei-ro, Seodaemun-gu, Seoul 03722, Republic of Korea. [2]Department of Urology, Severance Hospital, Urological Science Institute, Yonsei University College of Medicine, 50-1, Yonsei-ro, Seodaemun-gu, Seoul 03722, Republic of Korea.

References

1. Binder J, Kramer W. Robotically-assisted laparoscopic radical prostatectomy. BJU Int. 2001;87(4):408–10.
2. De Carlo F, Celestino F, Verri C, Masedu F, Liberati E, Di Stasi SM. Retropubic, laparoscopic, and robot-assisted radical prostatectomy: surgical, oncological, and functional outcomes: a systematic review. Urol Int. 2014;93(4):373–83.
3. Ficarra V, Novara G, Artibani W, Cestari A, Galfano A, Graefen M, et al. Retropubic, laparoscopic, and robot-assisted radical prostatectomy: a systematic review and cumulative analysis of comparative studies. Eur Urol. 2009;55(5):1037–63.
4. Coelho RF, Rocco B, Patel MB, Orvieto MA, Chauhan S, Ficarra V, et al. Retropubic, laparoscopic, and robot-assisted radical prostatectomy: a critical review of outcomes reported by high-volume centers. J Endourol. 2010; 24(12):2003–15.

5. Hsu EI, Hong EK, Lepor H. Influence of body weight and prostate volume on intraoperative, perioperative, and postoperative outcomes after radical retropubic prostatectomy1. Urology. 2003;61(3):601–6.
6. Frota R, Turna B, Santos BMR, Lin YC, Gill IS, Aron M. The effect of prostate weight on the outcomes of laparoscopic radical prostatectomy. BJU Int. 2008;101(5):589–93.
7. Link BA, Nelson R, Josephson DY, Yoshida JS, Crocitto LE, Kawachi MH, et al. The impact of prostate gland weight in robot assisted laparoscopic radical prostatectomy. J Urol. 2008;180(3):928–32.
8. Allaparthi SB, Hoang T, Dhanani NN, Tuerk IA. Significance of prostate weight on peri and postoperative outcomes of robot assisted laparoscopic extraperitoneal radical prostatectomy. Can J Urol. 2010;17(5):5383–9.
9. Boylu U, Turan T, Başataç C, Önol FF, Gümüş E. The effect of prostate weight on the outcomes of robot-assisted radical prostatectomy. Turkish J Urol. 2013;39(4):209.
10. Yasui T, Tozawa K, Kurokawa S, Okada A, Mizuno K, Umemoto Y, et al. Impact of prostate weight on perioperative outcomes of robot-assisted laparoscopic prostatectomy with a posterior approach to the seminal vesicle. BMC Urol. 2014;14(1):6.
11. Hirasawa Y, Ohno Y, Nakashima J, Shimodaira K, Hashimoto T, Gondo T, et al. Impact of a preoperatively estimated prostate volume using transrectal ultrasonography on surgical and oncological outcomes in a single surgeon's experience with robot-assisted radical prostatectomy. Surg Endosc. 2016;30(9):3702–8.
12. Labanaris AP, Zugor V, Witt JH. Robot-assisted radical prostatectomy in patients with a pathologic prostate specimen weight≥ 100 grams versus≤ 50 grams: surgical, oncologic and short-term functional outcomes. Urol Int. 2013;90(1):24–30.
13. Abboudi H, Khan MS, Guru KA, Froghi S, De Win G, Van Poppel H, et al. Learning curves for urological procedures: a systematic review. BJU Int. 2014;114(4):617–29.
14. Edge SB, Compton CC. The American joint committee on Cancer: the 7th edition of the AJCC cancer staging manual and the future of TNM. Ann Surg Oncol. 2010;17(6):1471–4.
15. Stephenson AJ, Kattan MW, Eastham JA, Dotan ZA, Bianco FJ Jr, Lilja H, et al. Defining biochemical recurrence of prostate cancer after radical prostatectomy: a proposal for a standardized definition. J Clin Oncol. 2006; 24(24):3973–8.
16. Lee YS, Ham WS, Kim WT, Joo HJ, Lee JS, Choi YD. Comparison of extraperitoneal and transperitoneal robot-assisted radical prostatectomy in prostate cancer: a single surgeon's experience. Korean J Urol. 2009;50(3):251–5.
17. Egevad L. Handling of radical prostatectomy specimens. Histopathology. 2012;60(1):118–24.
18. Kojima M, Troncoso P, Babaian RJ. Influence of noncancerous prostatic tissue volume on prostate-specific antigen. Urology. 1998;51(2):293–9.
19. Briganti A, Chun FK-H, Suardi N, Gallina A, Walz J, Graefen M, et al. Prostate volume and adverse prostate cancer features: fact not artifact. Eur J Cancer. 2007;43(18):2669–77.
20. Hong SK, Poon BY, Sjoberg DD, Scardino PT, Eastham JA. Prostate size and adverse pathologic features in men undergoing radical prostatectomy. Urology. 2014;84(1):153–7.
21. Min SH, Park YH, Lee SB, Ku JH, Kwak C, Kim HH. Impact of prostate size on pathologic outcomes and prognosis after radical prostatectomy. Korean J Urol. 2012;53(7):463–6.
22. Iversen P, Rasmussen F, Christensen IJ. Serum testosterone as a prognostic factor in patients with advanced prostatic carcinoma. Scand J Urol Nephrol Suppl. 1994;157:41–7.
23. Msezane LP, Gofrit ON, Lin S, Shalhav AL, Zagaja GP, Zorn KC. Prostate weight: an independent predictor for positive surgical margins during robotic-assisted laparoscopic radical prostatectomy. Can J Urol. 2007; 14(5):3697–701.
24. Yadav R, Tu JJ, Jhaveri J, Leung RA, Rao S, Tewari AK. Prostate volume and the incidence of extraprostatic extension: is there a relation? J Endourol. 2009;23(3):383–6.
25. Myers RP. Practical surgical anatomy for radical prostatectomy. Urol Clin North Am. 2001;28(3):473–90.
26. Madi R, Daignault S, Wood DP. Extraperitoneal v intraperitoneal robotic prostatectomy: analysis of operative outcomes. J Endourol. 2007;21(12):1553–8.
27. Boczko J, Erturk E, Golijanin D, Madeb R, Patel H, Joseph JV. Impact of prostate size in robot-assisted radical prostatectomy. J Endourol. 2007;21(2):184–8.

2

Extent of positive surgical margins following radical prostatectomy: Impact on biochemical recurrence with long-term follow-up

Yoann Koskas[1*], François Lannes[1], Nicolas Branger[1], Sophie Giusiano[2], Nicolas Guibert[3,5], Géraldine Pignot[4], Jochen Walz[4], Dominique Rossi[1] and Cyrille Bastide[1]

Abstract

Background: To assess the prognostic value of the extent of positive surgical margins (PSM) following radical prostatectomy (RP) on biochemical recurrence (BR) with long-term follow-up.

Methods: This retrospective study analyzed 1275 RPs performed between January 1992 and December 2013 in two university centers in Marseille (France). The inclusion criteria were: follow-up > 24 months, undetectable postoperative prostate-specific antigen (PSA), no seminal vesicle (SV) invasion, no lymph node invasion confirmed by surgery (pN0) or imaging (pNx), and no neoadjuvant or adjuvant treatment. BR was defined by PSA level ≥ 0.2 ng/mL on two successive samples. We included 189 patients, divided into two groups:
- Focal PSM (fPSM): single PSM (sPSM) ≤3 mm;
- Extensive PSM (ePSM): sPSM with linear length > 3 mm or several margins regardless of the length.

Results: The median follow-up was 101 months (18–283) and the median age was 63 years (46–76). BR occurred in only 12.1% (14/115) of cases involving fPSM and in 54.1% (40/74) of cases involving ePSM. In the multivariate model, ePSM patients were significantly associated with increased BR compared to fPSM (hazard ratio [HR] = 6.11; 95% confidence interval [CI] = 3.25–11.49). The ePSM significantly decreased BR-free survival ($p < 0.001$) for every patient and every subgroup (pT2, pT3a, pG ≤6, and pG ≥7). The median BR time following RP was significantly shorter for ePSM patients than fPSM (57.2 vs. 89.2 months $p < 0.001$).

Conclusion: With a median 8-year follow-up, ePSM was strongly associated with BR compared to fPSM. Therefore, it seems legitimate to monitor patients with fPSM. In cases of ePSM, adjuvant treatment appears effective.

Keywords: Prostate cancer, Radical prostatectomy, Biochemical recurrence, Positive surgical margins, Extent, Focal positive surgical margins

Background

The presence of positive surgical margins (PSM) following radical prostatectomy (RP) is a worrying for surgeons and patients alike as it represents an independent biochemical recurrence (BR) risk factor [1–8]. The rate of PSM is 5–30% for organ-confined prostate cancer and 17–65% for locally-advanced cancer [9–11].

* Correspondence: yoann.koskas@gmail.com
[1]Department of Urology, Hopital Nord, Chemin des Bourrely, 13015 Marseille, France
Full list of author information is available at the end of the article

A PSM means incomplete cancer resection and may lead to additional treatment, such as either adjuvant radiotherapy (AR) or chemical or surgical castration. These remedial treatments display side effects and affect patient quality of life [12]. However, despite the evidence that AR significantly reduces the BR risk in locally-advanced cancers [12], the optimal approach concerning PSM remains unclear. The strategy eventually employed varies according to institution, while often left to the surgeon's discretion or simply following each team's habitual practice.

Moreover, there is generally no evaluation of PSM characteristics (size, number, location, and focality) regarding these additional therapeutic decisions. This can be explained by the observation that there is no consensus yet taking into account these factors for the therapeutic decision.

One reason could be the lack of standardization of anatomopathological reports regarding PSM description, and thus a potential lack of information that could be detrimental to the therapeutic decision-making process. The College of American Pathologists recommends referring to the Gleason score of the margin [13].

Nevertheless, there are still no clear recommendations, especially regarding how to act depending on the PSM (length and number) extent. Lake et al. [14] reported that the extent of the margin significantly affects BR-free survival, which is improved in cases of fPSM (length ≤ 3 mm) compared to ePSM (multifocal PSM or length > 3 mm).

In another recent study based on a median 52-month follow-up, Lee et al. [15] demonstrated that ePSM can significantly affect BR-free survival compared to fPSM. It should, however, be noted that their study included patients classified N+ and/or pT3b, which could be confounding factors in the BR assessment. Similarly, Maxeiner et al. [16] reported that multiple PSM and those > 3 mm represented an independent BR factor, whereas these authors likewise included patients with potential confounding factors (N+, PT3b, PT4, or neoadjuvant treatment).

In our study involving a median 5-year follow-up, we sought to assess the BR risk in relation with PSM extent following RP for Stage ≤PT3a patients who had not received any neoadjuvant or adjuvant treatment. We also sought to determine the influence of other BR prognostic factors, such as PSM location within the prostate.

Methods

From January 1992 to December 2013, a total of 1275 patients underwent RP for prostate cancer in two university centers in Marseille (France). Using a prospective database, we retrospectively included patients exhibiting PSM who met the following criteria: follow-up > 18 months, undetectable postoperative PSA, no invasion of the SV, absence of lymph node invasion confirmed by surgery (pN0) or imaging (pNx), and no neoadjuvant or adjuvant treatment. The surgical techniques for RP differed among cases: open RP, laparoscopic RP (LP-RP), and robot-assisted laparoscopy (RALP-RP). Each intervention was conducted by experienced surgeons.

BR was defined as PSA level ≥ 0.2 ng/mL on two successive samples. The anatomopathological examination of all surgical specimens was performed according to the Stanford technique [17] up to 2009, and then as recommended by the ISUP from 2009 onwards [3]. A centralized reading of the slides was performed by the same pathologist. Positive margins were defined as the presence of cancerous tissue in contact with the inked surface of the prostatectomy specimen. Healthy tissue margins were considered negative margins.

The extent of the margin was assessed as follows:

- fPSM: single margin with a linear length ≤ 3 mm present on one cutaway view;
- ePSM: single margin with a linear length > 3 mm present on one cutaway view, single margin (regardless of the length) present on several cutaway views, or multiple margins present on one or more cutaway views.

For each patient, the location of the PSM *vis-a-vis* the prostate was likewise recorded and classified as follows: bladder neck PSM, basis PSM, posterolateral PSM, anterior PSM, and apex PSM. Additionally, the weight and volume of the prostate were listed.

We were then able to evaluate BR-free survival and BR risk depending on the PSM extent and search for other BR risk factors, such as the preoperative PSA level, Gleason score on the specimen, tumor stage (pT), and PSM location.

All statistical analyses were performed using the statistical software R Version 2.5.3. The statistical tests were bilateral and p-values ≤0.05 were considered significant. The comparisons of percentages were performed using the Chi-squared test, comparisons of means using Student's t-test, and comparisons of survival using either the LogRank test for bivariate situations or the Cox model for multivariate situations. Survival curves were plotted according to the Kaplan-Meier method.

Results

Overall, 189 patients exhibiting PSM who met the inclusion criteria were included in the study. The median follow-up was 101 months, while median age and preoperative PSA were 63 and 7.7 ng/mL, respectively. In total, 25% of patients were pT3a, and the remainder in pT2. Only 7% had a Gleason score ≥ 8, the majority (63%) were pG = 7. According to the D'Amico classification, 55% were low-risk, 34.4% intermediate-risk, and only 10.6% high-risk.

No differences regarding Gleason score, pT stage, or surgical technique were observed between the two subgroups. Lymph node dissection was performed on 117 patients (61.9%), whereas the others were classified as cNO based on imaging.

Table 1 Clinical and histological characteristics of patients according to the extent of positive surgical margin (PSM)

	Total cohort n (%)	fPSM n (%)	ePSM n (%)	p
Patients (n)	189	115 (60.9)	74 (39.1)	
Mean age (standard deviation)	71.8 (+/−6.3)	70.3 (+/−7.5)	74.1 (+/−8.3)	0.006
Mean PSA (standard deviation)	8.8 (+/−4.3)	8.1 (+/−3.6)	10.0 (+/−4.9)	0.003
Gleason Score (pG)				0.14
≤ 6	63 (33.3)	43 (37.4)	20 (27)	
7	119 (63)	68 (59.1)	51 (68.9)	
3 + 4	96 (49.2)	57 (49.6)	36 (48.6)	
4 + 3	23 (13.8)	11 (9.6)	15 (20.3)	
≥8	7 (3.7)	4 (3.5)	3 (4)	
pT Stage				0.61
T2a	15 (7.9)	9 (7.8)	6 (8.1)	
T2b	24 (12.7)	16 (13.9)	8 (10.8)	
T2c	101 (53.4)	64 (55.6)	37 (50)	
T3a	49 (25.9)	26 (22.6)	23 (31.1)	
Median follow-up (months)	101.1	95.3	110.3	0.08

fPSM focal positive surgical margin, *ePSM* extensive positive surgical margin, *PSA* prostate-specific antigen

The most often-performed RP technique was open RP (127 patients, 67.7%), with RALP RP performed on 61 patients (32.3%), and LP RP on only one case. The clinical and histological patient characteristics patients have been summarized in Table 1.

BR was observed in only 54 patients (28.6%). In the fPSM group, 14 (12.2%) suffered from recurrence, compared to 40 (54%) in the ePSM group. The clinical and histological features of these patients have been detailed in Table 2.

BR-free survival at 5 years was 86.8% for patients with fPSM versus 49.4% for those with ePSM, and at 8 years 85.1 and 44.8%, respectively (Fig. 1). Patients with ePSM were significantly more likely to develop BR ($p < 0.0001$), regardless of the subgroup. This significant relationship was found even for patients classified as pT3a or pG ≥7, albeit less pronounced.

Table 2 Clinical and histological characteristics of patients exhibiting biochemical recurrence (BR)

	Total PSM	fPSM	ePSM	p
N	54	14	40	
Mean PSA	9.0	6.4	9.5	0.001
pT Stage				
pT2 n (%)	31 (57.4)	9 (64.3)	22 (55.0)	0.081
pT3a n (%)	23 (42.6)	5 (35.7)	18 (45.0)	0.010
Gleason score pG				
pG ≤ 6 n (%)	17 (31.5)	2 (14.3)	15 (37.5)	0.002
pG = 3 + 4 n (%)	19 (35.2)	6 (42.9)	13 (32.5)	0.023
pG = 4 + 3 n (%)	13 (24.0)	4 (28.6)	9 (22.5)	0.097
pG ≥ 8 n (%)	5 (9.3)	2 (14.2)	3 (7.5)	0.174

fPSM focal positive surgical margin, *ePSM* extensive positive surgical margin, *PSA* prostate-specific antigen

In the univariate and multivariate models (Table 3), ePSM was strongly and significantly associated with BR, compared to fPSM (HR = 6.11; 95% CI = 3.25–11.49 on multivariate analysis). There was likewise a link between pT stage and BR occurrence: pT3a stages were associated with a higher risk of recurrence compared to pT2 stages (HR = 2.14; 95% CI = 1.20–3.81 on multivariate analysis). The preoperative PSA > 10 was not significantly associated with BR (HR = 1.33; 95% CI = 0.74–2.39) as well as Gleason score (pG > 6) on multivariate analysis. On univariate analysis, pG = 4 + 3 and pG ≥8 was significantly associated with BR (2.54 [1.23, 5.23] and 2.77 [1.02, 7.52], respectively).

In the multivariate model, an interaction between Gleason score (pG) and the PSM extent was tested, as well as between pT stage and the PSM extent. In both cases, the correlations were found to be not significantly different from 1.This observation suggests that the effect of the PSM extent on BR does not depend on the Gleason score or pT stage.

Concerning the loco-regional and remote evolution of the disease, 1/189 patients with fPSM became metastatic 16 years following RP, while 1 patient became lymph-node metastatic after 6 years.

Median BR time was significantly shorter for patients with ePSM compared to those with fPSM: 89.2 months in the fPSM group versus 57.2 months in the ePSM group.

Regarding the PSM characteris, the most common location was apical, exhibited in 99 patients (53%) The

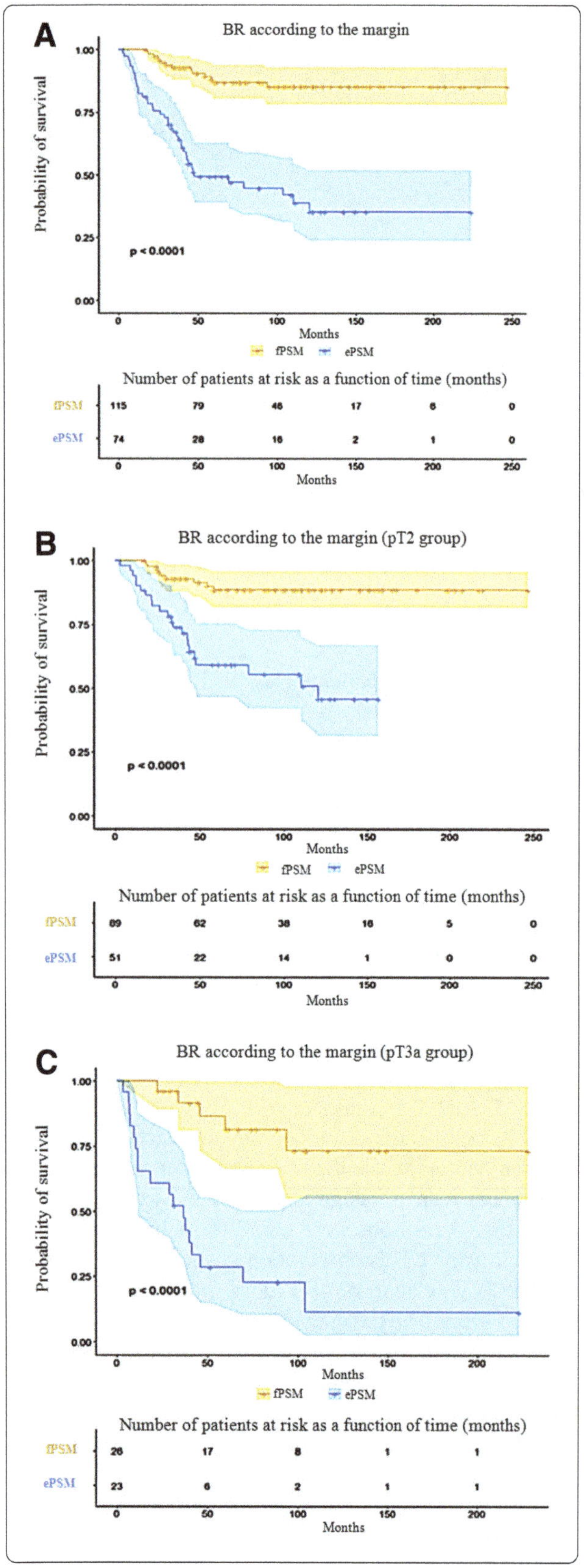

Fig. 1 Kaplan-Meier curves showing biochemical recurrence (BR)-free survival following. **a** All patients. **b** pT2 Stage. **c** pT3a Stage. Legends: fPSM: focal positive surgical margin; ePSM: extensive positive surgical margin

posterolateral location was the second most common, involving 79 patients (42%). For the basal PSM, 37 patients (20%) exhibited this location associated or not with another. Anterior and bladder-neck PSMs were significantly less frequent, with 1.5% exhibiting bladder-neck PSM and 2% anterior PSM. Multiple PSMs significantly decreased BR-free survival compared to single PSM locations.

No single PSMs significantly affected BR-free survival, although basal PSMs tended to decrease BR-free survival compared to the apical and posterolateral PSMs [22-24]

Discussion

To our knowledge, this is the first study with a median follow-up of 8 years that found no association between fPSM and BR in patients who had received no neoadjuvant or adjuvant treatment and exhibited slightly locally-advanced disease (<pT3b and N0).

This long-term data taken from a selected population enabled us to evaluate the PSM on BR. In this multicenter study with an 8-year median follow-up, we demonstrated that men with ePSM following prostatectomy were significantly more likely to develop BR than those with fPSM. Additionnally, the more extended the PSM, the shorter the BR time.

Other studies in the literature specifically analyzed the prognostic value of the PSM extent following prostatectomy for patients followed-up for prostate cancer.

Sooriakumaran et al. [18] analyzed a large series of 189 patients with PSM involving a minimum follow-up of 5 years. These authors reported that patients with PSM > 3 mm had significantly higher risk of developing BR. This study excluded patients who had neoadjuvant or adjuvant treatment, yet did include pT3b patients. This a potential confounding factor. For this reason we have deliberately excluded all potential confounders of RB.

Therefore, we intentionally excluded patients with locally-advanced disease (lymph node or seminal vesicle invasion) in order to better select patients whose BR was most likely to be linked to PSM. For patients with locally-advanced disease, BR is most likely a reflection of micro-metastatic systemic disease, meaning the PSM status in these cases would have a very limited influence on BR [19, 20].

An analysis of a large cohort identifying 498 patients with PSM reinforced this hypothesis [21], demonstrating

Table 3 Univariate and multivariate model and hazard ratio calculations for variables associated with biochemical recurrence

Variables	Univariate		Multivariate	
PSA (PSA > 10 vs ≤ 10)	1.45 (0.82–2.58)	0.205	1.33 (0.74–2.39)	0.339
pT (pT3a vs pT2)	2.58 (1.5–4.44)	< 0.001	2.14 (1.2–3.81)	0.01
pG ≤6	Reference		Reference	
pG = 3 + 4	NS		NS	
pG = 4 + 3	2.54 (1.23–5.23)	0.012	1.15 (0.53–2.47)	0.724
pG ≥8	2.77 (1.02–7.52)	0.046	1.41 (0.5–3.99)	0.513
PSM (ePSM vs fPSM)	6.05 (3.29–11.15)	< 0.001	6.11 (3.25–11.49)	< 0.001

The multivariate model includes all variables in this table, the age when the RP was performed and the year of treatment
HR hazard ratio, *CI* confidence interval, *fPSM* focal positive surgical margin, *ePSM* extensive positive surgical margin, *PSA* prostate-specific antigen

in multivariate analysis that PSM was an independent factor of BR for patients classified as pT2 and pT3a ($p < 0.001$; HR = 3.81; $p = 0.001$; HR = 2.09, respectively), whereas this was not so for pT3b and pT4 patients ($p = 0.196$ and $p = 0.061$, respectively).

All in all, for patients with lymph node or seminal vesicle invasion, the prognosis does not really seem related to PSM changes, but rather to the existence of micro-metastases responsible for the systemic spread of the disease. This is why we excluded these patients from our study.

Moreover, even if this hypothesis proved inaccurate, the postoperative measures would be the same. With or without PSM, it is still recommended to perform adjuvant therapy in patients classified as pT3b and pT4 [12]. It is therefore of little interest to focus on patients with locally-advanced disease in a study of PSM, as long as the results do not impact or only slightly impact the measures to be taken.

Regarding the length of the PSM, other studies have analyzed the effect, though often their populations were not selected to eliminate potential confounder BR factors.

Nevertheless, in large series of 501 patients, Stephenson [26] showed that the number of PSM was a significant predictor of BR, with multiple PSM resulting in worse prognosis compared to a solitary PSM (adjusted HR = 1.4, 95% CI: 1.1–1.8, $p = 0.002$). In parallel to this, ePSM was associated with BR, versus fPSM (adjusted HR = 1.3, 95% CI: 1.1–1.6, $p = 0.004$).

BR free-survival was significantly worse for patients with ePSM than those with fPSM (49.4 and 86.8%, respectively at 5 years, $p < 0.0001$) in our study. This result is widely found in other studies (Table 4).

One limitation of our study was the retrospective nature of our analysis.

In addition, while the number of patients analyzed was lower than that of some studies, we voluntarily restricted the study population (N +, ≥ T3b, adjuvant or neoadjuvant excluded) in order to get a selected population that could clearly reflect the effects of PCM. Only very few authors have investigated a population equally absent of BR confounders.

Lastly, we did not adjust our results according to tumor volume and the surgeon's experience, though these two variables constitute established risk factors for BR [25].

Also, in terms of limits, the Gleason score of the PSM could have been analyzed in order to reveal any possible link with BR. However, within the Marseille centers involved in our study, the Gleason score is either barely or not at all analyzed on PCMs.

Nevertheless, in agreement with a recent review, the impact of the Gleason score of PSM on BR is not currently acknowledged since too few studies have analyzed this factor [10]. We need better accuracy in analysis of PSM by pathologists if we are to move forward on this issue.

Regarding the primary endpoint, we choose the BR. This criterion is the most widely used in the literature for this type of analysis and certainly a relevant criterion when it comes to assessing disease recurrence. Nevertheless, the consideration of other criteria, such as metastasis-free survival, resistance to castration, or specific mortality to prostate cancer, would also be of value. In our study, only one patient (0.5%) developed metastatic recurrence after 16 years of follow-up, and no patients died from prostate cancer.

In a recent study, Mauermann investigated these factors in a cohort of 1712 patients, including 591 patients with PSM [8]. Patients with PSM were divided into two groups: single margin (regardless of size) and multiple margins. In total, 1.3% became metastatic, 1% became resistant to castration, and 1% died of prostate cancer. In the multivariate model, PSM (single or multiple) were never significantly associated with metastatic disease, resistance to castration, or specific mortality. In contrast, PSM (single and multiple) were a risk factor for BR. Again, this study included patients classified as pT3b, pT4, and N +, which likely accounts for this lack of significance.

Finally, the question remains whether treatment deferral should be recommended only when BR

Table 4 Hazard ratios of biochemical recurrence (BR) in multivariate model and BR-free survival following radical prostatectomy in men with fPSM or ePSM

Study	Year	n	fPSM no. (%)	ePSM no. (%)	Median follow-up, yr.	HR for BR (95% CI) ePSM vs fPSM *p* value	BR-free survival at 5 years for fPSM (%)	BR-free survival at 5 years for ePSM (%)	Including ≥pT3b, N+, neo or adjuvant treatment
Lake et al. [14]	2010	2022	344 (17.0)	99 (4.9)	4.1	NR	72	62	Yes
Lee e al [15]	2015	1733	114 (6.6)	359 (20.7)	4	NR	83	54	Yes
Sooriakumaran et al. [25]	2013	893	100 (11.2)	81 (9.1)	5	2.43 (1.14–5.18) < 0.05	81	65	Yes
Stenphenson et al. [27]	2009	1501	983 (65.5)	518 (34.5)	7	1.3 (1.1–1.6) *0.004*	63	43	No
May et al. [28]	2011	1036	122 (11.8)	145 (14.0)	4.3	1.0 (0.66–1.55) 0.96	49	51	No
Porpiglia et al. [29] [a]	2012	300	48 (16.0)	20 (6.7)	5.1	5.7 (1.5–2.17) 0.01	77	55	Yes
Ochiai et al. [30]	2007	117	81 (69.2)	32 (27.4)	3.6	NR	84	52	Yes
Van Oort et al. [31]	2010	174	NR	NR	3.6	2.15 (1.12–4.2) 0.02	NR	NR	Yes

In all studies, the cut-off for fPSM was the same as in our study (single margin ≤ 3 mm), except for Porpiglia et al.[a] (≤2.8 mm)
NR not reported, *HR* hazard ratio, *CI* confidence interval, *fPSM* focal positive surgical margin, *ePSM* extensive positive surgical margin, *PSA* prostate-specific antigen

occurs. This can prevent a number of patient side effects, for example in our study, 49.4% of patients with ePSM exhibited no BR with a median follow-up of 8 years.

Three large randomized trials compared AR vs. wait and see policy following prostatectomy for high-risk prostate cancer. The European Organization for Research and Treatment of Cancer (EORTC 22,911) and the German Cancer Society (ARO 96–02) trial (31, 32) reported a significantly improved 10-year cumulative BR-free survival for the postoperative irradiation group vs. the observation group. Overall survival and clinical progression were not significantly affected. The Southwest Oncology Group (SWOG) 8794 trial reported greater metastasis-free survival and overall survival in the postoperative radiotherapy arm (33). It should be note that in these three trials, patients in the wait and see arm who presented with BR did not undergo radiotherapy early on (early salvage radiation therapy), meaning this treatment was less effective due to being performed late.

Also, Briganti [25] studied this very point in a series of 390 patients. His objective was to evaluate BR-free survival in patients receiving AR versus observation only, followed by early salvage radiotherapy in cases of relapse in patients undergoing RP for pT3, pN0, and R0–R1 disease. There was no difference found between the two groups. It is important to note that the margin was not taken into account in this analysis, however.

A French study is currently in progress (GETUG/AFU 17) that could perhaps give more precise results in this matter.

In the end, the therapeutic dilemma for patients with PSMs following radical prostatectomy is to distinguish those who need adjuvant therapy from those for whom simple monitoring would suffice. While it is still unclear what the best treatment is for patients with PSMs, our data may provide beneficial information regarding how to best proceed, particularly for patients with fPSM.

Conclusion

Our study strongly suggests that the PSM extent should be taken into account in therapeutic decisions following radical prostatectomy. The existence of fPSM does not constitute a poor prognosis factor, as it was very rarely found associated with BR in our study. Therefore, it seems legitimate for us to propose close monitoring in these cases.

For patients with ePSM, however, the question remains whether early treatment would be beneficial. Our study clearly indicates that these patients much more frequently suffer BR, with 45% recurrence at 8 years, and it would thus appear essential to treat them early. Nevertheless, in these cases we believe it essential that the final therapeutic decision integrate the other prognostic factors (Gleason, preoperative PSA, pT) and life expectancy in order to treat these patients as well as possible. Further studies are now required to determine whether early salvage RT or RT associated with chemical castration are an equivalent alternative.

Abbreviations

AR: Adjuvant radiotherapy; BR: Biochemical recurrence; ePSM: Extensive positive surgical margin; fPSM: Focal positive surgical margin; LP-RP: Laparoscopic radical prostatectomy; PSA: Prostate-specific antigen; PSM: Positive surgical margin; RALP-RP: Robot-assisted laparoscopy radical prostatectomy; RP: Radical prostatectomy; sPSM: Single positive surgical margin; SV: Seminal vesicle

Acknowledgments
The authors thank all the administrative staff of the urology department of the North Hospital in Marseille which facilitated the collection of data.

Authors' contributions
YK: Project development, Data collection, Data analysis, Manuscript writing. FL: Project development, Data collection. NB: Data collection, Data analysis. SG: Data management. NG: Data analysis. GP: Data analysis. JW: Data management, Data collection. DR: Protocol development, Manuscript writing. CB: Protocol development, Data analysis, Manuscript writing. The authors have read and approved this information. All authors read and approved the final manuscript.

Author details
[1]Department of Urology, Hopital Nord, Chemin des Bourrely, 13015 Marseille, France. [2]Department of Anatomic Pathology, Hôpital nord, Chemin des Bourrely, 13015 Marseille, France. [3]Centre hospitalier universitaire de Lyon, Lyon, France. [4]Departement of urology, Institut Paoli-Calmettes, 13008 Marseille, France. [5]Hopital Edouard Herriot, 69003 Lyon, France.

References

1. Yossepowitch O, Briganti A, Eastham JA, Epstein J, Graefen M, Montironi R, et al. Positive surgical margins after radical prostatectomy: a systematic review and contemporary update. Eur Urol. 2014;65(2):303–13.
2. Chalfin HJ, Dinizo M, Trock BJ, Feng Z, Partin AW, Walsh PC, et al. Impact of surgical margin status on prostate-cancer-specific mortality. BJU Int. 2012; 110(11):1684–9.
3. Tan PH, Cheng L, Srigley JR, Griffiths D, Humphrey PA, Van Der Kwast TH, et al. International Society of Urological Pathology (ISUP) consensus conference on handling and staging of radical prostatectomy specimens. Working group 5: surgical margins. Mod Pathol. 2011;24(1):48–57.
4. Pfitzenmaier J, Pahernik S, Tremmel T, Haferkamp A, Buse S, Hohenfellner M. Positive surgical margins after radical prostatectomy: do they have an impact on biochemical or clinical progression? BJU Int. 2008;102(10):1413–8.
5. Wright JL, Dalkin BL, True LD, Ellis WJ, Stanford JL, Lange PH, et al. Positive surgical margins at radical prostatectomy predict prostate cancer specific mortality. J Urol. 2010;183(6):2213–8.
6. Novara G, Ficarra V, Mocellin S, Ahlering TE, Carroll PR, Graefen M, et al. Systematic review and meta-analysis of studies reporting oncologic outcome after robot- assisted radical prostatectomy. Eur Urol. 2012;62(3): 382–404.
7. Boorjian SA, Karnes RJ, Crispen PL, Carlson RE, Rangel LJ, Bergstralh EJ, et al. The impact of positive surgical margins on mortality following radical prostatectomy during the prostate specific antigen era. J Urol. 2010;183(3): 1003–9.
8. Mauermann J, Fradet V, Lacombe L, Dujardin T, Tiguert R, Tetu B, et al. The impact of solitary and multiple positive surgical margins on hard clinical end points in 1712 adjuvant treatment–naive pT2-4 N0 radical prostatectomy patients. Eur Urol. 2013;64(1):19–25.
9. Swindle P, Eastham JA, Ohori M, Kattan MW, Wheeler T, Maru N, et al. Do margins matter? The prognostic significance of positive surgical margins in radical prostatectomy specimens. J Urol. 2005;174(3):903–7.
10. Fontenot PA, Mansour AM. Reporting positive surgical margins after radical prostatectomy: time for standardization. BJU Int. 2013;111(8):E290–9.
11. Han M, Partin AW, Chan DY, Walsh PC. An evaluation of the decreasing incidence of positive surgical margins in a large retropubic prostatectomy series. J Urol. 2004;171(1):23–6.
12. Thompson IM, Tangen CM, Paradelo J, Lucia MS, Miller G, Troyer D, et al. Adjuvant radiotherapy for pathologically advanced prostate cancer: a randomized clinical trial. Jama. 2006;296(19):2329–35.
13. Srigley JR, Humphrey PA, Amin MB, Chang SS, Egevad L, Epstein JI, et al. Protocol for the examination of specimens from patients with carcinoma of the prostate gland. Arch Pathol Lab Med. 2009;133(10):1568–76.
14. Lake AM, He C, Wood DP. Focal positive surgical margins decrease disease-free survival after radical prostatectomy even in organ-confined disease. Urology. 2010;76(5):1212–6.
15. Lee S, Kim KB, Jo JK, Ho J-N, Oh JJ, Jeong SJ, et al. Prognostic value of focal positive surgical margins after radical prostatectomy. Clin Genitourin Cancer. 2015.
16. Maxeiner A, Magheli A, Jöhrens K, Kilic E, Braun TL, Kempkensteffen C, et al. Significant reduction in positive surgical margin rate after laparoscopic radical prostatectomy by application of the modified surgical margin recommendations of the 2009 International Society of Urological Pathology consensus. BJU Int. 2016;118:750–7.
17. Stamey TA, Sozen TS, Yemoto CM, McNEAL JE. Classification of localized untreated prostate cancer based on 791 men treated only with radical prostatectomy: common ground for therapeutic trials and TNM subgroups. J Urol. 1998;159(6):2009–12.
18. Sooriakumaran P, Ploumidis A, Nyberg T, Olsson M, Akre O, Haendler L, et al. The impact of length and location of positive margins in predicting biochemical recurrence after robot-assisted radical prostatectomy with a minimum follow-up of 5 years. BJU Int. 2015;115(1):106–13.
19. Salomon L, Anastasiadis AG, Levrel O, Katz R, Saint F, de la Taille A, et al. Location of positive surgical margins after retropubic, perineal, and laparoscopic radical prostatectomy for organ-confined prostate cancer. Urology. 2003;61(2):386–90.
20. Sofer M, Savoie M, Kim SS, Civantos F, Soloway MS. Biochemical and pathological predictors of the recurrence of prostatic adenocarcinoma with seminal vesicle invasion. J Urol. 2003;169(1):153–6.
21. Ploussard G, Agamy MA, Alenda O, Allory Y, Mouracade P, Vordos D, et al. Impact of positive surgical margins on prostate-specific antigen failure after radical prostatectomy in adjuvant treatment-naïve patients. BJU Int. 2011; 107(11):1748–54.
22. Eastham JA, Kuroiwa K, Ohori M, Serio AM, Gorbonos A, Maru N, et al. Prognostic significance of location of positive margins in radical prostatectomy specimens. Urology. 2007;70(5):965–9.
23. Meeks JJ, Eastham JA. Radical prostatectomy: positive surgical margins matter. In: Urologic oncology: seminars and original investigations: Elsevier; 2013. p. 974–9.
24. Dev HS, Wiklund P, Patel V, Parashar D, Palmer K, Nyberg T, et al. Surgical margin length and location affect recurrence rates after robotic prostatectomy. In: Urologic oncology: seminars and original investigations: Elsevier; 2015.
25. Briganti A, Wiegel T, Joniau S, Cozzarini C, Bianchi M, Sun M, et al. Early salvage radiation therapy does not compromise cancer control in patients with pT3N0 prostate cancer after radical prostatectomy: results of a match-controlled multi-institutional analysis. Eur Urol. 62(3):472–87.
26. Stephenson AJ, Wood DP, Kattan MW, et al. Location, extent and number of positive surgical margins do not improve accuracy of predicting prostate cancer recurrence after radical prostatectomy. J Urol. 2009;182(4):1357–63.
27. May M, Brookman-May S, Weißbach L, et al. Solitary an small (≤ 3 mm) apical positive surgical margins are related to biochemical recurrence after radical prostatectomy. Int J Urol. 2011;18(4):282–9.
28. Porpiglia F, Fiori C, Manfredi M, et al. Surgical margin status of specimen and oncological outcomes after laparoscopic radical prostatectomy: experience after 400 procedures. World J Urol. 2012;30(2):245–50.
29. Ochiai A, Sotelo T, Troncoso P, et al. Natural history of biochemical progression after radical prostatectomy based on length of a positive margin. Urology. 2008;71(2):308–12.
30. Oort V, Inge M, Bruins HM, Kiemeney LA, et al. The length of positive surgical margins correlates with biochemical recurrence after radical prostatectomy. Histopathology. 2010;56(4):464–71.
31. Van Oort IM, Bruins HM, Kiemeney LA, Knipscheer BC, Witjes JA, & Hulsbergen-van de Kaa CA. The length of positive surgical margins correlates with biochemical recurrence after radical prostatectomy. Histopathology. 2010;56(4):464–71.

3

Pediatric testicular torsion: Does patient transfer affect time to intervention or surgical outcomes at a rural tertiary care center?

Tyler Overholt[1], Morris Jessop[2], John Barnard[2*] and Osama Al-Omar[2]

Abstract

Background: Testicular torsion (TT) is a urologic emergency that requires prompt surgical intervention. In rural Appalachia, patients are often transferred from surrounding communities due to lack of urologic care. We hypothesized that those transferred would have delayed intervention and higher rates of orchiectomy when compared to those who presented directly to our hospital.

Methods: We performed a retrospective review of patient charts with an ICD-9 diagnosis of TT from 2008 to 2016. Patients met inclusion criteria if diagnosis was confirmed by operative exploration. We compared rate of testicular loss and time until surgical intervention between groups.

Results: Twenty-three patients met inclusion criteria (12 transferred, 11 direct). Patient demographics did not significantly differ between groups. Transferred patients had a higher orchiectomy rate (33% v 22%, $p = 0.41$) although this was not statistically significant. Time to surgery from symptom onset was significantly longer in those transferred (12.9 h) compared to those not transferred (6.9 h, $p = 0.02$). Distance of transfer was not correlated with time of delay ($r^2 = 0.063$).

Conclusions: Transferred patients with TT have numerically higher rates of orchiectomy which may reach significance in an appropriately powered study, and relative delays in surgical intervention. This study highlights the need for improved access to urologic care in rural areas.

Keywords: Testicular torsion, Rural, Patient transfer, Orchiectomy

Background

Testicular torsion (TT) is a urologic emergency where prompt surgical intervention is necessary to prevent testicular loss. TT can occur in male patients at any age, but there is a bimodal distribution which has been described with peaks within the first year of life and between ages 13–16 years old [1]. The etiology of TT can be further classified into two broad categories: intravaginal and extravaginal [2]. Intravaginal TT occurs when the testis twists completely within the tunica vaginalis [3]. This mechanism is the most common etiology and is usually seen in individuals with a bilateral anatomic defect known as the bell clapper deformity [3, 4]. In extravaginal TT, there is a loose attachment between the tunica vaginalis and the scrotal wall early in prenatal development that increases the likelihood of the tunica vaginalis and its contents to twist around the spermatic cord, most commonly in the neonatal period [5, 6].

Management is centered around prompt surgical exploration for every patient with a definitive diagnosis as well as those with inconclusive imaging due to the morbidity associated with delay in management [7]. Delayed intervention can result in permanent ischemic injury of the testis that can lead to long term consequences including testicular loss and infertility [8–10]. Irreversible ischemia from torsion begins in 6 h from symptom onset and the likelihood of testicular salvage is the highest within the first 6 hours [7, 11]. Based on prior literature, treatment with 6 h of symptom onset correlates with

* Correspondence: jbarnar4@hsc.wvu.edu
[2]Department of Urology, West Virginia University, Morgantown, USA
Full list of author information is available at the end of the article

90–100% chance of testicular salvage [12]. However, treatment within 6–12 h decreases salvage rates to 20–50%, and treatment in the 12–24 h range affords only a 0–10% chance of testicular salvage [12]. If surgery is delayed more than 24 h following symptom onset, testicular non-viability is almost inevitable even if the testicular tissue appears viable during surgical exploration [13]. Due to factors such as patient preference, hospital capacity, and access to health care providers capable of managing TT, over 1/3rd of patients with suspected TT are transferred to a tertiary care facility for management, which increases total time of ischemic damage and morbidity [11].

In rural West Virginia, patients often need to be transferred from far distances to seek care from West Virginia University Hospitals due to the lack of Urologic care availability in many areas of the state. This issue is present in rural areas all throughout Appalachia and the rural United States as a whole. Patients with testicular torsion who have to travel from rural areas to facilities capable of managing torsion can be at increased risk for adverse outcomes including orchiectomy. The aim of our study was to look at the relationships between transferring from outside facilities prior to presentation at our facility and the rate of complications and delays in care. We hypothesized that those transferred to our hospital would have a relative delay in surgical intervention and higher rates of orchiectomy compared to those who presented directly to our hospital.

Methods

After Institutional Review Board approval, a retrospective analysis of patient charts at Ruby Memorial Hospital (RMH) was performed using ICD-9 diagnosis of testicular torsion from 2008 to 2016. For each TT patient, the primary metrics were the surgical outcomes, including rate of orchiectomy between transferred and non-transferred patients, time from symptom onset to presentation, time from symptom onset to surgical intervention, and time from presentation to surgical intervention. We also aimed to characterize laterality of the affected testicle, if imaging was obtained prior to surgical management, and the mean total symptom duration. In TT patients who were transferred from outside facilities, we also aimed to characterize the mode of transfer, the distance of transfer, and relative delay in surgical intervention caused by transfer.

Criteria for inclusion were met if the patient had a diagnosis of testicular torsion that was confirmed by operative exploration. Patients were excluded from the study if suffering from neonatal torsion or if the symptoms were present for over 24 h. Multiple patients were also excluded due to poor documentation of symptom duration.

Patients were separated into those transferred and those who presented directly to our hospital. One hundred and eight patients with testicular torsion were revealed from the ICD-9 search and of those, 23 met inclusion criteria. Twelve patients were transferred from another hospital and sent to RMH due to lack of urologic care at outside facilities and 11 of these patients presented directly to RMH.

Graphpad and Microsoft Excel were utilized for statistical analysis. Normal distribution of data was confirmed using the Shapiro Wilk test. Statistical analyses performed include chi-squared tests for categorical variable data and two-tailed simple t-tests for continuous variable data. Statistical significance was determined by a threshold p value < 0.05.

Results

Mean age of patients was 17.11 ± 5.88 years. 69.6% of patients in the study were Caucasian, 13.0% were Black, 4.4% were Hispanic, and 13.0% were unspecified. 47.8% of patients were affected on the right testicle and 42.2% were affected on the left testicle. Doppler ultrasound was performed in all 23 patients prior to surgical intervention. Mean duration of symptoms for all patients was 10.0 h. Demographic characteristics did not significantly differ between the two patient groups (Table 1).

The mean time to surgical incision from symptom onset in patients who transferred from another facility was 12.9 h. The mean time to surgical incision from symptom onset in patients who presented directly to our tertiary hospital was 6.9 h. Time to surgery from symptom onset was significantly longer in those transferred ($p = 0.02$).

Among transferred patients, 33% underwent orchiectomy on surgical exploration. Of those presenting directly to our hospital, 22% underwent orchiectomy. No statistically significant difference in rate of orchiectomy between the two patient groups was identified ($p = 0.41$).

The mean time to surgical incision from presentation at RMH in patients who transferred from another facility was 2.6 h. The mean time to surgical incision from presentation in those who presented directly to RMH was 3.8 h. Time from presentation to RMH to surgical incision was significantly less in those who transferred than those who presented directly to RMH ($p = 0.013$).

Overall, 73% of patients that were transferred to RMH were transferred by ambulance. The mean distance of transfer was 23.8 miles. The mean delay in care from the time of presentation to outside facility to presenting at RMH for all transferred patients was 9.8 h. Distance of transfer was not correlated with the time of delay ($r^2 = 0.063$)(Fig. 1).

Approximately 83% of patients who transferred from another facility received follow up care and 91% of patients who presented directly to RMH received follow up care. The mean number of days to receive follow up care in patients who were transferred was 171 days. The mean number of days to receive follow up care in

Table 1 Demographic and clinical characteristics of study participants

Characteristics	Patients transferred to RMH	Patients directly presented to RMH
Age	15.12 ± 5.30	19.29 ± 5.92
Ethnicity		
White	11/12 (91.67%)	5/11 (45.45%)
Hispanic	0/12 (0%)	1/11 (9.09%)
Black	0/12 (0%)	3/11 (27.27%)
Unknown	1/12 (8.33%)	2/11 (18.18%)
Mode of transport		
Ambulance	8/12 (72.73%)	
Air	1/12 (8.33%)	N/A
Unknown	3/12 (25%)	
Laterality	5/12 (41.67%) Right	6/11 (54.55%) Right
	7/12 (58.33%) Left	5/11 (45.45%) Left
Doppler US prior to surgical intervention	12/12 (100%)	11/11 (100%)

patients who presented directly to RMH was 71 days. There was not a statistically significantly difference in number of follow up days between the two patient groups ($p = 0.49$).

Discussion

This study focuses on the relationships between patient transfer from rural areas throughout West Virginia to RMH and the clinical and surgical outcomes in patients with testicular torsion. The hypothesis that those transferred to our hospital would have a longer delay in surgical intervention and a higher numerical rate of orchiectomy was supported. There was a statistically significant delay from onset of testicular torsion symptoms to surgical intervention in the patients who were transferred to RMH compared to those who presented to RMH directly. These results suggest that patients who live in rural areas and present to rurally located hospitals first require transfer and travel time that is more likely to result in delays in definitive management. The rate of orchiectomy was 11% higher in patients who transferred to RMH than in the patients who presented to RMH directly. Although this number did not reach statistical significance, most likely due to small sample size of patients, these results suggest that delays in surgical intervention for testicular torsion patients are more likely to be associated with the need for orchiectomy.

Testicular torsion patients who were transferred to RMH had a significant decrease in time from presentation at RMH to surgical incision than patients who presented directly to RMH. There are multiple possible explanations for why these results were seen. One such explanation could be appropriate communication between facilities prior to arrival at RMH to ensure expeditious management. Another explanation may be that diagnostic criteria were completed at the outside hospital, expediting the process at RMH. Other studies have recognized the importance of shorter times from arrival to the operating rooms in patients who have already experienced delays in management due to the need for

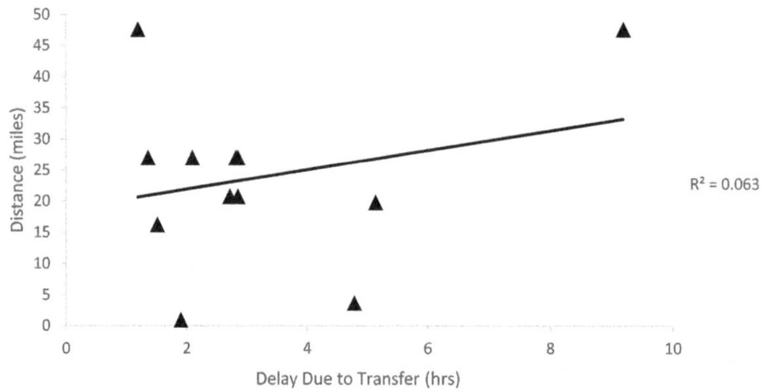

Fig. 1 Relationship between delays of care and transfer distances in patients transferred from outside facilities to RMH

hospital transfer. One study implemented a standardized track called "Straight to the Operating Room" with a goal of reducing time to surgery, decreased hospitalization costs, and less overall testicular loss [14]. While they did not see a statistically significant reduction in testicular loss, the STOR track did significantly decrease time to surgery and hospitalization cost for affected patients [14]. Additionally, the distance that patients had to travel was not statistically correlated with amount of delay. These results, along with the finding that 73% of patients were transferred via ambulance, suggest that transportation distance itself was not associated with delays in care. Other studies have also shown that travel distance was not statistically correlated with total delay time. One study found that in patients traveling from distances all over 40 miles away, there was no difference in surgical outcomes between patients who travelled by car, ambulance, or helicopter [15].

Patients who transferred to RMH were 8% less likely to receive follow up than those who presented directly to our facility. Although this number did not reach statistical significance, the mean number of days to follow up care was 99.73 days longer in patients who transferred to RMH than patients who presented directly to RMH. These results suggest that geographic proximity to our facility may play a role in receiving follow up care, but due to many factors including post-surgical counseling and communication with patients and their families, a large percentage of the patients are receiving the follow up care that they need.

Fourteen total patients were excluded from this study solely due to symptom duration in excess of 24 h. Of these patients, 11 (78.6%) were transferred from outside facilities and all 14 patients (100%) had an orchiectomy as their surgical outcome. These results suggest the need for community and rural clinician education on recognizing the signs and symptoms of testicular torsion.

Conclusions

These results imply that patients who live in rural areas may have an increased likelihood to face negative outcomes than patients who live in close enough proximity to a facility with adequate care. This is in conjunction with other studies about delays in care for patients in rural settings. In a study assessing the health status of cancer survivors in rural areas versus urban areas throughout the United States, patients who lived in rural areas were more likely to have poor outcomes including additional comorbidities, worse overall physical and mental health, difficulties with maintaining jobs due to their health [16]. Similar data has been shown for trauma patients where individuals who experience traumas in rural areas have a 50% higher mortality than individuals in urban areas [17]. In a retrospective study looking at prehospital causes of rural fatality rates following motor vehicle crashes in Alabama, it was found that longer emergency medical service response time, longer time on the scene, and longer distances to travel to the scene were all associated with increased mortality in rural trauma patients [18]. Individuals from rural areas face challenges of difficult travel, lack of access to health care facilities, and lack of access to specialty care [19, 20].

This study demonstrated that patients with testicular torsion who transferred from an outside facility prior to presentation at RMH had higher rates of orchiectomy, relative delays in surgical care, less follow up care, and longer times to receive follow up care. This study also highlights the prevalence of delays in diagnosis and presentation, which could be due to gaps in primary care recognition of this urologic emergency.

Delays in management of testicular torsion can result in life long complications and adverse outcomes for individuals affected. In addition to its retrospective design, limitations of the study also include small sample size. However, inclusion and exclusion criteria were formed to be as specific as possible to minimize bias from confounding factors. Future studies may be aimed at looking at testicular torsion patients in rural Appalachia as a whole. This study highlights the need for streamlined access to prompt urologic care in rural areas to minimize the morbidity associated with delay.

Abbreviations

RMH: Ruby Memorial Hospital; TT: Testicular Torsion

Acknowledgements

Not applicable.

Authors contributions

TO – Primary Author, Data Collection, Data Analysis, Writing. MJ – Co-Author, Data Collection, Data Analysis, Writing. JB – Co-Author, Writing, Formatting, Submission. OA – Principle Investigator, Revision. All authors have reviewed and are in agreement with the manuscript. All authors read and approved the final manuscript.

Author details

[1]School of Medicine, West Virginia University, Morgantown, USA.
[2]Department of Urology, West Virginia University, Morgantown, USA.

References

1. Pogorelić Z, Mustapić K, Jukić M, Todorić J, Mrklić I, Mešštrović J, Jurić I, Furlan D. Management of acute scrotum in children: a 25-year single center experience on 558 pediatric patients. Can J Urol. 2016;23(6):8594–601.
2. Kapoor S. Testicular torsion: a race against time. Int J Clin Pract. 2008;62(5): 821–7.
3. Lin EP, Bhatt S, Dubens DJ, Dogra VS. Testicular torsion: twists and turns. Semin Ultrasound CT MR. 2007;28:317–28.
4. Caesar RE, Kaplan GW. Incidence of the bell-clapper deformity in an autopsy series. J Urol. 1994;44(1):114–6.
5. Hazeltine M, Panza A, Ellsworth P. Testicular torsion: current evaluation and management. Int J Urol Nurs. 2017;37(2):61–71, 93.
6. Nebot S, Salvador RI, Aliaga SP, Inigo EG. Perinatal testicular torsion: ultrasound assessment and differential diagnosis. Radiology. 2017;59(5):391–400.

7. Bowlin PR, Gatti JM, Murphy JP. Pediatric testicular torsion. Surg Clin. 2017; 97(1):161–72.
8. Nussambaum Blask AR, Bulas D, Shalaby-Rana E, Rushton G, Shao C, Maid M. Color Doppler sonography and scintography of the testis: a prospective, comparative analysis in children with acute scrotal pain. Pediatr Emerg Care. 2002;18:67–71.
9. McAndrew HF, Pemberton R, Kikiros CS, Gollow I. The incidence and investigation of acute scrotal problems in children. J Pediatr Surg. 2002;18: 435–7.
10. Visser AJ, Heyns CF. Testicular function after torsion of the spermatic cord. Br J Urol. 2003;92:200–3.
11. Arevalo MK, Sheth KR, Menon VS, Ostrov L, Hemnes H, Singla N, Koral K, Schlomer BJ, Baker LA. Straight to the operating room: an emergency surgery track for acute testicular torsion transfers. J Pediatr. 2018;129:178–83.
12. Pogorelić Z, Mrklić I, Jurić I, Biočić M, Furlan D. Testicular torsion in the inguinal canal in children. J Pediatr Urol. 2013;9(6):793–7.
13. Lian BY, Ong CP, Chiang LW, Rai R, Nah SA. Factors predicting testicular atrophy after testicular salvage following torsion. J Pediatr Surg. 2016;26(1):17–21.
14. Arevalo MK, Sheth KR, Menon VS, Ostrov L, Hennes H, Singla N, Koral K, Schlomer BJ, Baker LA. Straight to the operating room: an emergent surgery track for acute testicular torsion transfers. J Pediatr. 2018;192:178–83.
15. Weiss DA, Tsarouhas N, Carr MC, Kalmus A, Zderic SA. How do they get here: does the method of transportation impact salvage for patients with testicular torsion? J Pediatr Urol. 2017;13(3):281.e1–5.
16. Weaver KE, Geiger AM, Lingyi L, Douglas Case L. Rural-urban disparities in health status among US cancer survivors. J Cancer. 2013;119(5):1050–7.
17. Baker SP, O'Neil B, Ginsburg MJ, Li G. The injury fact book, 2nd Edition. New York: Oxford University Press Inc.; 1992;26–28, 52:65–70.
18. Gonzalez RP, Cummings G, Mulekar M, Rodning C. Increased mortality in rural vehicular trauma: identifying contributing factors through data linkage. J Trauma. 2006;6(12):404–9.
19. Beck SI, Towsley GL, Caserta MS, Lindau K, Dudley WN. Symptom experiences and quality of life of rural and urban older adult cancer survivors. Cancer Nurs. 2009;32:359–69.
20. Arcury TA, Preisser JS, Gesler WM, Powers JM. Access to transportation and health care utilization in a rural region. J Rural Health. 2005;21:31–8.

4

The comparison of the effect of phenylephrine and epinephrine on penile spongy tissue in rats after experimental hypospadias surgery: A quantitative stereological study

Mehdi Shirazi[1,2], Mohammad-Bagher Rajabalian[1], Ali Noorafshan[2,3], Saied Karbalay-Doust[2,3*], Zahra Jahanabadi[1] and Faisal Ahmed[1]

Abstract

Background: Many factors including vasoconstrictor agents can interfere with wound healing process. This study aimed to compare the histopathological outcome of injection of two sympathomimetic drugs used during urologic surgery, including phenylephrine and epinephrine, on the structure of spongy tissue and urethra in a rat model of experimental hypospadias repair using stereological methods.

Methods: Male rats were allocated into three groups. The first group underwent surgery without using any agents. The second and third groups underwent surgery with diluted phenylephrine (1:5000) and diluted epinephrine (1: 100000) injection in the urethral plate before operation, respectively. Quantitative histological evaluation of all penises was performed after 3 weeks.

Results: The results indicated no significant differences among the three groups regarding the vessels and urethral lumen and epithelium. However, the volumes of the spongy tissue and collagen bundles and the number of fibroblasts were significantly higher (35–55%) in surgery + phenylephrine and surgery + epinephrine groups in comparison to the surgery group ($p < 0.05$), with no preferences.

Conclusions: Hypospadias repair using phenylephrine and epinephrine injection showed no adverse effects. Furthermore, they might lead to better postoperative structural outcomes without any preferences. However, further experimental and human studies are required to draw a firm conclusion.

Keywords: Epinephrine, Hypospadias repair, Phenylephrine, Stereology, Rat

Background

The reconstruction procedure in hypospadias might be associated with some complications, such as dehiscence, urethrocutaneous fistulas, proximal strictures, diverticula, meatal stenosis, and bleeding [1]. Bleeding from the site of incision is one of the most important challenges during hypospadias repair. Early postoperative bleeding or oozing from the site of surgery may require immediate exploration and treatment. In some circumstances, hematoma formation at the site of operation may lead to cosmetic problems and even surgery failure [2]. However, the best method for inducing effective homeostasis without permanent tissue injury during hypospadias surgery has not been determined yet [3]. Various techniques have been used to manage this problem, including tourniquet application, use of bipolar electrocautery, and injection of vasoconstrictor agents into the site of incision. Tourniquet application and monopolar electrocautery have some

* Correspondence: karbalas@sums.ac.ir
[2]Histomorphometry and Stereology Research Center, Shiraz University of Medical Sciences, Zand Ave., Shiraz 71348-45794, Iran
[3]Anatomy Department, School of Medicine, Shiraz University of Medical Sciences, Shiraz, Iran
Full list of author information is available at the end of the article

limitations that could lead to pressure injury, vascular and thermal damages, scarring of the affected penile skin, and ischemic damages [3–5]. Epinephrine is a vasoconstrictor, which is commonly used to prevent or minimize bleeding during hypospadias surgery. Phenylephrine is another vasoconstrictor with more specific actions on vessels and fewer systemic adverse effects. However, administration of phenylephrine in hypospadias surgery has received less attention [6]. It has been demonstrated that applying homeostasis techniques during hypospadias repair might lead to ischemia and tissue damage on the urethral wall [3]. There is also concern that application of vasoconstrictor agents might interfere with wound repair. Therefore, the present study aims to evaluate the effects of injection of two vasoconstrictor agents, namely phenylephrine and epinephrine, on the structure of the urethra and corpus spongiosum in a rat model of hypospadias repair using stereological methods.

Methods

Animals

In this trial, 15 male adult Sprague-Dawley rats with average body weight of 200–220 g were prepared from the Center of Comparative and Experimental Medicine of the University. The rats were maintained in cages with a 12/12-h light-dark cycle, room temperature of 22–24 °C, humidity of 50%, and access to water and food. All animals were kept according to the Animal Care and Ethics Committee of the University (agreement license No. 1396-01-01-14,119).

Experimental design

The animals were randomly divided into three groups ($n = 5$ per group). According to standard stereological articles, five animals were sufficient in each group [7]. The first group underwent surgery without any hemostasis techniques. The second and third groups underwent surgery with preoperative phenylephrine and epinephrine injection into the incision site, respectively.

Vasoconstrictors

Diluted epinephrine (1:100000) and diluted phenylephrine (1:5000) were applied in this study as vasoconstrictor agents. Equal volumes (less than 0.1 ml) of the designated diluted vasoconstrictors were injected in the incision sites in the experimental groups before proceeding to surgery [6].

Urethral incision and repair

All rats were anesthetized using intramuscular injection of ketamine (10–15 mg/kg) and xylazine (6–10 mg/kg). The site of operation was well shaved and disinfected by povidone-iodine topical solution. Then, it was draped with sterile sheets. External genitalia were exposed and a urethral catheter (24 g-yellow angiocath) was inserted into the urethra. Prior to the operation, diluted phenylephrine and epinephrine were injected under to the urothelium beside the incision line in groups 2 and 3, respectively [3]. Then, under sterile conditions, a longitudinal incision was made on the ventral surface of the penis over the mid raphe line from base to glans to open the corpus spongiosum and urethra. Afterwards, urethral repair was done with running suture (Vicryl 7–0). At the end of the procedure, the catheter was removed and oxytetracycline spray was used in place to prevent wound infection [8].

Tissue preparation

Three weeks after the surgery, the rats after deep anesthesia by an intraperitoneal injection ketamine (100 mg/kg of body weight) and xylazine (8 mg/kg of body weight) were euthanized and the body of the penis, including two corpora cavernous and the corpus spongiosum that envelops the urethra, was cut from the basal part and was deposited in buffered formaldehyde. The length and weight of the penis were calculated and its volume "V (penis)" was measured by the immersion technique [8]. Then, according to the length of the penis, eight to twelve transverse slabs with equal distances were sectioned. After tissue processing, all slabs were embedded in paraffin. At this stage, 4 and 25 μm sections were obtained by a microtome. Then, the sections were stained with hematoxylin, eosin, and Heidenhain's azan trichrome.

Estimation of the volume of penile corpus spongiosum

The volume of corpus spongiosum was estimated under stereo-microscopy from the basal part to the glans of the penis. It should be noted that all penis sections were studied at the magnification of 64×. The whole volume of the corpus spongiosum was calculated using "Cavalieri's method" [9]. Accordingly, the stereological probe (point grid) was superimposed over the image of penis sections viewed on the monitor. Then, the areas of corpus spongiosum sections "ΣA" were multiplied by the penis sections thickness (T). After all, the area was estimated by the stereology software and the volume was estimated by the following formula:

$$V\,(\text{corpus spongiosum}) = \sum A\,(\text{corpus spongiosum}) \times T$$

Estimating the volume density

The volume density of the penis sections was analyzed using a video microscopy system. Then, the stereological probe (point grid) was superimposed on the live microscopic image on a monitor by the software designed at the Histomorphometry and Stereology Research Center of the University. The volume density "*Vv* (structure/corpus spongiosum)" of the spongy tissue, urethra (lumens and epithelium), vessels, and collagen bundles was estimated by the "point-counting technique" [8, 10, 11]. The following formula was employed:

$$Vv\ (\text{structure/corpus spongiosum}) = \text{P}\ (\text{structure})/\text{P}\ (\text{corpus spongiosum})$$

Where 'P(structure)' was the number of test points falling on the structures (spongy tissue, urethral lumens, urethral epithelium, vessels, and collagen bundles) and 'P (corpus spongiosum)' was the total number of points put on the reference space (corpus spongiosum). The total volume of each structure was also estimated by the following formula:

$$\text{V}\ (\text{structure}) = Vv\ (\text{structure/corpus spongiosum}) \times \text{V}\ (\text{corpus spongiosum})$$

Estimating the number of corpus spongiosum fibroblasts

The number and numerical density of corpus spongiosum fibroblasts were calculated using thick sections (25 μm) via the optical disector technique [12, 13]. The optical disector including a microscope (Numerical Aperture (*NA*) of 1.40, 100×) and a microcator with digital readout (MT12, Heidenhain, Traunreut, Germany) was set for estimating motion in the Z-direction. Every fibroblast nucleus that came into focus within the "disector height" was chosen if it was placed completely or slightly in the counting frame and did not contact the forbidden line. The fibroblasts' density was estimated using the following formula:

$$NV\ (\text{fibroblast/corpus spongiosum}) = \sum \text{Q}/\left[\sum \text{P} \times a\ (f) \times \text{h}\right]$$

Where ΣQ was the number of fibroblasts computed inside the sampling frame, ΣP was number of disectors, $a\ (f) = 774\ \mu m^2$ was the region of the unbiased counting frame, and $h = 15\ \mu m$ was the altitude of the disector. Indeed, the upper and lower 4 μm of each section were considered as guard zones by a microcator. The total number of the fibroblasts was estimated by multiplying the numerical density by V (corpus spongiosum). The fibroblasts were studied under the magnification of 1560× using a 40× oil immersion lens.

Statistical analysis

The data were analyzed using one-way Analysis of Variance (ANOVA) followed by Tukey's post-hoc test. *P*-values < 0.05 were considered to be statistically significant. All statistical analyses were performed using the SPSS statistical software, version 20.0 (IBM, Armonk, NY, USA program).

Results

Quantitative changes

The total volume of the spongy tissue and collagen bundles increased by respectively 35 and 42% in the surgery + phenylephrine group and 35 and 40% in the surgery + epinephrine group in comparison to the surgery group ($p < 0.05$) (Fig. 1).

The total number of the fibroblasts increased by 37% in the surgery + phenylephrine group and by 55% in the surgery + epinephrine group in comparison to the surgery group ($p < 0.05$) (Fig.1).

The data showed that the volumes of the microvessels and urethral lumen and epithelium remained constant in the surgery, surgery + phenylephrine, and surgery + epinephrine groups ($p > 0.05$) (Fig.1). However, no significant differences were found between the surgery + phenylephrine and surgery + epinephrine groups regarding the volumes of spongy tissue, vessels, urethral lumen and epithelium, and collagen bundles and the number of fibroblasts ($p > 0.05$) (Fig.1).

Qualitative changes

Qualitative evaluation of the spongy tissue and the urethra has been presented in Fig. 2. After experimental hypospadias surgery, higher volumes of collagen bundles and larger populations of fibroblasts were seen in the histological sections of the surgery + phenylephrine and surgery + epinephrine groups compared to the surgery group.

Discussion

The surgical procedure performed to treat hypospadias must provide the basic expectations, such as a vertical meatus in the middle aspect of the glans, directed urinary stream, and a straightened penis at the time of erection. Yet, maintaining the healthy structure of the penis should be the main goal [14, 15].

Providing a bloodless operative field for the surgeon is a great challenge during hypospadias repair. If this goal is achieved, it will result in a better cosmetic outcome and decrease the failure of surgery. Various techniques, such as the use of tourniquet, cauterization, and injection of vasoconstrictor agents into the site of incision, are available to manage this problem [16–18]. Kajbafzadeh et al. evaluated the effects of different hemostasis techniques on the urethral wall structure in a rabbit model of hypospadias repair. Their assessment on ultra-structural injuries, apoptotic damages, and tissue fibrosis indicated that ultrastructural and cellular damage in the urethral wall were more prominent following epinephrine hemostasis [3]. Cakmak et al. also compared tourniquet application and epinephrine injection to penile skin and concluded that epinephrine injection to penile skin might exert a deleterious effect on wound healing [19]. However, the present study findings showed that epinephrine usage in

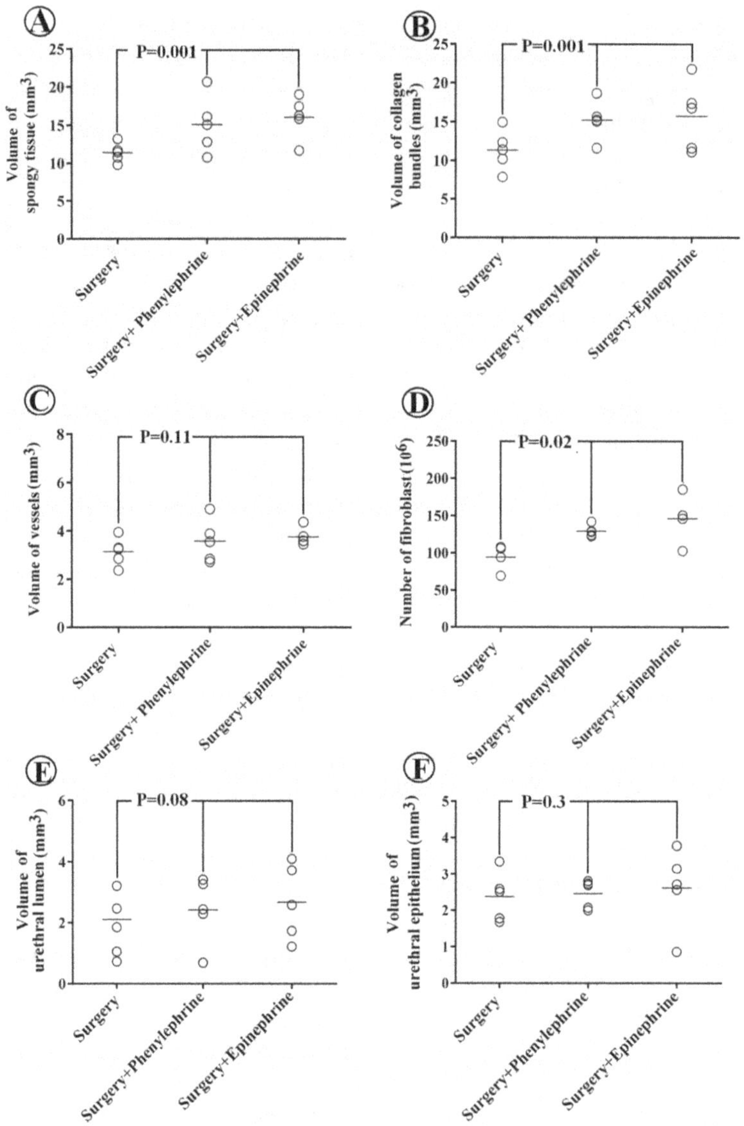

Fig. 1 The aligned dot plot of the volumes of the spongy tissue (**a**), collagen bundles (**b**), and vessels (**c**), number of fibroblasts (**d**), and volumes of urethral lumen (**e**) and urethral epithelium (**f**) in the surgery, surgery + phenylephrine, and surgery + epinephrine groups. Each dot represents an animal and the horizontal bar is the average of the mentioned parameters in the experimental groups ($p < 0.05$ or $p > 0.05$)

hypospadias surgery improved some stereological parameters, including a greater number of fibroblasts and collagen bundles in the spongy tissue postoperatively. Another study by Alizadeh et al. also revealed that epinephrine injection decreased bleeding without any significant harmful effects on postoperative clinical outcomes in hypospadias surgery [17].

The current study demonstrated the advantages of using injected vasoconstrictor agents to obtain a better stereological outcome compared to the surgery group following hypospadias surgery in rats. Vasoconstrictor drugs constrict blood vessels and decrease perfusion to the site of injection. Thus, bleeding decreases at their administration site [6]. In the present study, epinephrine and phenylephrine were applied as vasoconstrictors. Epinephrine is a vasoconstrictor used commonly for preventing or minimizing bleeding during surgical procedures. Epinephrine has agonist effects on both alpha and beta adrenergic receptors, but it exerts its vasoconstrictor action through affecting alpha adrenergic receptors. When epinephrine tissue levels decrease over time, the primary effect on the vessels will revert to vasodilation, as beta effects predominate. This may lead to increased postoperative blood loss. On the other hand, phenylephrine is a vasoconstrictor with almost pure alpha agonist effects, resulting in few systemic side effects. Indeed, phenylephrine has a long duration of action compared to epinephrine. Therefore, the postoperative period passes with less bleeding and total blood loss is usually lower when

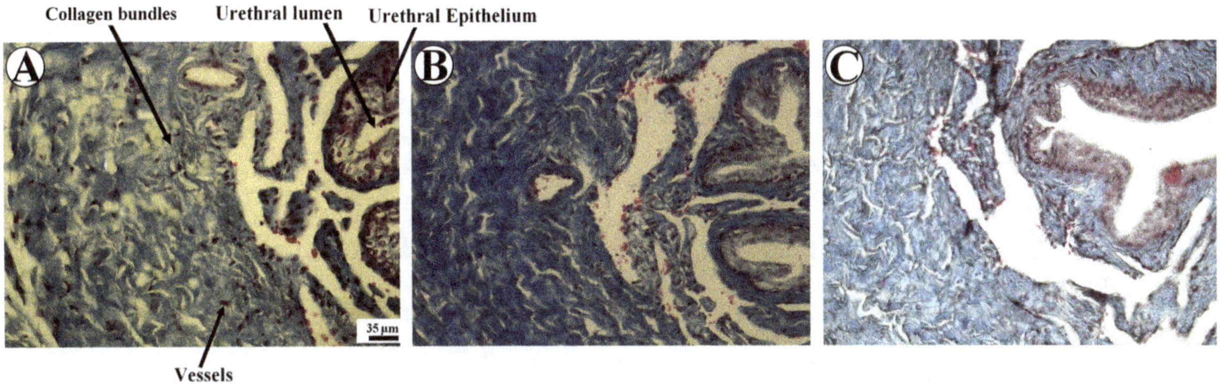

Fig. 2 The micrographs of the penis sections in the experimental hypospadias (surgery, (**a**)), surgery + phenylephrine (**b**), and surgery + epinephrine (**c**) groups. Greater volumes of collagen bundles were observable in the surgery + phenylephrine and surgery + epinephrine groups. The microvessels and urethral lumen and epithelium have been shown on the figure. Scale bars = 35 μm. Heidenhain's azan trichrome stain

phenylephrine is used [6]. Unfortunately, less attention has been paid to the use of phenylephrine in hypospadias surgery. However, it is used in priapism treatment in which vasoconstrictor effect is required. Burnett and Bivalaqua reported that phenylephrine was the preferred vasoconstrictor for treatment of priapism because of its lower risk profile for systemic cardiovascular adverse effects [20]. Moreover, Montague et al. recommended that if phenylephrine was unavailable for treatment of priapism, other alpha adrenergic agonists, such as epinephrine, norepinephrine, and ephedrine, could be used [21].

The present study compared the histopathological outcomes of injecting phenylephrine and epinephrine on the spongy tissue and the urethra. According to the results, phenylephrine and epinephrine injection led to a better stereological outcome compared to the surgery group following hypospadias surgery in rats. Similarly, Najeh et al. demonstrated that epinephrine solution 1:100000 was safe and decreased bleeding and wound hematoma in hypospadias surgery. It also eliminated the need for tourniquet, reduced the use of bipolar cautery, and decreased the duration of operation and admission [2].

The current study had some limitations. Firstly, the animals undergoing surgery did not have hypospadias. Therefore, actual hypospadias models were not available and normal urethras were incised. Secondly, clinical outcomes, such as total bleeding during surgery, wound hematoma, and urethrocutaneous fistula formation, were not assessed after the surgery. Thirdly, adverse effects, including tachycardia and hypertension, were not evaluated. Finally, the utilized method was not compared to other hemostasis techniques, such as tourniquet application. Thus, further experimental and human studies are needed to draw firm conclusions. Future evaluations may also be required to compare phenylephrine and epinephrine in terms of systemic adverse effects and clinical outcomes in hypospadias surgery in order to determine which one can be the best option for achieving hemostasis during this surgery.

Conclusions

The study findings revealed that hypospadias repair using the aforementioned vasoconstrictors resulted in better postoperative stereological outcomes compared to surgery without using any hemostasis techniques. Besides, no stereological differences were observed between phenylephrine and epinephrine.

Acknowledgements

This work was performed at the Histomorphometry and Stereology Research Center, Shiraz University of Medical Sciences, Shiraz, Iran. This article was a part of the thesis written by Dr. Mohammad-Bagher Rajabalian for the Specialty Degree in Urology awarded by Shiraz University of Medical Sciences. Hereby, the authors would like to thank Ms. A. Keivanshekouh at the Research Improvement Center of Shiraz University of Medical Sciences for improving the use of English in the manuscript.

Authors' contributions

MS, ZJ, and AN designed the study, analyzed the data, and drafted the manuscript. MBR and FA took part in animal experiments, did the data analysis, and contributed to drafting the manuscript. SK took part in data analysis and contributed to drafting the manuscript. All authors read and approved the final manuscript.

Author details

[1]Department of Urology, Shiraz University of Medical Sciences, Shiraz, Iran. [2]Histomorphometry and Stereology Research Center, Shiraz University of Medical Sciences, Zand Ave., Shiraz 71348-45794, Iran. [3]Anatomy Department, School of Medicine, Shiraz University of Medical Sciences, Shiraz, Iran.

References

1. Fisch M. Urethral reconstruction in children. Curr Opin Urol. 2001;119(3): 253–5 Review.
2. Al-Omari N, Treef W, Daradka I, Nabulsi B, Sarrayra M, Idamat A. Safety and efficacy of topical epinephrine solution 1/100,000 in hypospadias surgery. JRMS. 2009;16:30–3.
3. Kajbafzadeh AM, Payabvash S, Tavangar SM, Salmasi AH, Sadeghi Z, Elmi A, Tirgari F, Razavi AE. Comparison of different techniques for hemostasis in a rabbit model of hypospadias repair. J Urol. 2007;178(6):2555–60.

4. Fang DB, Shen YH, Zhu XW, Fang JJ, Mao QQ, Chao-Jun W, Tan FQ, He QW, Shen BH, Xie LP. Penile necrosis resulting from post-circumcision microwave diathermy: A report of 9 cases. Zhonghua Nan Ke Xue. 2015;21(5):428–31.
5. Frenkl TL, Agarwal S, Caldamone AA. Results of a simplified technique for buried penis repair. J Urol. 2004;171(2 Pt 1):826–8.
6. Malamed S. Handbook of local anesthesia. 6th ed. St. Louis: Elsevier Health Sciences; 2012.
7. Hyde DM, Tyler NK, Plopper CG. Morphometry of the respiratory tract: avoiding the sampling, size, orientation, and reference traps. Toxicol Pathol. 2007;35(1):41–8.
8. Shirazi M, Noorafshan A, Serhan A. Effects of different suture materials used for the repair of hypospadias: a stereological study in a rat model. Urol Int. 2012;89(4):395–401. https://doi.org/10.1159/000343423.
9. Khoshvakhti H, Yurt KK, Altunkaynak BZ, Türkmen AP, Elibol E, Aydın I, Kıvrak EG, Önger ME, Kaplan S. Effects of melatonin on diclofenac sodium treated rat kidney: a stereological and histopathological study. Ren Fail. 2015;37(8): 1379–83. https://doi.org/10.3109/0886022X.2015.1073556.
10. Costa WS, Rebello SB, Cardoso LE, Cavalcanti AG, Sampaio FJ. Stereological and biochemical analysis of muscular and connective tissue components in the penile corpus cavernosum adjacent to the fibrous plaque of Peyronie's disease. BJU Int. 2009;103(2):212–6. https://doi.org/10.1111/j.1464-410X.2008.08023.x.
11. Ferreira FT, Dambros M, Bisogni S, Dambros MC, Scolfaro MR, Palma PC. Effects of testosterone supplementation on prevention of age-related penile remodeling. Aging Male. 2014;17(1):12–7. https://doi.org/10.3109/13685538.2013.873784.
12. Kristiansen SL, Nyengaard JR. Digital stereology in neuropathology. APMIS. 2012;120(4):327–40. https://doi.org/10.1111/j.1600-0463.2012.02889.x Review.
13. Mahmoudi R, Honarmand Z, Karbalay-Doust S, Jafari-Barmak M, Nikseresht M, Noorafshan A. Using curcumin to prevent structural impairments of testicles in rats induced by sodium metabisulfite. EXCLI J. 2017;16:583–92. https://doi.org/10.17179/excli2017-143.
14. Weber DM, Landolt MA, Gobet R, Kalisch M, Greeff NK. The penile perception score: an instrument enabling evaluation by surgeons and patient self-assessment after hypospadias repair. J Urol. 2013;189(1):189–93. https://doi.org/10.1016/j.juro.2012.08.178.
15. Hansson E, Becker M, Aberg M, Svensson H. Analysis of complications after repair of hypospadias. Scand J Plast Reconstr Surg Hand Surg. 2007;41(3):120–4.
16. Canning DA. Re: A comparison between tourniquet application and epinephrine injection for hemostasis during hypospadias surgery: the effect on bleeding and postoperative outcome. J Urol. 2017;198(4): 733. https://doi.org/10.1016/j.juro.2017.07.023.
17. Alizadeh F, Fakoor A, Haghdani S. A comparison between tourniquet application and epinephrine injection for hemostasis during hypospadias surgery: the effect on bleeding and postoperative outcome. J Pediatr Urol. 2016;12(3):160.e1–5. https://doi.org/10.1016/j.jpurol.2016.02.005.
18. Van Savage JG, Palanca LG, Slaughenhoupt BL. A prospective randomized trial of dressings versus no dressings for hypospadias repair. J Urol. 2000; 164(3):981–3.
19. M C, F C, U K, O B, A S, O C. Tourniquet application and epinephrine injection to penile skin: is it safe? Urol Res. 2002;30(4):268–72.
20. Burnett AL, Bivalacqua TJ. Priapism: current principles and practice. Urol Clin North Am. 2007;34(4):631–42 viii. Review.
21. Montague DK, Jarow J, Broderick GA, Dmochowski RR, Heaton JP, Lue TF, Nehra A, Sharlip ID, Members of the erectile dysfunction guideline update panel. Americal urological association. J Urol. 2003;170(4 Pt 1):1318–24.

5

Dissection of the inferior mesenteric vein versus of the inferior mesenteric artery for the genitourinary function after laparoscopic approach of rectal cancer surgery

Anna Pallisera-Lloveras[1*], Paula Planelles-Soler[2], Naim Hannaoui[2], Laura Mora-López[1], Jesús Muñoz-Rodriguez[2], Sheila Serra-Pla[1], Arturo Dominguez-Garcia[2], Joan Prats-López[2], Salvador Navarro-Soto[1], Xavier Serra-Aracil[1] and on behalf of Tauli-Colorectal Cancer Study Group

Abstract

Background: Total Mesorectal Excision (TME) is the standard surgical technique for the treatment of rectal cancer. However, rates of sexual dysfunction ofup to 50% have been described after TME, and rates of urinary dysfunction of up to 30%. Although other factors are involved, the main cause of postoperative genitourinary dysfunction is intraoperative injury to the pelvic autonomic nerves. The risk is particularly high in the inferior mesenteric artery (IMA). The aim of this study is to compare pre- and post-TME sexual dysfunction, depending on the surgical approach usedin the inferior mesenteric vessels: either directly on the IMA, or from the inferior mesenteric vein (IMV) to the IMA.

Methods: Prospective, randomized,controlled study of patients with rectal adenocarcinoma with neoadjuvant chemoradiotherapy, who will be randomly assigned to one of two groups depending on the surgical approach to the inferior mesenteric vessels. The main variable is pre- and postoperative sexual dysfunction; secondary variables are visualization and preservation of the pelvic autonomic nerves, pre- and postoperative urinary dysfunction, and pre- and postoperative quality of life. The sample will comprise 90 patients, 45 per group.

Discussion: The aim is to demonstrate that the dissection route from the IMV towards the IMA favors the preservation of the pelvic autonomic nerves and thus reducesrates of sexual dysfunction post-surgery.

Keywords: Genitourinary dysfunction, Injury to the pelvic autonomic nerves, Total Mesorectal excision, Rectal cancer

* Correspondence: apallill@gmail.com; apallisera@tauli.cat
[1]Coloproctology Unit, General and Digestive Surgery Department, Parc Taulí University Hospital, Sabadell, UniversitatAutònoma de Barcelona, Parc Taulí s/n. 08208 Sabadell, Barcelona, Spain
Full list of author information is available at the end of the article

Background

Despite the advances in adjuvant and neoadjuvant chemotherapy (QT) and radiotherapy (RT) for colorectal cancer, surgery remains the only curative treatment [1]. Since its first description by Heald in 1982 [2, 3], Total Mesorectal Excision (TME) has been the standard surgical technique for the treatment of rectal cancer, and has brought about significant improvement in oncological results in terms of both survival and local recurrence [4].

However, the literature describes post-TME rates of urinary dysfunction (urinary incontinence, difficulty in voiding or neurogenic bladder) of up to 30% [5, 6]. The prevalence of sexual dysfunction is above 50%; in men, it includeserectile dysfunction and ejaculation problems, and in women, decreased vaginal lubrication, dyspareunia and difficulty reaching orgasm [5, 6]. For this reason, the study of functional results such as genitourinary function, fecal continence and quality of life in general is taking on increasing importance [1].

Although other factors may be responsible for postoperative genitourinary dysfunction, the main cause is intraoperative injury to the pelvic autonomic nerves [1, 6]. This inadvertent lesion usually occurs due to a lack of anatomical knowledge or due to poor visualization of the nerves [6]. Minimally invasive techniques such as laparoscopic colorectal surgery and robotic surgery have improved surgical technique and surgical visibility, that helps in recognizing the inferior hypogastric plexus [7]. Moreover, a thorough acquaintance with anatomical reference points and experience ofthe dissection during TME reduces the risk of injuring the autonomic nerves, and leaves the mesorectal fascia intact. Indeed, proficient TME technique helps to preserve the autonomic nerves, lowering the incidence of urinary dysfunction from 10 to 30% to 0–12% and sexual dysfunction from 40 to 60% to 10–35% [5, 6]. Table 1 shows the genitourinary dysfunction after TME surgery, with the preservation of the pelvic autonomic nerves [8–10].

In rectal cancer surgery particular attention must be paid to certain areas, due to the risk of autonomic nerve damage [6]. Figure 1 depicts the surgical anatomy of the pelvic region and the key points where the risk of injury increases during surgery (Table 2) [5, 6, 11–14]. As described in the table, one of the regions with the highest risk of injury is the inferior mesenteric artery (IMA).

Recently, Melani [15] described a new laparoscopic approach for the release of the splenic flexure, in which a dissection of the mesenteric vessels is performed from the inferior mesenteric vein (IMV) to the IMA. This route presents a dissection plane that follows the anatomical peritoneal sheets of the retroperitoneum and improves the visualization of the pelvic autonomic nerves from their origin. Compared with the standard approach to the inferior mesenteric vessels (i.e., directly on the IMA), we believe thatthe approach from the IMV to the IMA will improve nerve preservation and thus reduce the incidence of sexual and urinary dysfunction.

Hypothesis and objectives

Hypothesis

The hypothesis is that the dissection route from the IMV to the IMA favors the preservation of the pelvic autonomic nerves, and thus reduces genitourinary dysfunction in patients after laparoscopic TME.

Objectives

The main objective is to determine the pre- and post-TME rates of sexual dysfunction in patients with rectal cancer randomly assigned to one of two nerve preservation techniques.

In both groups, the secondary objectives are to assess: urinary dysfunction pre- and post-TME; the visualization

Table 1 Genitourinary dysfunction after TME surgery with preservation of the pelvic autonomic nerves

Author (year)	Surgical approach	N	Measurement methods	Time of measurement	Urinary dysfunction (%)	Sexual dysfunction (%)
Dulskas A, et al. [1] (2016)	Open	108	Urinary: IPSS, BFLUTS Sexual: IIEF, FSFI	Pre-IQ and 6 m postIQ	Men 8.3% Women 11.1%	Men 27.8% Women 11.1%
Pontallier A, et al. [7] (2016)	Lap Transanal	34 38	Urinary: IPSS Sexual: IIEF, FSFI	12 months after closure of the stoma	23.5% 31.5%	61% 29%
Liu Z, et al. [8] (2016)	Lap	518	Own scale	At discharge and 6 months postIQ	NE	Ejaculation 42.5% Erection 41.9%
Adam JP, et al. [9] (2016)	Lap	169	Urinary: IPSS Sexual: IIEF, FSFI	Pre-treatment, post-QTRT and 3,6 and 12 months postIQ	17%	Men: Erection 43% Ejaculation 68% Women: Lubrication 62% Dyspareunia 42% Orgasm 57%

TME total mesorectal excision, *SP* surgical procedure, *IPSS* International Prostatic Symptom Score, *BFLUTS* Bristol Female Lower Urinary Tract Symptoms, *IIEF* International Index of Erectile Function, *FSFI* Female Sexual Function Index. QTRT: chemoradiotherapy

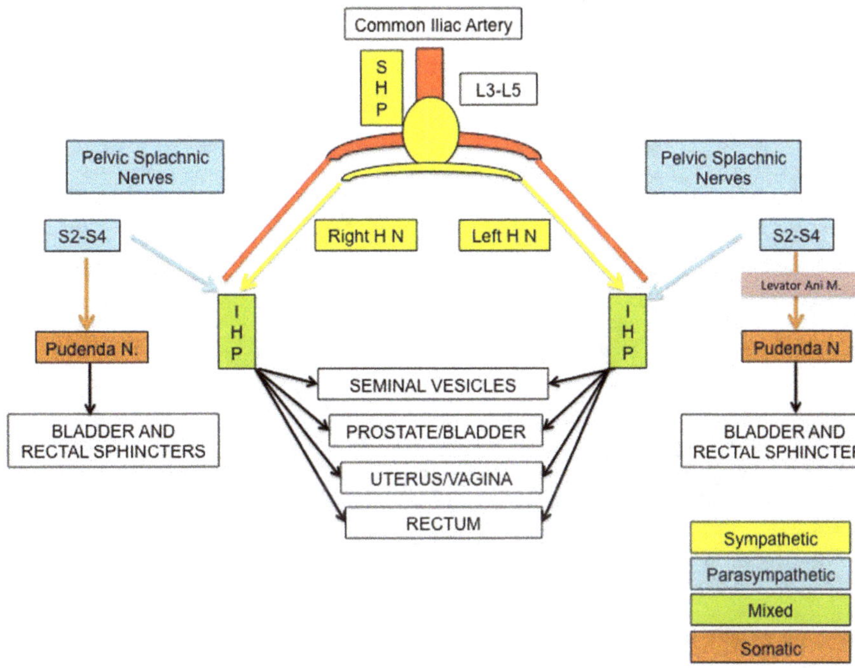

Fig. 1 Outline of the pelvic autonomic nerves and their target organs

and preservation of the superior hypogastric plexus (SHP), the hypogastric nerves, the inferior hypogastric plexus (IHP) and the Bundle of Walsh; and the impact of genitourinary dysfunction on patients' quality of life.

Methods/design

Study design

In this prospective, controlled randomized study of patients undergoing laparoscopic TME for rectal cancer, with neoadjuvant chemoradiotherapy, patients will be assigned to one of two groups, in a 1:1 ratio: the intervention arm (dissection route from the IMV to the IMA), and the control arm (dissection route directly to the IMA).

Study area and participants

The study will be carried out at the ParcTaulí University Hospital of Sabadell (Sabadell, Barcelona, Spain), which has a specialized unit for Colorectal Surgery, Urology, Radiodiagnosis, Oncology, and Radiotherapy.

The study population will comprise patients diagnosed with rectal cancerundergoing total colonoscopy with multifocal biopsy, rectoscopy with endorectal ultrasound (ERUS), pelvic magnetic resonance imaging (MRI) and thoraco-abdominal computed tomography (CT). All patients will be evaluated by the multi-disciplinary committee of colorectal tumors and must comply with the following criteria:

Inclusion criteria

Male sex; age 18 years or over; diagnosis of rectal adenocarcinoma ≤10 cm from the anal verge, measured by rigid rectoscopy, candidate to TME; candidate for neoadjuvant treatment (chemoradiotherapy); scheduled laparoscopic radical TME surgery carried out by colorectal surgeons; ASA I, II or III; provision of signed informed consent.

Exclusion criteria

Female sex; age under 18; not candidate for neoadjuvant treatment and/or adenocarcinoma > 10 cm from the anal verge candidate to partial TME; abdominoperineal resection (APR); emergency surgery; recurrent tumor; cT4; history of infra-abdominal or pelvic prostate procedures; radiotherapy prior to the current process; patients with severe sexual or urinary dysfunction before surgery; no provision of signed informed consent.

Criteria for withdrawal

Patients who do not attend the subsequent follow-up.

Definitions

Sexual dysfunction (SD) is defined as difficulty at any stage of sexual intercourse (which includes desire, arousal, orgasm and resolution) that prevents the individual or their partner from enjoyingsexual activity [16]. Erectile dysfunction (ED) is defined as the persistent inability to reach and maintain an erection sufficient to allow satisfactory sexual performance, which mayhave a physical and psychological effect on health and have a significant impact on the quality of life of patients and their respective partners [17].

Table 2 Areas with risk of lesion in the main autonomic nerves, and their effects

Nerve injured	Area of risk	Urinary dysf.	Sexual dysf.
SHP (sympathetic) 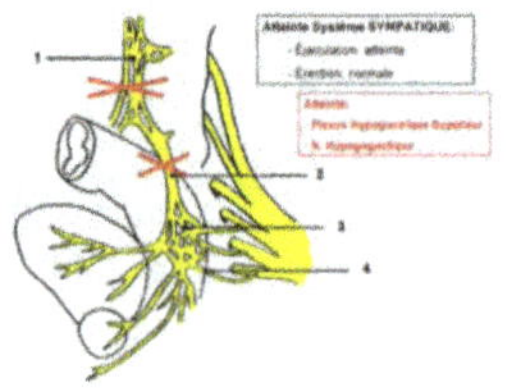	Dissection and ligature of IMA	Stress urinary incontinence	Retrograde ejaculation
Hypogastric nerves	Posterior dissection		Alteration in ejaculation (no alteration erection)
Splanchnic nerves (parasympathetic) 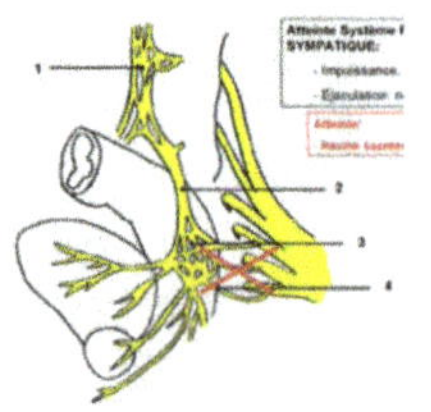	Rare in TME In radical lymph node dissections	Neurogenic bladder	Men: alteration erection Women: Dyspareunia
IHP (mixed) 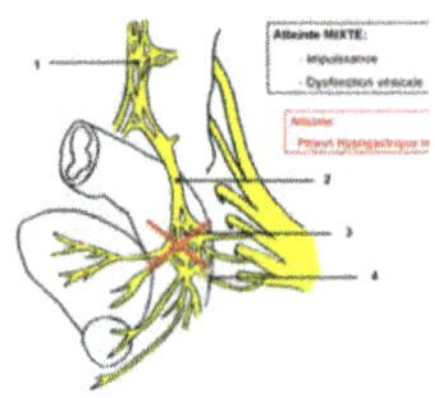	Lateral dissection	Incontinence Difficulty voiding	Problems with ejaculation and erection
- IHP one-sided		Difficulty voiding	Men: Ejaculation and erection problems Women: Problems with genital lubrication
- IHP two-sided		Bladder denervation	Men: impotence Women: dyspareunia and ↓ability to reach orgasm
Neurovascular bundle of Walsh and cavernous nerve	Anterior dissection		Men: impotencia and erectile dysfunction Women:dispareunia and reduced genital lubrication
Pudendo nerve and levator ani	Perineal stage of Miles APR	Urinary incontinence	Sexual sensorial impotence

According to the *2017 European* Association of *Urology* (EAU) *guidelines*, the diagnostic evaluation should be carried out with a correct anamnesis, the use ofvalidated questionnaires such as the International Index of Erectile Function or IIEF-5[18] and the Erection Hardness Score (EHS) [19], a full physical examination and basic analytical parameters such as total testosterone levels [17]. In addition, Doppler ultrasound of the penis is recommended, with the aim of recording objective parameters of induced erection so as to identify the cause of ED [17].

The IIEF-5 questionnaire consists of five questions that are scored from 0 to 5. Scores of 21 or lower are considered to indicateED. The test also classifies the severity of the ED as mild (score 17–21), mild to moderate (score 12–16), moderate 8–11 or severe (score 1–7) [18].

The EHS classifies erections in four grades: grade 1 or severe (does not allow penetration); grade 2 or moderate (increased circumference, relatively rigid, but not enough to achieve penetration); grade 3 or mild (increased length and circumference to allow penetration, but not enough to be satisfactory); grade 4 (maximum dimensions in terms of length and strength to achieve satisfactory penetration) [19].

Urinary or voiding dysfunction is defined as any alteration in the correct functioning in the storage or periodic emptying of urine, either in isolation or simultaneously [20]. To measure the severity of symptoms and the impact on the quality of life, or to monitor the response to a particular treatment, the ICIQ-SF (International Consultation on Incontinence Questionnaire) is used [21]. The ICIQ-SF consists of three questions, with a total score of 1 to 21; a score higher than 0 is considered a diagnosis of urinary incontinence.

The IPSS (International Prostate Syndrome Score) [22] consists of seven questions that assess voiding, frequency, intermittency, urgency, weak stream and effort. Each question is scored from 0 to 5: an overall score of 1 to 7 reflects mild symptomatology, one from 8 to 19 moderate, and from 20 to 35 severe. However, the only method that can objectively evaluate the filling and emptying phase, and therefore diagnose the presence and type of urinary dysfunction, is the urodynamic study [20].

Informed consent and legal considerations

Patients will be informed, both orally and in writing, of the objective and duration of the study. It will be made clear that participation is voluntary and they will be informed of all the possible risks and associated complications. Patients who meet the inclusion criteria and sign informed consent will enter the randomization process. They may withdraw their consent to participate at any time.

The variables described are recorded in a computerized database (Microsoft® Acces 2003). The data will be introduced in a protected format to avoid (as far as possible) the entry of out-of-range or anomalous values. The patients' data will berecorded anonymously and in accordance with the Spanish legislation on data protection (LOPD, 1999) [23].

The study protocol, the patients'data and the informed consent documents have been approved by the Clinical Research Ethics Committee in accordance with the 2015 Royal Decree on medical trials with drugs. The Parc Taulí's ethics committee will serve as the reference (ID: 2017/315). The study has been registered in the ClinicalTrials.gov database (ID: NCT03520088).

The trial will be carried out in accordance with the 7th Revision of the Declaration of Helsinki [24] and follows the guidelines of the 2013 SPIRIT Standard Protocols for Clinical Trials [25],CONSORT 2010 for Clinical Trials [26],and the Spanish Agency for Medicines and Health Medical Products).

Description of the randomization

A simple randomization system will be used, in which the selected patients will be randomly assigned by a computer program in a 1:1 ratio to one of two study arms: the intervention arm (dissection route from the IMV to the IMA) and the control arm (dissection route directly to the IMA).

Blinding

Neither the patient nor the urologist performing the sexual and urinary function study will have access to any surgical data; nor will they know which arm of the study the patient belongs to.

Trial interventions

Patients who meet the inclusion criteria and sign the informed consent document will be referred to the urologist for functional study after 8–10 weeks of neoadjuvant treatment, before surgery (Fig. 2).

The study consists of: a) an anamnesis with medical and psychosexual history; b) total testosterone level (ng/dL); c) Erection Hardness Score (EHS) [19]; d)IIEF-5 [18];e) I-PSS [22]; f)ICIQ-SF [21]; g) the European Organization for Research and Treatment of Cancer Quality-of-Life questionnaire (EORTC-QLQ C30) [27]; h) Doppler ultrasound of the penis; i) Urodynamic study.

For the Doppler ultrasound of the penis, a baseline study will be carried out to assess the ultrasound structure of the scrotal wall, both corpora cavernosa and the corpus spongiosum, the presence of calcifications or plaques of fibrosis, and their location. Subsequently, 15 mg of prostaglandin E1, a vasodilator agent that induces erection,will be applied to one of the corpora cavernosa (the sidechosen for the injection is irrelevant). After 20 min of the application the ultrasound provides dorsal and transversal measurements during the initial phases, and oblique-longitudinal measurements once tumescence begins, of the diameter of both cavernous arteries, their peak systolic flow velocity (cm/s) and their flow velocity at the end of diastole (cm/s) [28].

For the urodynamic study a flowmetry will be performed, recording: maximum urine volume (mL), maximum flow (mL/s), average flow (mL/s), and urination time (s)) and subsequently an ultrasound evaluation of postvoid residue (mL) [20].

Subsequently, patients undergo surgery after being randomly assigned to one of the two study arms. Before surgery, all patients will undergo mechanical colon preparation with antibiotic and thromboembolic prophylaxis, in accordance with the center's protocol.

Surgical technique

The surgery performed will be TME, using laparoscopic low anterior resection (LAR) approach or transanal TME (TaTME) [29], combining a laparoscopic approach and Transanal endoscopic operation (TEO).

The surgery is performed only by 5 surgeons, who are part of the colorectal unit. All of them experts in laparoscopic surgery and they have training on both techniques (intervention and control arm).

The surgery is performed laparoscopically with the patient in the Lloyd-Davies position. If release and mobilization of the splenic angle is necessary the Melani technique is applied [15], with the subsequent dissection of the IMA according to the randomization schedule, as follows:

a) Control group, with direct dissection of the IMA. Opening of the mesosigma peritoneum, laterally separating the SHP and hypogastric nerves.

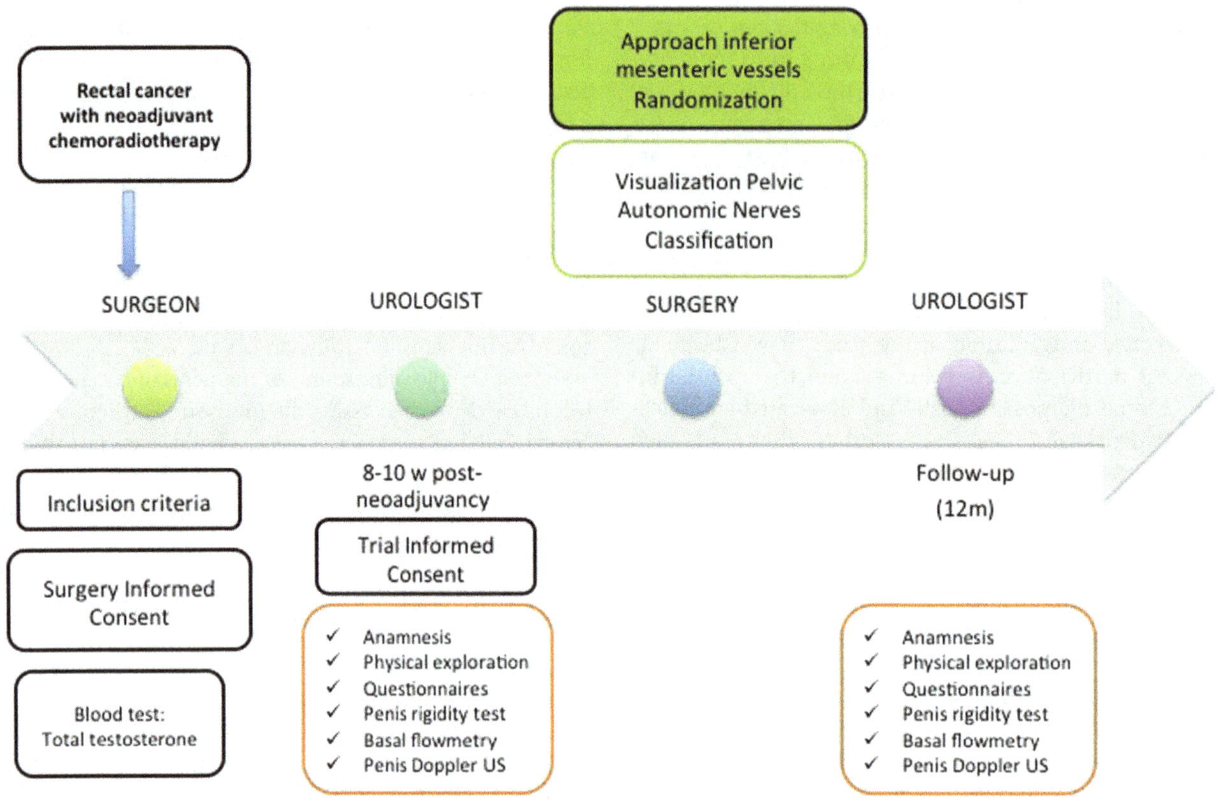

Fig. 2 Proposed study schedule

Visualization and preservation of the ureter, left primitive iliac vessels and the left gonadal vessels, and maintaining Gerota's fascia intact. High ligation of the IMA is performed about 1.5-2 cm from its origin in the aorta. The medial-to-lateral dissection proceeds, as far as the dissection of the splenic angle mobilization;

b) Intervention group, with dissection of the IMV to the IMA. Release of the splenic angle is followed by medial to lateral dissection from the IMV to the IMA, and a high ligation is performed about 1.5-2 cm from its origin in the aorta. Subsequently, the dissection follows the plane of the retroperitoneum from cranial to caudal and medial to lateral as far as the mesosigma.

The surgery continues with the following standardized steps: opening of the left Told's Fascia; mesorectal dissection immediately posterior to the superior rectal artery, following the plane anterior to the presacral parietal fascia; bilateral dissection, avoiding traction and blunt dissection that might damage the nerves or the integrity of the mesorectum; the anterior dissection is performed after completing the posterior dissection as far as the pelvic floor, leaving the Denonvilliers fascia intact, and following the avascular plane.

In the case of laparoscopic LAR, a Pfannenstiel incision is made toextract the specimen with the subsequent mechanical end-to-end colorectal anastomosis with EEA™ Auto suture 28 (Covidien™, Dublin, Ireland).

In transanal TME [29],TEO equipment is used (Karl Storz GmbH, Tüttlingen, Germany), and a pouch is made to close the distal rectum at least 1 cm below the visualization of the lesion. The area of the sectionis marked 1 cm from the pouch and transanal dissection of the mesorectal is carried out until reaching the dissection performed by laparoscopy. The lateral anterior dissection continues, leaving the Denonvilliers fascia intact.

In the case of an end colostomy is required, a colostomy orifice is performed in a previously marked site, sectioning the proximal colon with a scalpel and performing an end colostomy, with placement of a prophylactic mesh using the modified Sugarbaker technique [30, 31].

Follow-up

The patient will be referred again to the urologist to repeat the genitourinary dysfunction study 12 months after surgery: Doppler ultrasound of the penis, baseline flowmetry, EHS and the IIEF-5, I- PSS, ICIQ-SF and EORTC-QLQ C30 questionnaires.

Study variables

Main variable

Preoperative, post-neoadjuvant and postoperative sexual dysfunction at 12 months in all intervened patients will be determined by the urologist, based on the results of the IIEF-5 questionnaire and/or Doppler ultrasound (peak systolic velocity, tele-diastolic velocity and response to vasodilator agent). Scores of 21 or below on the IIEF-5 questionnaire will be taken to indicate sexual dysfunction. The ultrasound will confirm or rule out the presence of sexual dysfunction generated by the test: an adequate response to thevasodilator agent, with blood flow above 35 cm/s in a patient with an altered IIEF-5 or EHS test will be considered a diagnostic criterion for ED of a neurogenic cause.

Secondary variables

- Preoperative, post-neoadjuvant and postoperative erection hardness at 12 months;
- Preoperative, post-neoadjuvant and postoperative urinary dysfunction at 12 months, determined based on the results of the ICIQ-SF, IPSS and baseline flowmetry questionnaires (maximum urine volume, maximum flow, mean flow and urination time) with postvoid residue (mL). The presence of urinary dysfunction will be suspected if the patient has a score of 1 or aboveon the ICIQ-SF questionnaire, a score of 7 or above in the IPSS questionnaire or alterations in the flowmetry parameters: a maximum flow below 15 mL/s, a urinary volume less than 150 mL and/or a postvoid residue greater than 20% will be considered abnormal.
- Quality of life post-neoadjuvancy and 12 months after surgery will be assessed using the EORTC QLQ-C30 questionnaire.
- Visualization and preservation of the SHP, hypogastric nerves, the IHP and the neurovascular bundle of Walsh, during surgery (for each of these nerves), classified into: a) visualization and preservation of the nerves; b) visualization but no preservation; c) no visualization. This variable will be determined by the surgical team that performs the procedure. It will be taken into account that some patients may need the nerve resection for oncological purposes. The intervention will be recorded so that a surgeon not participating in the procedure can classify the nerve injury, as described above, and independently from the main surgeon. If there is disagreement between the two surgeons, the evaluation of a third external reviewer will be requested.

Other variables

Preoperative: age (years), body mass index (BMI) (kg/m2), smoking (packets/year), Charlson comorbidity index (CCI), previous pelvic surgeries, previous radiotherapy, Briganti criteria (low /intermediate/high risk), total testosterone levels (ng/dL). Characteristics of the tumor: height of the lesion (cm) by rectoscopy, location of the tumor (anterior, posterior, right or left lateral), cTNM staging.

Surgical Type of surgical technique (LAR, NOTES-hybrid), surgical time.

Postoperative Morbidity at 30 days (according to the Clavien-Dindo classification [32]), 30-day mortality, CCI [33], hospital stay. Definitive pathological anatomy: Size of the lesion (mm), pTNM and the completeness of mesorectal excision,according to the Quirke classification.

Statistical analysis

Sample size

With an α risk of 0.05 (5%), a one-sided hypothesis and a βriskof 0.1 (power of 90%), taking into account that the prevalence of post-TME sexual dysfunction is 50% and intending to reduce the figure to 20%,it will be necessary to include 41 patients in the two groups. Estimating a possible loss to follow-up of 10%, the total sample required will be 90 patients: 45 per group.

In our hospital rectal surgery for cancer is expected between 60 and 70/year, with inclusion criteria, we think that about 45–50 could be included. That means, that probabibly in two years, the recruitment should be finished.

Analysis of patients by intention to treat, per protocol, and patients lost

Patients will be analysed by intention to treat (ITT), per protocol, andlost patients.

The intention to treat analysis will be applied to all randomized patients.

The per protocol analysis will include part of the group in which direct dissection of the IMA is performed, and all the group that undergo dissection from the IMV to the IMA. Statistical analysis of the lost patients will be performed.

Monitoring

Monitoring will be carried out by a data manager. The variables will be recorded on an Access database which the data manager will manage via the various hospitals.

Statistical analysis

To evaluate the main objective of the study, the reduction in sexual dysfunction achieved by the preservation of the pelvic autonomic nerves, we will use the method based on the one-sided confidence interval at 95% of the difference in sexual dysfunction between the two groups

[34, 35], in both the intention to treat and per protocol samples.

The quantitative variables will be described giving values of mean and standard deviation, or medians, interquartile interval and range, as appropriate. The categorical variables will be described in absolute numbers and percentages.

The statistical analysis of the quantitative variables, with independent groups, will be performed with the parametric Student's T-test, provided that its conditions of application are met; otherwise, the non-parametric Mann-Whitney U test will be used.

In the statistical analysis for categorical variables, the Pearson X^2 test or the Fisher exact test will be used.

These methods will be used to compare the baseline characteristicsof the two groups in order to assess whether the randomization has been effective.

Statistical significance will be set at a p value of less than 0.05.

Discussion

In our study, only men, submitted to TME and candidate for neoadjuvant treatment (chemoradiotherapy) are included, so that the sample is more homogeneous in terms of final results.

TME, performed by minimally invasive surgery through laparoscopic or robotic approaches and/or TaTME, reduces morbidity and accelerates postoperative recovery. Improved quality of life in the medium and long term continues to be one of the main objectives of TME.

Some authors have shown better functional results with the robotic approach due to the superior movements of the wristed instruments that facilitate fine dissection, coupled with a stable and magnified view that helps in recognizing the inferior hypogastric plexus [7]. Due to the lack of experience in robotic surgery and our long experience in laparoscopic surgery, the design of our study has been made only in laparoscopic approach, to avoid the learning curve bias.

It is known, that quality of life and sexual dysfunction rates are not similar among patients submitted to LAR and APR. In our study, only patients submitted to LAR are included, in order to have a more homogeneous sample.

Different definitions of the concept of "quality of life" have been proposed and perhaps no single definition is fully satisfactory. The best one may be: "a state of general satisfaction, derived from the realization of the potential of the person. It has subjective aspects and objective aspects. It is a subjective feeling of physical, psychological and social well-being. It includes, as subjective aspects, intimacy, emotional expression, perceived safety, personal productivity and objective health. As objective aspects, material well-being, harmonious relationships with the physical and social environment and with the community, and health objectively perceived". As early as 1986, the European Organization for Research and Treatment of Cancer (EORTC) launched a program to assess the quality of life of patients participating in international clinical trials. This is why we have chosen the questionnaire validated by this organization, the EORTC-QLQ C30 [27], to evaluate the quality of life in our study.

Quality of life in our patients is defined by the need for an ostomy orby the presence ofsexual and urinary dysfunctions. Data on these dysfunctions are generally compiled through the use of questionnaires, which all present subjective limitations. As described above, sexual dysfunction is the difficulty at any stage of sexual intercourse (including desire, arousal, orgasm and resolution) that prevents the individual or their partner from enjoying sexual activity [5]. As detailed in the material and methods section, we have followed the indications of the EAU *guidelines (2017)* for the study of sexual dysfunction. The reason for adding the Doppler ultrasound study is to evaluate the cavernous arteries and their spectral evolution, in order to record objective parameters of induced erection and thus to identify the cause of the erectile dysfunction [17]. In addition, there is no reference in the literature of the study of SD in TME with the Doppler and that will give us objective data about it. Clearly, anxiety, psychological strain and any adrenergic stimulus may lead to false positive results, but with the exception of these cases, an altered result can be attributed to a neurogenic cause of erectile dysfunction in patients with a history of nerve damage [36]. Urinary dysfunction is defined as any alteration in the correct functioning in the storage or periodic voiding of urine, either in isolation or simultaneously. The tests used in the study are, once again, the ones recommended in the EAU *guidelines*; however, the only method able to objectively evaluate the presence and type of urinary dysfunction is urodynamic study by means of flowmetry [20].

The rationale for our study is the belief that the dissection routefrom the IMV to the IMA can improve nerve preservation of the nerves. The reason is anatomical, because this approach route follows the plane of dissection of the peritoneal sheets of the retroperitoneum, favoring visualization (and therefore a better preservation) of the pelvic autonomic nerves from their origin.

We hope that our study will show that the approach from the IMV to the IMA can increase the preservation of the pelvic autonomic nerves, and can thuslower the rates of sexual dysfunctionto a figure around 20%.

In parallel, though this is not the objective of our study, we believe that the detection of possible presurgical sexual dysfunction can promote prompt treatment of this dysfunction after surgery. Previous studies in the setting of prostate adenocarcinoma surgery have shown that the selection of the patient (according to age and preoperative sexual function, measured with the IIEF), as well as the surgical technique (in the case of radical prostatectomies, the preservation of the neurovascular bundles) are the main determinants of postoperative erectile function [37]. Correct stratification of patients is vital to patient assessment and to the selection of the most appropriate postoperative treatment strategy. These studies conclude that when patients are correctly stratified and selected, a high recovery rate of erectile function can be expected after radical prostatectomy with neurovascular preservation.

If our hypothesis is supported, we believe that the change in approach proposed here will help to improve quality of life in patients undergoing surgery for rectal cancer with neoadjuvant radiotherapy.

Acknowledgements

We thank the members of the colorectal tumor multidisciplinary committee at the Parc Taulí University Hospital for their participation. We also thank Michael Maudsley for helping with the English.

Tauli-Colorectal Cancer Study Group. From Parc Tauli University Hospital. Coloproctology Unit. General and Digestive Surgery Department: Anna Pallisera-Lloveras, Laura Mora-López, Sheila Serra-Pla, Salvador Navarro-Soto, Xavier Serra-Aracil, Marta Hidalgo[2] Urology Department: Paula Planelles-Soler, NaimHannaoui, Jesús Muñoz-Rodriguez, Arturo Dominguez-Garcia, Joan Prats-López. [3]Ostomy Nurse and Case Manager: Carmen Del Pino. Medical Oncology Department: Carles Pericay, Ismael Macias. [5]Radiology Department: Eva Ballesteros. Pathology Department: Àlex Casalots. Digestive Department: Eva Martinez-Bauer.

E-mail addres of authors: Anna Pallisera-Lloveras (apallill@gmail.com), Paula Planelles-Soler (paula.planelles@gmail.com), Naim Hannaoui (NHannaoui@-tauli.cat), Laura Mora-López (mora.lopez.laura@gmail.com), Jesús Muñoz-Rodriguez (JMUNOZR@tauli.cat), Sheila Serra-Pla (sheilaserrapla@gmail.com), Arturo Dominguez-Garcia (arturodom1980@hotmail.com), Joan Prats-López (JPrats@tauli.cat), Salvador Navarro-Soto (SNavarro@tauli.cat), Xavier Serra-Aracil (xserraa@gmail.com).

Tauli-Colorectal Cancer Study Group. Coloproctology Unit. General and Digestive Surgery Department: Anna Pallisera-Lloveras, Laura Mora-López, Sheila Serra-Pla, Salvador Navarro-Soto, Xavier Serra-Aracil, Marta Hidalgo (mhidalgo@tauli.cat). [2]Urology Department: Paula Planelles-Soler, Naim Hannaoui, Jesús Muñoz-Rodriguez, Arturo Dominguez-Garcia, Joan Prats-López. [3]Ostomy Nurse and Case Manager: Carmen Del Pino (CDelPino@tauli.cat). Medical Oncology Department: Carles Pericay (CPericay@tauli.cat), Ismael Macias (imacias@tauli.cat). [5]Radiology Department: Eva Ballesteros (EBallesteros@tauli.cat). Pathology Department: Àlex Casalots (ACasalots@tauli.cat). Digestive Department: Eva Martinez-Bauer (EMartinezB@tauli.cat).

Authors' contributions

All authors contributed to the design and writing of the paper. All authors have read and approved the final manuscript.

Author details

[1]Coloproctology Unit, General and Digestive Surgery Department, Parc Taulí University Hospital, Sabadell, UniversitatAutònoma de Barcelona, Parc Taulí s/n. 08208 Sabadell, Barcelona, Spain. [2]Urology Department, Parc Taulí University Hospital, Sabadell, Universitat Autònoma de Barcelona, Parc Taulí s/n 08208, Sabadell, Barcelona, Spain.

References

1. Dulskas A, Samalavicius NE. A prospective study of sexual and urinary function before and after total mesorectal excision. Int J Color Dis. 2016;31: 1125–30.
2. Heald RJ, Husband EM, Ryall RD. The mesorectum in rectal cancer surgery-the clue to pelvic recurrence? Br J Surg. 1982;69:613–6 PMID: 6751457.
3. Heald RJ. The "holy plane" of rectal surgery. J R Soc Med. 1988;81:503–8.
4. Heald RJ, Ryall RD. Recurrence and survival after total mesorectal excision for rectal cáncer. Lancet. 1986;1(8496):1479–82 PMID: 2425199.
5. Dulskas A, Miliauskas P, Tikuisis R, Escalante R, Samalavicius NE. The functional results of radical rectal cancer surgery: review of the literature. Acta Chir Belg. 2016;116:1–10.
6. Kim NK, Kim YW, Cho MS. Total mesorectal excision for rectal cancer with emphasis on pelvic autonomic nerve preservation: expert technical tips for robotic surgery. Surg Oncol. 2015;24(3):172–80.
7. Morelli L, Di Franco G, Guadagni S, Rossi L, Palmeri M, Furbetta N, Gianardi D, Bianchini M, Caprili G, D'Isidoro C, Mosca F, Moglia A, Cuschieri A. Robot-assisted total mesorectal excision for rectal cancer: case-matched comparison of short-term surgical and functional outcomes between the da Vinci xi and Si. Surg Endosc. 2018;32(2):589–600.
8. Pontallier A, Denost Q, Geluwe BV, Adam JP, Celerier B, Rullier E. Potential sexual function improvement by using transanal mesorectal approach for laparoscopic low rectal cancer excision. SurgEndosc. 2016;30(11):4924–33.
9. Liu Z, Huang M, Kang L, Wang L, Lan P, Cui J, Wang J. Prognosis and postoperative genital function of function-preservative surgery of pelvic autonomic nerve preservation for male rectal cancer patients. BMC Surg. 2016;16:12.
10. Adam JP, Denost Q, Capdepont M, van Geluwe B, Rullier E. Prospective and longitudinal study of urogenital dysfunction after proctectomy for rectal cancer. Dis Colon Rectum. 2016;59:822–30.
11. Havenga K, Grossmann I, DeRuiter M, Wiggers T. Definition of Total Mesorectal excision, including the perineal phase: technical considerations. Dig Dis. 2007;25:44–50.
12. Chew MH, Yeh YT, Lim E, Seow-Choen F. Pelvic autonomic nerve preservation in radical rectal cancer surgery: changes in the past 3 decades. Gastroenterol Rep. 2016;4(3):173–85.
13. Moszkowicz D, Alsaid B, Bessede T, Penna C, Nordlinger B, Benoît G, Peschaud F. Where does pelvic nerve injury occur during rectal surgery for cancer? Color Dis. 2011;13(12):1326–34.
14. Clausen N, Wolloscheck T, Konerding MA. How to optimize autonomic nerve preservation in total mesorectal excision: clinical topography and morphology of pelvic nerves and fasciae. World J Surg. 2008;32:1768–75.
15. Komolafe OO, Melani AG, Véo CA, Denadai MV, de Oliveira JC. Laparoscopic mobilization for resection of the transverse colon for cancer: a simple, reproducible method. Surg Laparosc Endosc Percutan Tech. 2012;22(5): e267–70.
16. López-Ibor J. DSM-IV-TR: diagnostic and statistical manual of mental disorders. San Francisco: American Psychiatric Association; 2013. p. 600–3.
17. Salonia A, Eardley I, Giuliano F, Hatzichristou D, Moncada I, Vardi Y, Wespes E, Hatzimouratidis K, European Association of Urology. European Association of Urology guidelines on priapism. Eur Urol. 2014;65:480–9.
18. Rosen RC, Riley A, Wagner G, Osterloh IH, Kirkpatrick J, Mishra A. The international index of erectile function (IIEF): a multidimensional scale for assessment of erectile dysfunction. Urology. 1997;49:822–30.
19. Mulhall JP, Goldstein I, Bushmakin AG, Cappelleri JC, Hvidsten K. Validation of the erectionhardnessscore. J Sex Med. 2007;4:1626–34.
20. Groen J, Pannek J, Castro Diaz D, Del Popolo G, Gross T, Hamid R, Karsenty G, Kessler TM, Schneider M, 't Hoen L, Blok B. Summary of European Association of Urology (EAU) Guidelines on Neuro-Urology. Eur Urol. 2006; 69:324–33.
21. Bright E, Cotterill N, Drake M, Abrams P. Developing and validating the InternationalConsultation on IncontinenceQuestionnaire bladder diary. Eur Urol. 2014;66(2):294–300.
22. Barry MJ, Fowler FJ Jr, O'Leary MP, Bruskewitz RC, Holtgrewe HL, Mebust WK, Cockett AT. The American urological association symptom index for benign prostatic hyperplasia. The measurement Committee of the American Urological Association. J Urol. 1992;148:1549–57 discussion 1564.
23. Ley orgánica 15/1999 de 13 de diciembre de protección de datos de carácter personal (LOPD). BOE n° 298 de 14 /12/1999.

24. Emanuel EJ. Reconsidering the declaration of Helsinki. Lancet. 2013;381: 1532–3.
25. Chan A-W, Tetzlaff JM, Altman DG, Laupacis A, Gøtzsche PC, Krleža-Jerić K, Hróbjartsson A, Mann H, Dickersin K, Berlin JA, Doré CJ, Parulekar WR, Summerskill WS, Groves T, Schulz KF, Sox HC, Rockhold FW, Rennie D, Moher D. SPIRIT 2013 statement: definingstandardprotocolitemsforclinicaltrials. Ann InternMed. 2013;158:200–7.
26. Schulz KF, Altman DG, Moher D, for the CONSORT Group. CONSORT 2010 Statement: updated guidelines for reporting parallel group randomised trials. Int J Surg. 2011;9:672–7.
27. Aaronson NK, Ahmedzai S, Bergman B, Bullinger M, Cull A, Duez NJ, Filiberti A, Flechtner H, Fleishman SB, de Haes CJ, Kaasa S, Klee M, Osoba D, Razavi D, Rofe PB, Schraub S, Sneeuw K, Sullivan M, Takeda F. The European Organization for Research and Treatment of Cancer QLQ-C30: a quality-of-life instrument for use in international clinical trials in oncology. J Natl Cancer Inst. 1993;85:365–76.
28. Sarteschi LM, Montorsi F, MenchiniFabris F, Guazzoni G, Lencioni R, Rigatti P. Cavernous arterial and arteriolar circulation in patients with erectile dysfunction: a power Doppler study. J Urol. 1998;159:428–32.
29. Serra-Aracil X, Mora-Lopez L, Casalots A, Pericay C, Guerrero R, Navarro-Soto S. Hybrid NOTES: TEO fortransanal total mesorectalexcision: intracorporealresection and anastomosis. Surg Endosc. 2016;30:346–54.
30. Serra-Aracil X, Bombardo-Junca J, Moreno-Matias J, Darnell A, Mora-Lopez L, Alcantara-Moral M, Ayguavives-Garnica I, Navarro-Soto S. Randomized, controlled, prospective trial of the use of a mesh to prevent parastomal hernia. Ann Surg. 2009;249:583–7.
31. López-Cano M, Serra-Aracil X, Mora L, Sánchez-García JL, Jiménez-Gómez LM, Martí M, Vallribera F, Fraccalvieri D, Serracant A, Kreisler E, Biondo S, Espín E, Navarro-Soto S, Armengol-Carrasco M. Preventing Parastomal hernia using a modified Sugarbaker technique with composite mesh during laparoscopic abdominoperineal resection: a randomized controlled trial. Ann Surg. 2016;264:923–8.
32. Dindo D, Demartines N, Clavien P-A. Classification of surgical complications. A new proposal with evaluation in a cohort of 6336 patients and results of a survey. Ann Surg. 2014;240:205–13.
33. Slankamenac K, Graf R, Barkun J, et al. The comprehensive complication index: a novel continuous scale to measure surgical morbidity. Ann Surg. 2013;258:1–7.
34. Kaul S, Diamond GA. Goodenough: a primer ontheanalysis and interpretation of noninferioritytrials. Ann InternMed. 2006;4(145):62–9.
35. Piaggio G, Elbourne DR, Altman DG, Pocock SJ, Evans SJ, CONSORT group. Reporting of noninferiority and equivalencerandomizedtrials: anextension of the CONSORT statement. JAMA. 2006;295:1152–60.
36. de la Torre HP, Hernández Jover D, Martí Malet J, Ochoteco García JI. Valoración de la Disfunción Eréctil mediante ecografía Doppler-Duplex. ArchEspUrol. 2001;54:617–25.
37. Briganti A, Gallina A, Suardi N, Capitanio U, Tutolo M, Bianchi M, Passoni N, Salonia A, Colombo R, Di Girolamo V, Guazzoni G, Rigatti P, Montorsi F. Predicting erectile function recovery after bilateral nerve sparing radical prostatectomy: a proposal of a novel preoperative risk stratification. J Sex Med. 2010;7:2521–31.

6

Pathological upgrading in prostate cancer treated with surgery in the United Kingdom: Trends and risk factors from the British Association of Urological Surgeons Radical Prostatectomy Registry

Nicholas Bullock[1,2*], Andrew Simpkin[3], Sarah Fowler[4], Murali Varma[5], Howard Kynaston[1,2] and Krishna Narahari[2]

Abstract

Background: Accurate grading at the time of diagnosis if fundamental to risk stratification and treatment decision making in patients with prostate cancer. Whilst previous studies have demonstrated significant pathological upgrading and downgrading following radical prostatectomy (RP), these were based on historical cohorts and do not reflect contemporary patient selection and management practices. The aim of this national, multicentre observational study was to characterise contemporary rates and risk factors for pathological upgrading after RP in the United Kingdom (UK).

Methods: All RP entries on the British Association of Urological Surgeons (BAUS) Radical Prostatectomy Registry database of prospectively entered cases undertaken between January 2011 and December 2016 were extracted. Those patients with full preoperative PSA, clinical stage, needle biopsy and subsequent RP pathological grade information were included. Upgrade was defined as any increase in Gleason grade from initial needle biopsy to pathological assessment of the entire surgical specimen. Statistical analysis and multivariate logistic regression were undertaken using R version 3.5 (R Foundation for Statistical Computing, Vienna, Austria).

Results: A total of 17,598 patients met full inclusion criteria. Absolute concordance between initial biopsy and pathological grade was 58.9% (n = 10,364), whilst upgrade and downgrade rates were 25.5% (n = 4489) and 15.6% (n = 2745) respectively. Upgrade rate was highest in those with D'Amico low risk compared with intermediate and high-risk disease (55.7% versus 19.1 and 24.3% respectively, $P < 0.001$). Although rates varied between year of surgery and geographical regions, these differences were not significant after adjusting for other preoperative diagnostic variables using multivariate logistic regression.

Conclusions: Pathological upgrading after RP in the UK is lower than expected when compared with other large contemporary series, despite operating on a generally higher risk patient cohort. As new diagnostic techniques that may reduce rates of pathological upgrading become more widely utilised, this study provides an important benchmark against which to measure future performance.

Keywords: Gleason grade, Needle biopsy, Pathological, Prostate cancer, Radical prostatectomy

* Correspondence: bullocknp@cardiff.ac.uk
[1]Division of Cancer and Genetics, Cardiff University School of Medicine, Cardiff, UK
[2]Department of Urology, Cardiff and Vale University Health Board, University Hospital of Wales, Cardiff, UK
Full list of author information is available at the end of the article

Background

Despite first being described over fifty years ago, Gleason score has stood the test of time and remains one of the most powerful prognostic indicators in patients undergoing radical treatment with curative intent [1–5]. The Gleason grading system was updated in 2005 and again in 2014 following consensus conferences of the International Society of Urological Pathology (ISUP) [6, 7]. In the more recent update, the ISUP supported adoption of a validated Grade Group stratification system ranging from 1 (Gleason score ≤ 6) to 5 (Gleason score 9 or 10), to be used in conjunction with the overall Gleason system in order to simplify the number of grading categories and facilitate more accurate stratification of disease [6].

Despite advances in recent years, conventional diagnostic pathways employ transrectal ultrasound (TRUS) guided prostate biopsy to acquire systematic needle biopsies of the prostate, which has recently been shown to have a sensitivity of only 48% for the diagnosis of 'clinically significant' cancer, defined as Gleason score of at least 4 + 3 or a maximum core length of at least 6 mm [8]. Given the heterogeneity of disease it is not surprising that a significant proportion of cases are upgraded following radical prostatectomy (RP) compared with the initial TRUS biopsy [9–11]. This has wide ranging implications, as it may potentially lead to undertreatment of those that are undergraded by the initial biopsy, or conversely, overtreatment of those that have been overgraded. Furthermore, upgrading has been associated with adverse pathological outcomes, such as positive surgical margin status and biochemical recurrence [12, 13].

Whilst a small number of studies have reported pathological upgrading rates following RP in large patient populations, these utilised historical cohorts that underwent surgery prior to 2012 [10, 11]. Furthermore, neither involved participants from the United Kingdom (UK), thereby limiting the generalisability of findings to this patient population and the National Health Service. This is of particular importance as, owing to differences in screening practices across Europe and North America, a relatively high proportion of patients present with advanced disease at the time of diagnoses in the UK [14–18].

The objective of this large observational study was to characterise contemporary rates of pathological upgrading after RP in the UK and identify risk factors for upgrading within this population.

Methods

Case selection

Data for patients undergoing radical prostatectomy in the UK were uploaded prospectively by individual surgeons or institutions onto the British Association of Urological Surgeons (BAUS) Radical Prostatectomy Registry database. All patients that underwent RP between 1st January 2011 and 31st December 2016 were eligible for inclusion. Patients with missing data for key variables such as preoperative Prostate Specific Antigen (PSA), initial biopsy Gleason grade, clinical T stage or final RP Gleason grade were excluded, as were those that underwent salvage surgery.

Pathological assessment

The time from initial biopsy to RP was not recorded in the database. However, in the UK the National Health Service Cancer Reform Strategy states that patients diagnosed with cancer should receive definitive treatment within 31 days of the decision to do so. This means that most patients will have undergone surgery within 1–2 months of the initial biopsy, thereby ameliorating potential for genuine grade progression between histological assessment of the biopsy and surgical specimen.

Whilst the exact type of initial prostate biopsy was not recorded, TRUS guided biopsy utilising an extended sampling approach was standard practice across the UK during the study period. All biopsies were evaluated and reported by a Consultant Pathologist with or without expertise in urological pathology. Almost all RP specimens were examined and reported by a Consultant Pathologist with expertise in urological pathology. No cases were re-reviewed for the purposes of this study. The primary outcome was upgrading, defined as any increase in Gleason grade between the initial biopsy and final RP histology.

Statistical analysis

Continuous variables were reported using mean, median and range, and categorical variables as percentages. For unadjusted comparison between upgraded and non-upgraded cases, Chi-squared and t-tests were used to assess for statistically significant differences in categorical and continuous variables respectively. Logistic regression was used to formally determine the association of key preoperative variables and upgrading, with the odds ratio for each being reported alongside a 95% confidence interval and p-value. D'Amico risk category was not included in the mutually adjusted model, since it is a composite variable derived from PSA, clinical T-stage and biopsy Gleason grade (all of which were included in the model). All analyses were performed in R v3.5 (R Core Team (2018). R: A language and environment for statistical computing. R Foundation for Statistical Computing, Vienna, Austria).

Results

Patient demographics

17,598 of 30,424 patients that were entered onto the registry between 1st January 2011 and 31st December 2016 met full inclusion criteria. Table 1 demonstrates

Table 1 Patient, disease and operative characteristics

Patient and disease characteristics	
Age (years)	
Mean	63.22
Median	64
Range	35–92
Preoperative PSA (ng/ml)	
Mean	10.06
Median	7.85
Range	0–181
Preoperative biopsy ISUP Grade Group (%)	
1	3914 (22.2)
2	8328 (47.3)
3	2893 (16.4)
4	1427 (8.1)
5	1036 (5.9)
Preoperative clinical stage (%)	
T1	5435 (30.9)
T2	8311 (47.2)
T3	3839 (21.8)
T4	13 (0.10
Preoperative D'Amico risk group (%)	
Low risk	1766 (10.0)
Intermediate risk	6563 (37.3)
High risk	9269 (52.7)
Operative characteristics	
Year of surgery (%)	
2011	1001 (5.7)
2012	1159 (6.6)
2013	2259 (12.8)
2014	3783 (21.5)
2015	4566 (25.9)
2016	4830 (27.4)
Region (%)	
A	79 (0.4)
B	701 (4.0)
C	1653 (9.4)
D	2081 (11.8)
E	706 (4.0)
F	2084 (11.8)
G	1315 (7.5)
H	29 (0.2)
I	67 (0.4)
J	2093 (11.9)
K	1885 (10.7)
L	1736 (9.9)
M	745 (4.2)
N	1798 (10.2)
O	324 (1.8)
P	302 (1.7)

the patient and operative characteristics. Mean age and preoperative PSA were 63.2 years and 10.06 ng/ml respectively. The majority of cases were performed for D'Amico high risk disease (52.7%; n = 1766), with only 10% (n = 1766) for low risk disease. The proportion of cases performed each year increased from 2011 to 2016, owing to both a yearly increase in the number of cases entered onto the registry together with a reduction in the number of cases excluded on account of missing data each year.

Pathological upgrade rates

Absolute concordance between initial biopsy and pathological Gleason grade was 58.9% (n = 10,364), whilst upgrade and downgrade rates were 25.5% (n = 4489) and 15.6% (n = 2745) respectively. Table 2 demonstrates concordance between the initial biopsy and final RP histology as stratified by ISUP Grade Groups. Concordance was lowest in those patients with Grade Group 1 and 4 on initial biopsy (39.6 and 25.4% respectively), whilst highest in those patients with Grade Group 2 (76.6%). An increase by one ISUP Grade Group (for example, from Grade Group 1 on initial biopsy to Grade Group 2 on final RP histopathology) constituted the majority of upgrading events, with 319 (8.2%), 286 (3.4%) and 181 (6.3%) cases being upgraded by two or more Grade Groups in patients with Grade Group 1, 2 and 3 on initial biopsy respectively.

Risk factors for pathological upgrading

Table 3 provides the association between patient and operative characteristics and pathological upgrading. Upgrading was associated with a higher preoperative PSA (10.8 ng/ml versus 9.81 ng/ml; $p < 0.001$) and reduced over time, with 30.6% of cases being upgraded in 2011 compared with 23.2% in 2016 (Fig. 1a; $p < 0.001$). Of note, upgrade rate was highest in those with D'Amico low risk compared with intermediate and high-risk disease (Fig. 1b; 55.7% versus 19.1 and 24.3% respectively, $P < 0.001$). There was considerable variation in upgrading between regions, with rates ranging from 13.9% in region A to 37.9% in region H (Fig. 1c; $P < 0.001$).

Table 4 gives the results of the mutually adjusted logistic regression analysis for upgrading. After adjusting for differences in other characteristics, both increased age and preoperative PSA were associated with increased

Table 2 Concordance between the initial biopsy and final RP histology when stratified by ISUP Grade Groups

RP ISUP Grade Group	Biopsy ISUP Grade Group									
	1 (≤6)		2 (3 + 4)		3 (4 + 3)		4 (8)		5 (9–10)	
	No.	%	No.	%	No.	%	No.	%	No.	%
1 (≤6)	1550	39.6	430	5.2	38	1.3	21	1.5	2	0.2
2 (3 + 4)	2045	52.2	6381	76.6	955	33.0	351	24.6	103	9.9
3 (4 + 3)	235	6.0	1231	14.8	1579	54.6	486	34.1	227	21.9
4 (8)	52	1.3	165	2.0	140	4.8	363	25.4	73	7.0
5 (9–10)	32	0.8	121	1.5	181	6.3	206	14.4	631	60.9
Total	3914	100	8328	100	2893	100	1427	100	1036	100

odds of pathological upgrading (OR 1.022; $p < 0.001$ per year and OR 1.026; $p < 0.001$ per ng/ml respectively). Higher initial biopsy ISUP Grade Groups were associated with lower odds of upgrading, whilst clinically T2 and T3 tumours had the highest odds of upgrading. Those cases performed in more recent years were associated with reduced odds of upgrading when compared with 2011, although all failed to reach significance. Likewise, despite apparent regional differences, almost all failed to reach significance.

Discussion

This is the largest study to date exploring pathological upgrading after radical prostatectomy, as well as the first of its kind conducted within a large contemporary UK patient cohort. There are several potential reasons for differences occurring between initial biopsy Gleason grade and that of the RP specimen. Whilst genuine grade progression in the time between initial biopsy and RP is possible, this is unlikely and thus the majority of discrepancy occurs as a result of either sampling error or variation in pathological reporting.

Sampling error occurs when an area of high-grade tumour is missed by the initial needle biopsy, leading to undergrading. Conversely, the biopsy may oversample the high-grade component of a tumour. This scenario is well described, with many studies demonstrating conventional TRUS guided prostate biopsy to be poor at localising the index tumour and/or estimating true tumour grade [9–11, 19].

Variation in pathological reporting may result from the inherent subjectivity of tumour grading, microscopic interpretation issues and differences in rules used to report the Gleason score. Tumour grade is a morphological and biological continuum with arbitrary cut-offs, so a degree of variation is inevitable in borderline cases. Microscopic interpretation such as distinction between poorly formed glands of pattern 4 and tangential sectioning of pattern 3 glands is also subjective [10].

A number of authors have therefore sought to quantify the level of inter-observer agreement among pathologists [20, 21], with one recent study demonstrating kappa values of 0.61 for needle biopsies and 0.37 for RP specimens between the original pathology report and a 'gold standard' report issued by expert urological pathologists [22]. This study also recognised that the accuracy of Gleason grading may depend on the level of experience and training of the reporting pathologist [22]. Whilst the differing service structure means the findings of many of these US based studies cannot be completely applied to the UK, inter-observer variability will no doubt be partially responsible for some of the grade changes seen in the current series. For example, whilst several cases were upgraded following RP, a significant number were also downgraded, most notably from ISUP Grade Group 3 to 2 and from Grade Group 4 to either 3 or 2. In the UK many initial needle biopsies are reported in smaller District General Hospitals by pathologists who may or may not have expertise in urological pathology, whilst almost all RP specimens are reported in larger tertiary referral centres by expert urological pathologists. It is therefore possible that some of the observed overcalling of Gleason pattern 4 may have arisen due to lack of awareness among general UK pathologists of the 2014 ISUP consensus conference recommendation that occasional/seemingly poorly formed or fused glands are insufficient for a diagnosis of pattern 4 [6]. Finally, even when pathologists agree on the grade, they may report the Gleason score differently. For example, when cores show different Gleason scores, contemporary practice varies with either the overall (global) or worst Gleason score recorded for each biopsy series [7, 23, 24].

In this cohort of 17,598 patients we found overall upgrade and downgrade rates of 25.5 and 15.6% respectively. Interestingly upgrade rate was highest in those patients undergoing RP for low risk prostate cancer, as classified using D'Amico criteria that are widely used in UK practice [25]. Whilst this is somewhat expected given that this group comprises patients with Gleason 3 + 3 = 6 disease on initial biopsy, for whom the only change in grade can be upgrading, the rate of 55.7% is higher than reported in other comparable series. Whilst

Table 3 Association between patient, disease and operative characteristics and pathological upgrading after RP

Characteristic	No upgrade (*n* = 13,109)	Upgrade (*n* = 4489)	*p*-value
Age (years)	63.2 (6.56)	63.3 (6.44)	0.159
Preoperative PSA (ng/ml)	9.81 (7.93)	10.8 (8.94)	< 0.001
Preoperative biopsy ISUP Grade Group			< 0.001
1	1550 (39.6%)	2364 (60.4%)	
2	6811 (81.8%)	1517 (18.2%)	
3	2572 (88.9%)	321 (11.1%)	
4	1213 (85.0%)	214 (15.0%)	
5	963 (93.0%)	73 (7.05%)	
Preoperative clinical stage			< 0.001
T1	3957 (72.8%)	1478 (27.2%)	
T2	6350 (76.4%)	1961 (23.6%)	
T3	2792 (72.7%)	1047 (27.3%)	
T4	10 (76.9%)	3 (23.1%)	
Preoperative D'Amico risk group			< 0.001
Low risk	782 (44.3%)	984 (55.7%)	
Intermediate risk	5307 (80.9%)	1256 (19.1%)	
High risk	7020 (75.7%)	2249 (24.3%)	
Year of surgery			< 0.001
2011	695 (69.4%)	306 (30.6%)	
2012	848 (73.2%)	311 (26.8%)	
2013	1602 (70.9%)	657 (29.1%)	
2014	2835 (74.9%)	948 (25.1%)	
2015	3420 (74.9%)	1146 (25.1%)	
2016	3709 (76.8%)	1121 (23.2%)	
Region			< 0.001
A	68 (86.1%)	11 (13.9%)	
B	544 (77.6%)	157 (22.4%)	
C	1239 (75.0%)	414 (25.0%)	
D	1643 (79.0%)	438 (21.0%)	
E	552 (78.2%)	154 (21.8%)	
F	1536 (73.7%)	548 (26.3%)	
G	1020 (77.6%)	295 (22.4%)	
H	18 (62.1%)	11 (37.9%)	
I	49 (73.1%)	18 (26.9%)	
J	1553 (74.2%)	540 (25.8%)	
K	1382 (73.3%)	503 (26.7%)	
L	1301 (74.9%)	435 (25.1%)	
M	505 (67.8%)	240 (32.2%)	
N	1246 (69.3%)	552 (30.7%)	
O	226 (69.8%)	98 (30.2%)	
P	227 (75.2%)	75 (24.8%)	

this may have implications for counselling men with low risk disease that are considering surveillance, we must be wary not to extrapolate this figure to all patients. In the UK, recent years have seen a reduction in the number of men with low risk disease that undergo radical treatment [14], which is reflected within our cohort (n =

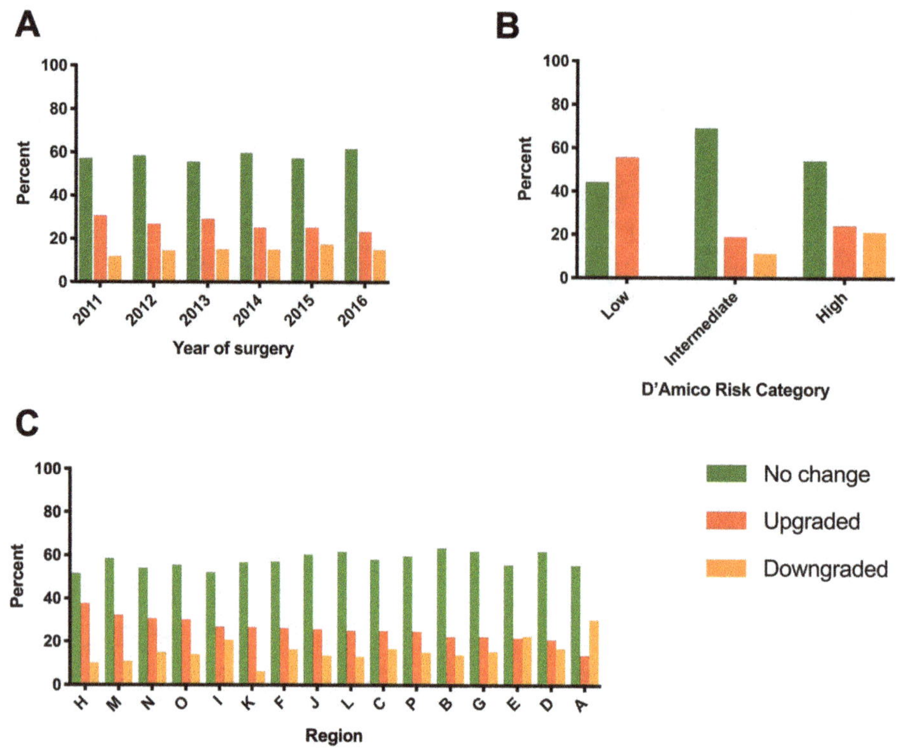

Fig. 1 Grade change according to: **a**, year of surgery. **b**, D'Amico risk category. **c**, anonymised region, ranked in order of upgrade rate

1766; 10%). This means those patients with low risk disease that undergo RP are likely to have other 'high risk' features, such as large volume tumour.

This study also demonstrated a reduction in upgrading in more recent years, with the rate falling from 30.6% in 2011 to 23.2% in 2016. Furthermore, we also identified variation in upgrading between geographical regions, with rates ranging from 13.9% in region A to 37.9% in region H. However, when adjusting for differences in other preoperative variables, almost all differences between regions and years of surgery failed to reach significance. Collectively this means that such differences can be explained by variation in other factors such as increasing age, preoperative PSA and clinical stage, as well as decreasing biopsy ISUP Grade Group, all of which were found to be significant risk factors for upgrading in our mutually adjusted logistic regression model.

Whilst TRUS guided biopsy utilising an extended sampling approach was standard practice across the UK during the study period, the exact biopsy technique utilised in each case was not recorded in the registry. Recent years have seen a trend towards increased uptake of prebiopsy mpMRI and contemporary diagnostic techniques such as mpMRI influenced biopsy strategy, template guided transperineal biopsy and mpMRI-TRUS fusion biopsy, which have been shown to reduce pathological upgrading after surgery [26–28]. Furthermore, these techniques have also been shown to reduce diagnosis of 'clinically insignificant' cancers, such as those that are Gleason 3 + 3 [29]. Collectively this may explain the trend towards a reduction in upgrading in seen in more recent years in this series. Furthermore, as these techniques continue to become more widely utilised, future rates of pathological upgrading are likely to decrease, thereby rendering this study an important benchmark against which to measure performance.

A number of other studies have explored upgrading and downgrading following RP. Whilst many of these utilised small historical cohorts, the results of the two largest and most recent series may be compared to the findings presented here. The first of these, published by Epstein et al. in 2012, reported grade change in 7643 US patients that underwent surgery between 2002 and 2010 [10]. Although similar in terms of age, the cohort had a lower PSA and higher proportion of T1 and Gleason 6 disease, thus representing a lower risk population. Interestingly the authors report an upgrade rate of 36.3% from Gleason 5–6 to a higher grade after RP, representing a higher concordance in this group compared with the present study (63.7% versus 39.6% respectively). The reasons for these differences are likely multifactorial but may be due to the small proportion of patients with initial biopsy Gleason 6 undergoing surgery within our cohort, along with the likelihood of this group possessing

Table 4 Mutually adjusted logistic regression analysis for pathological upgrading after RP

Characteristic	Odds ratio (95% confidence interval)	*p*-value
Age	1.022 (1.016–1.028)	< 0.001
Preoperative PSA	1.026 (1.022–1.031)	< 0.001
Preoperative biopsy ISUP Grade Group		
1 (reference)	1	
2	0.123 (0.112–0.135)	< 0.001
3	0.057 (0.049–0.065)	< 0.001
4	0.085 (0.072–0.101)	< 0.001
5	0.030 (0.023–0.039)	< 0.001
Preoperative clinical stage		
T1 *(reference)*	1	
T2	1.231 (1.120–1.353)	< 0.001
T3	1.990 (1.774–2.232)	< 0.001
T4	1.199 (0.275–5.237)	0.809
Year of surgery		
2011 *(reference)*	1	
2012	0.930 (0.749–1.156)	0.514
2013	1.084 (0.896–1.311)	0.408
2014	0.851 (0.710–1.021)	0.082
2015	0.935 (0.782–1.118)	0.462
2016	0.908 (0.759–1.086)	0.289
Region		
A	0.792 (0.403–1.556)	0.498
B	1.077 (0.857–1.353)	0.526
C	1.071 (0.906–1.265)	0.421
D	0.980 (0.834–1.152)	0.808
E	0.886 (0.704–1.115)	0.303
F	1.152 (0.984–1.348)	0.078
G	0.891 (0.743–1.068)	0.210
H	1.980 (0.840–4.669)	0.118
I	1.299 (0.688–2.452)	0.420
J *(reference)*[a]	1	
K	0.830 (0.706–0.976)	0.024
L	0.863 (0.731–1.020)	0.084
M	0.837 (0.678–1.033)	0.098
N	1.132 (0.963–1.330)	0.133
O	0.995 (0.741–1.338)	0.976
P	0.654 (0.477–0.897)	0.008

[a]Region J chosen as a reference owing to largest number of patients

additional high-risk features that would have favoured this treatment approach. However, despite these differences, there was agreement that both increasing age and preoperative PSA were predictors of upgrading [10].

More recently, Danneman et al. reported upgrading within a cohort of 15,598 patients from the Swedish National Prostate Cancer Register that underwent RP between 2000 and 2012 [11]. Inclusion criteria restricted analysis to patients less than 70 with T1–2 disease and a serum PSA of < 20 ng/ml, thereby again comprising a lower risk population than represented here. The authors report an upgrade rate of 35% from Gleason 2–6 to a higher grade after RP, giving a concordance of 65% in this group. Once again this is much higher than the present study and may similarly be due to differences in patient demographics.

The strengths of this study lie in the large cohort and its origin from a national level data registry. Furthermore, unlike similar studies, all patients were treated between 2011 and 2016, thereby representing more contemporary patient selection and management practices. This is particularly relevant to the UK, where reducing numbers of patients with low risk disease are undergoing radical intervention each year [14].

This study does however have a number of limitations, including the surgeon/institution reported nature of the data registry. Although a large proportion of the total number of patients that undergo RP in UK are entered, some regions report few numbers and it is possible there are differences between those patients that are entered and those that are not. Another limitation is the amount of missing preoperative data, which led to the exclusion of a number of cases from the full analysis. This is a recognised issue with the BAUS Radical Prostatectomy Registry that must be acknowledged but has not prevented meaningful observations being reported [30, 31]. The type of initial biopsy performed was also unclear, as was whether the overall or worst Gleason score had been recorded in each case. However, these scores are different in only a minority of cases and previous studies have demonstrated that both are clinically comparable [32]. Finally, the registry lacked additional pathological parameters that have previously been linked to risk of upgrading, including prostate size [10, 12] and extent of cancer in the biopsy [10, 13].

Conclusions

Pathological upgrading after RP remains an important consideration in the management of patients with prostate cancer. This large study demonstrates that overall upgrading in the UK is lower than expected, with risk factors including increasing age, preoperative PSA, and clinical stage. As new diagnostic techniques that may reduce rates of pathological upgrading become more widely utilised, this study will provide an important benchmark against which to measure performance.

Abbreviations

BAUS: British Association of Urological Surgeons; ISUP: International Society of Urological Pathology; mpMRI: multi-parametric magnetic resonance imaging; PSA: Prostate Specific Antigen; RP: Radical prostatectomy;

TRUS: Transrectal ultrasound; UK: United Kingdom; US: United States of America

Acknowledgements
The authors would like to acknowledge the BAUS Section of Oncology for allowing access to the data for the purposes of this study, as well as all of the UK Urological Surgeons who contribute to the BAUS Radical Prostatectomy Registry.

Authors' contributions
KN and NB were responsible for study inception and design. SF was responsible for data acquisition and NB, AS and KN undertook the subsequent analysis. NB, KN, HK and MV were responsible for interpretation of the data and drafting of the manuscript. All authors approved the final manuscript version prior to submission.

Author details
[1]Division of Cancer and Genetics, Cardiff University School of Medicine, Cardiff, UK. [2]Department of Urology, Cardiff and Vale University Health Board, University Hospital of Wales, Cardiff, UK. [3]School of Mathematics, Statistics and Applied Mathematics, National University of Ireland, Galway, Ireland. [4]British Association of Urological Surgeons, London, UK. [5]Department of Cellular Pathology, Cardiff and Vale University Health Board, University Hospital of Wales, Cardiff, UK.

References

1. Mellinger GT, Gleason D, Bailar J III. The histology and prognosis of prostatic cancer. J Urol. 1967;97:331–7.
2. Epstein JI, Partin AW, Sauvageot J, Walsh PC. Prediction of progression following radical prostatectomy: a multivariate analysis of 721 men with long-term follow-up. Am J Surg Pathol. 1996;20:286–92.
3. Albertsen PC, Hanley JA, Gleason DF, Barry MJ. Competing risk analysis of men aged 55 to 74 years at diagnosis managed conservatively for clinically localized prostate cancer. JAMA. 1998;280:975–80.
4. Egevad L, Granfors T, Karlberg L, Bergh A, Stattin P. Prognostic value of the Gleason score in prostate cancer. BJU Int. 2002;89:538–42.
5. Barry MJ, Albertsen PC, Bagshaw MA, Blute ML, Cox R, Middleton RG, Gleason DF, Zincke H, Bergstralh EJ, Jacobsen SJ. Outcomes for men with clinically nonmetastatic prostate carcinoma managed with radical prostactectomy, external beam radiotherapy, or expectant management: a retrospective analysis. Cancer. 2001;91:2302–14.
6. Epstein JI, Egevad L, Amin MB, Delahunt B, Srigley JR, Humphrey PA. The 2014 International Society of Urological Pathology (ISUP) consensus conference on Gleason grading of prostatic carcinoma. Am J Surg Pathol. 2016;40:244–52.
7. Epstein JI, Allsbrook WC Jr, Amin MB, Egevad LL, ISUP Grading Committee. The 2005 International Society of Urological Pathology (ISUP) consensus conference on Gleason grading of prostatic carcinoma. Am J Surg Pathol. 2005;29:1228–42.
8. Ahmed HU, Bosaily AE-S, Brown LC, Gabe R, Kaplan MK, Collaco-Moraes Y, Ward K, Hidley RG, Freeman A, Kirkham AP, Oldroyd R, Parker C, Emberton M. PROMIS study group. Diagnostic accuracy of multi-parametric MRI and TRUS biopsy in prostate cancer (PROMIS): a paired validating confirmatory study. Lancet. 2017;389:815–22.
9. Cohen MS, Hanley RS, Kurteva T, Ruthazer R, Silverman ML, Sorcini A, Hamawy K, Roth RA, Tuerk I, Libertino JA. Comparing the Gleason prostate biopsy and Gleason prostatectomy grading system: the Lahey Clinic Medical Center experience and an international meta-analysis. Eur Urol. 2008;54:371–81.
10. Epstein JI, Feng Z, Trock BJ, Pierorazio PM. Upgrading and downgrading of prostate cancer from biopsy to radical prostatectomy: incidence and predictive factors using the modified Gleason grading system and factoring in tertiary grades. Eur Urol. 2012;61:1019–24.
11. Danneman D, Drevin L, Delahunt B, Samaratunga H, Robinson D, Bratt O, Loeb S, Stattin P, Egevad L. Accuracy of prostate biopsies for predicting Gleason score in radical prostatectomy specimens: nationwide trends 2000–2012. BJU Int. 2017;119:50–6.
12. Davies JD, Aghazadeh MA, Phillips S, Salem S, Chang SS, Clark PE, Cookson MS, Davis R, Herrell SD, Penson DF, Smith JA, Barocas DA. Prostate size as a predictor of Gleason score upgrading in patients with low risk prostate cancer. J Urol. 2011;186:2221–7.
13. Freedland SJ, Kane CJ, Amling CL, Aronson WJ, Terris MK, Presti JC, SEARCH Database Study Group. Upgrading and downgrading of prostate needle biopsy specimens: risk factors and clinical implications. Urology. 2007;69:495–9.
14. National Prostate Cancer Audit. Patient Summary 2018 - Fourth Year Annual Report. London: Royal College of Surgeons of England. 2018:1–6.
15. Helgstrand JT, Røder MA, Klemann N, Toft BG, Lichtensztajn DY, Brooks JD, Brasso K, Vainer B, Iversen P. Trends in incidence and 5-year mortality in men with newly diagnosed, metastatic prostate cancer—A population-based analysis of 2 national cohorts. Cancer. 2018;124:2931–8.
16. Brawley OW. Trends in prostate cancer in the United States. J Natl Cancer Inst Monogr. 2012;2012:152–6.
17. Zakaria AS, Dragomir A, Brimo F, Kassouf W, Tanguay S, Aprikian A. Changes in the outcome of prostate biopsies after preventive task force recommendation against prostate-specific antigen screening. BMC Urol. 2018;18:69.
18. Jegerlehner S, Chiolero A, Aujesky D, Rodondi N, Germann S, Konzelmann I, Bulliard JL, NICER. Working Group. Recent incidence and surgery trends for prostate cancer: Towards an attenuation of overdiagnosis and overtreatment? PLoS One. 2019;14:e0210434.
19. Sinnott M, Falzarano SM, Hernandez AV, Jones JS, Klein EA, Zhou M, Magi-Galluzzi C. Discrepancy in prostate cancer localization between biopsy and prostatectomy specimens in patients with unilateral positive biopsy: implications for focal therapy. Prostate. 2012;72:1179–86.
20. Allsbrook WC Jr, Mangold KA, Johnson MH, Lane RB, Amin MB, Bostwick DG, Humphrey PA, Jones EC, Reuter VE, Sakr W, Sesterhenn IA, Troncoso P, Wheeler TM, Epstein JI. Interobserver reproducibility of Gleason grading of prostatic carcinoma: urologic pathologists. Hum Pathol. 2001;32:74–80.
21. Melia J, Moseley R, Ball R, Griffiths DF, Grigor K, Harnden P, Jarmulowicz M, McWilliam LJ, Montironi R, Waller M, Moss S, Parkinson MC. A UK-based investigation of inter-and intra-observer reproducibility of Gleason grading of prostatic biopsies. Histopathology. 2006;48:644–54.
22. Goodman M, Ward KC, Osunkoya AO, Datta MW, Luthringer D, Young AN, Marks K, Cohen V, Kennedy JC, Harber MJ, Amin MB. Frequency and determinants of disagreement and error in gleason scores: A population-based study of prostate cancer. Prostate. 2012;72:1389–98.
23. Varma M, Berney D, Oxley J, Trpkov K. Gleason Score assignment is the sole responsibility of the pathologist. Histopathology. 2018;73:5–7.
24. The Royal College of Pathologists. Datasets for histopathology reports for prostatic carcinoma. Standards and datasets for reporting cancers. London: Royal College of Pathologists. 2016:60.
25. D'amico AV, Whittington R, Malkowicz SB, Schultz D, Blank K, Broderick GA, Tomaszewski JE, Renshaw AA, Kaplan I, Beard CJ, Wein A. Biochemical outcome after radical prostatectomy, external beam radiation therapy, or interstitial radiation therapy for clinically localized prostate cancer. JAMA. 1998;280:969–74.
26. Huo AS, Hossack T, Symons JL, PeBenito R, Delprado WJ, Brenner P, Stricker PD. Accuracy of primary systematic template guided transperineal biopsy of the prostate for locating prostate cancer: a comparison with radical prostatectomy specimens. J Urol. 2012;187:2044–50.
27. Calio BP, Sidana A, Sugano D, Gaur S, Maruf M, Jain AL, Merino MJ, Choyke PL, Wood BJ, Pinto PA, Turkbey B. Risk of upgrading from prostate biopsy to radical prostatectomy pathology—does saturation biopsy of index lesion during multiparametric magnetic resonance imaging-transrectal ultrasound fusion biopsy help? J Urol. 2018;199:976–82.
28. Kim SP, Karnes RJ, Mwangi R, van Houten H, Gross CP, Gershman B, Leapman MS, Shah ND. Contemporary Trends in Magnetic Resonance Imaging at the Time of Prostate Biopsy: Results from a Large Private Insurance Database. Eur Urol Focus. 2019. https://doi.org/10.1016/j.euf.2019.03.016.
29. Kasivisvanathan V, Rannikko AS, Borghi M, Panebianco V, Mynderse LA, Vaarala MH, Briganti A, Budaus L, Hellawell G, Hindley RG, Roobol MJ, Eggener S, Ghei M, Villers A, Bladou F, Villeirs GM, Virdi J, Boxler S, Robert G, Singh PB, Venderink W, Hadaschik BA, Ruffion A, Hu JC, Margolis D, Crouzet S, Klotz L, Taneja SS, Pinto P, Gill I, Allen C, Giganti F, Freeman A, Morris S, Punwani S, Williams NR, Brew-Graves C, Deeks J, Takwoingi Y, Emberton M, Moore CM, PRECISION Study Group Collaboarators. MRI-targeted or standard biopsy for prostate-cancer diagnosis. N Engl J Med. 2018;378:1767–77.

30. Vesey SG, McCabe JE, Hounsome L, Fowler S. UK radical prostatectomy outcomes and surgeon case volume: based on an analysis of the British Association of Urological Surgeons Complex Operations Database. BJU Int. 2012;109:346–54.
31. Laird A, Fowler S, Good DW, Stewart GD, Srinivasan V, Cahill D, Brewster SF, McNeill SA. British Association of Urological Surgeons (BAUS). Contemporary practice and technique-related outcomes for radical prostatectomy in the UK: a report of national outcomes. BJU Int. 2015;115:753–63.
32. Tolonen TT, Kujala PM, Tammela TL, Tuominen VJ, Isola JJ, Visakorpi T. Overall and worst gleason scores are equally good predictors of prostate cancer progression. BMC Urol. 2011;11:21.

7

Surgical approaches for treatment of ureteropelvic junction obstruction

Annemarie Uhlig[1*], Johannes Uhlig[2,3], Lutz Trojan[1], Marc Hinterthaner[4], Alexander von Hammerstein-Equord[4†] and Arne Strauss[1†]

Abstract

Background: Multiple surgical treatment options are available for the treatment of ureteropelvic junction obstruction (UPJO). The aim of this study is to compare the most frequently used technics in a comprehensive network approach.

Methods: A systematic literature search of the EMBASE, MEDLINE and COCHRANE libraries was conducted in January 2018. Publications were included that evaluated at least two of the following surgical techniques: open pyeloplasty (OP), endopyelotomy (EP), laparoscopic (LP) and robot assisted pyeloplasty (RP). Main outcomes were operative success, complications, urinary leakage, re-operation, transfusion rate, operating time, and length of stay. Network meta-analyses with random effects models simultaneously assessed effectiveness of all surgical techniques.

Results: A total of 26 studies including 3143 patients were analyzed. Compared with RP, EP and LP showed lower operative success rates (EP: OR = 0.09, 95%CI:0.05–0.19; p < 0.001; LP: OR = 0.51, 95%CI:0.31–0.84; p = 0.008). Compared with OP, LP and RP had lower risk for complications (LP: OR = 0.62; 95%CI:0.41–0.95; p = 0.027; RP: OR = 0.41; 95%CI:0.22–0.79; p = 0.007). Compared with RP, no significant differences were detected for urinary leakage or re-operation, transfusion rates. Compared with EP, RP yielded longer operating time (mean = 102.87 min, 95%CI: 41.79 min–163.95 min, p = < 0.001). Further significant differences in operating times were detected when comparing LP to EP (mean = 115.13 min, 95%CI:65.63 min–164.63 min, p = < 0.001) and OP to EP (mean = 91.96 min, 95%CI:32.33 min–151.58 min, p = 0.003).

Conclusions: Multiple surgical techniques are available for treatment of UPJO. RP has the highest rates of operative success and as well as LP lower complication rates than OP. Although surgical outcomes are worse for EP, its operating time is shorter than OP, RP, and LP. Surgeons should consider these findings when selecting the optimal treatment method for individual patients.

Keywords: Endoscopy, Laparoscopy, Minimally invasive surgical procedures, Laparotomy, Network meta-analysis

* Correspondence: annemarie.uhlig@med.uni-goettingen.de
[†]Alexander von Hammerstein-Equord and Arne Strauss contributed equally to this work.
[1]Department of Urology, University Medical Center Goettingen, Goettingen, Germany
Full list of author information is available at the end of the article

Background

Surgical techniques for treatment of ureteropelvic junction obstruction (UPJO) have seen significant advancements during the last decades. From open approaches over laparoscopic techniques and endopyelotomy (EP) in the 1990s, robot assisted approaches have been introduced in 2002 [1, 2]. Currently, all of these techniques are clinically applied, although laparoscopic and robot assisted pyeloplasty (LP and RP) are often claimed to be superior to other approaches [3–7]. Several studies reported that minimal invasive treatment options outperform open pyeloplasty (OP) with respect to early recovery and lower complication rates, whereas OP operating time is shorter [3, 4]. Comparing LP and RP, length of hospital stay, operating and suturing time seem to be shorter for RP [8–11]. In one meta-analysis, operative success rate was significantly higher for RP [9]. While abdominal surgery is required for open, laparoscopic and robot assisted approaches, EP probably has the lowest invasiveness [12]. Even though EP has been replaced by other approaches in many institutions, several experts in the field still advocate this technique [13]; especially, as few literature is available summarizing the evidence on all approaches. Notwithstanding that meta-analyses have been published comparing individual studies for two treatment options, these provides limited guidance in the current situation with multiple approaches available for UPJO which must be evaluated against each another. The aim of this network-meat analysis is to provide a comprehensive overview for most frequently used techniques for treatment of UPJO and to compare their effectiveness regarding various clinically important outcomes.

Materials and methods

Search strategy

This study was registered a priori at PROSPERO (CRD42018085917). The systematic literature search using EMBASE, MEDLINE and COCHRANE libraries was performed in January 2018 and was unrestricted with respect to publication language and date. In addition, publication lists of reviews and included articles as well as conference proceedings were searched. Furthermore, we searched a registry for clinical trials (www.clinicaltrials.gov) to identify potentially unpublished studies. The full search strategy is available in the Additional file 1.

Criteria for study inclusion and exclusion

We included retro- and prospective studies comparing at least two of the following surgical approaches for the treatment of UPJO: OP, LP, RP and EP. Studies had to assess at least one of the following outcomes: operative success, operating time, suturing time, estimated blood loss, transfusion rate, conversion rate, re-operation rate, intra- and postoperative as well as overall complications, urinary leakage, deaths, length of hospital stay, time to return to normal activities, renal function, pain, analgesia requirement, survival time and costs. No minimum follow-up time was required for study inclusion. Of these, the following outcomes were statistically evaluated: operative success was examined as the total number of successes as defined by the authors; rates of transfusion, conversion, re-operation as well as intra- and postoperative complications, and urinary leakage were evaluated as total numbers as well. Reviews and meta-analyses were excluded as well as studies focusing on children or animals. In addition, we excluded studies which reported insufficient data on measures of dispersion or pooled outcome data of two surgical approaches. In case of more than one publication reporting on the same patient cohort, the more comprehensive one was selected in order to meet the assumption of independence for meta-analyses.

Definition of operative success

The authors of the papers used varying definitions for operative success: Objective success was reported by all authors and included mostly included patent ureteropelvic junction confirmed by radionuclide diuretic renogram or intravenous urography (IVU) and sometimes decrease in severity of hydronephrosis. Objective success was often defined as absence of symptoms or "significant" improvement with no further specification. If separate measures for subjective and objective success were reported instead of combined values, only success rates of objective measures were included in the in the statistical analysis to account for the subjectivity of perceived pain [14–16]. Measures for success of the surgical procedure e.g. whether a laparoscopic surgery could be performed without conversion, were not taken into account.

Data extraction

Publication titles identified via the literature search were independently screened by 3 blinded authors resulting in a selection for abstract and full text screening which was performed by 2 independent blinded authors. From the resulting list of publications suited for inclusion, data extraction was performed in the same manner. Disagreement was resolved by consultation of a third author and majority vote. As suggested by Rothman et al., a study was considered as prospective if data collection on interventions and covariates took place before the outcome occurred [17].

Assessment of study quality

Study quality assessment using the Downs and Black instrument was performed by two independent blinded authors resolving disagreement by consensus involving a third author [18]. The Downs and Black instrument rates the quality of randomized and non-randomized studies on a scale from 0 to 32 points (0 points for the worst and 32 for the best study quality) using a catalogue of 27 items. For each item 1 point is given except for the description of the distribution of principal confounders in each group of subjects where a maximum of 2 points can be reached and for the evaluation of study power for which a maximum of 5 points can be reached. For power evaluation study sizes were credited 1 up to 5 points for < 15, 15 to 44, 45 to 59, 60 to 100, > 100 patients according to the quartiles of sample sizes of included studies. Study quality was labeled "low" (1–10 points on Downs and Black instrument), "moderate" (11–21 points) and "high" (22–32 points). The Newcastle Ottawa Scale was used for additional study quality assessment. As suggested by the Cochrane handbook, study quality was separately assessed for each outcome [19].

Statistical analyses

For dichotomous outcomes, Odds Ratios (OR) were calculated from absolute numbers or percentage given in standard manner. Continuous outcomes such as operating time, estimated blood loss and length of hospital stay were compared as median or mean with standard deviation. If available, data from multivariable models was preferentially used [20, 21]. In case of two treatment for similar interventions e.g. endopyelotomy and acucise endopyelotomy, the results were pooled [22]. If only median and interquartile range (IQR) for continuous outcomes were reported, and a large sample size indicated the high probability of an underlying normal distribution, the standard deviation was calculated by dividing the IQR by 1.35 [16]. All outcomes were compared to endopyelotomy as the reference group. A network meta-analysis with random effects approach was used as statistical method for comparison. All outcomes were ranked by p-score methods to estimate the amount of certainty that a single treatment outperforms the average of competing interventions. The p-score ranges from 0 to 1, the latter indicating the highest certainty possible [23]. Study heterogeneity was evaluated by Higgins's I^2 considering percentages below 25% as of potentially low relevance, from 26 to 50% as "moderate", from 51 to 75% as "substantial", and from 76 to 100% as "considerable" heterogeneity [19]. The consistency assumption was evaluated via visual assessment of net heat plots and by Cochran's Q statistic. All pairwise comparisons of more than 10 studies were tested for publication bias using the weighted linear regression of the treatment effect on its standard error [24]. Sensitivity analyses were performed including only studies with at least 12 months follow-up time. The statistical analysis was performed using R version 3.4.2 with the packages "meta", "netmeta", and "metabias" as well as R Studio version 1.1.383. All p-values were calculated two-sided and an alpha-level of < 0.05 was considered statistically significant.

Results

Study characteristics

The systematic literature search yielded 3008 studies published between 1995 and 2017 of which 26 fulfilled the inclusion criteria [14–16, 20–22, 25–44]. Figure 1 depicts the selection process of the studies whereas Table 1 details the study characteristics. In total, 3143 patients were analyzed: 556 receiving OP, 1540 receiving LP, 798 receiving RP, and 249 receiving EP. Operative success and complications were evaluated by 24 studies each, whereas operating time was reported by 22 studies and length of hospital stay by 21 studies. Estimated blood loss was evaluated by 13 studies, postoperative complications by 10 studies, conversion rates by 9 studies and re-operation rates by 8 studies. Transfusion rates, intraoperative complications, urinary leakage and analgesia requirement were reported by 7 studies each. Four studies evaluated death rates, whereas suturing time and time to return to normal activities was reported by 3 studies each. Pain, renal function, and costs were evaluated by 1 study each whilst none of the included studies reported on survival time. Six studies were three-armed trials [14, 21, 25, 28, 30, 40]; the remaining 20 studies evaluated two of the 4 outcomes. Figure 2 details the number of comparisons for each end point. Only 3 congress abstracts provided sufficient data to meet the inclusion criteria [30, 31, 38]. Study design was retrospective in 18 studies, 1 study included pre- and retrospective data [40] and 5 studies explicitly stated a prospective design [27, 36, 38, 41, 44]. For 2 studies no information was available [31, 32]. Only one study had a randomized controlled design [38] and two further studies used multivariable adjustment methods to account for confounding [20, 21]. The mean follow up ranged from 1 month to greater than 6 years with the majority of the studies reporting follow-up times greater than 1 year. The study population consisted of adult patients in 15 of the included publications, whereas 8 studies reported on mixed cohorts of adults and children with the majority of patients being of age > 18 years in case of available information [30, 32–34, 41–44]. For 3 studies the inclusion criteria with respect to patient age were unclear [21, 31, 38]. The percentage of female patients ranged from 32 to 77% with 6 studies omitting this information [15, 16, 25, 26, 31, 38]. The geographic region of the study population was Asia in 8 cases [22, 30, 32, 34, 37, 40, 41, 43], Europe for 7 studies [15, 29, 31, 33, 35, 38, 42], and North America for 10 studies [16, 20, 21, 25–28, 36, 39, 44]. One study reported on a mixed Asian and North American population [14].

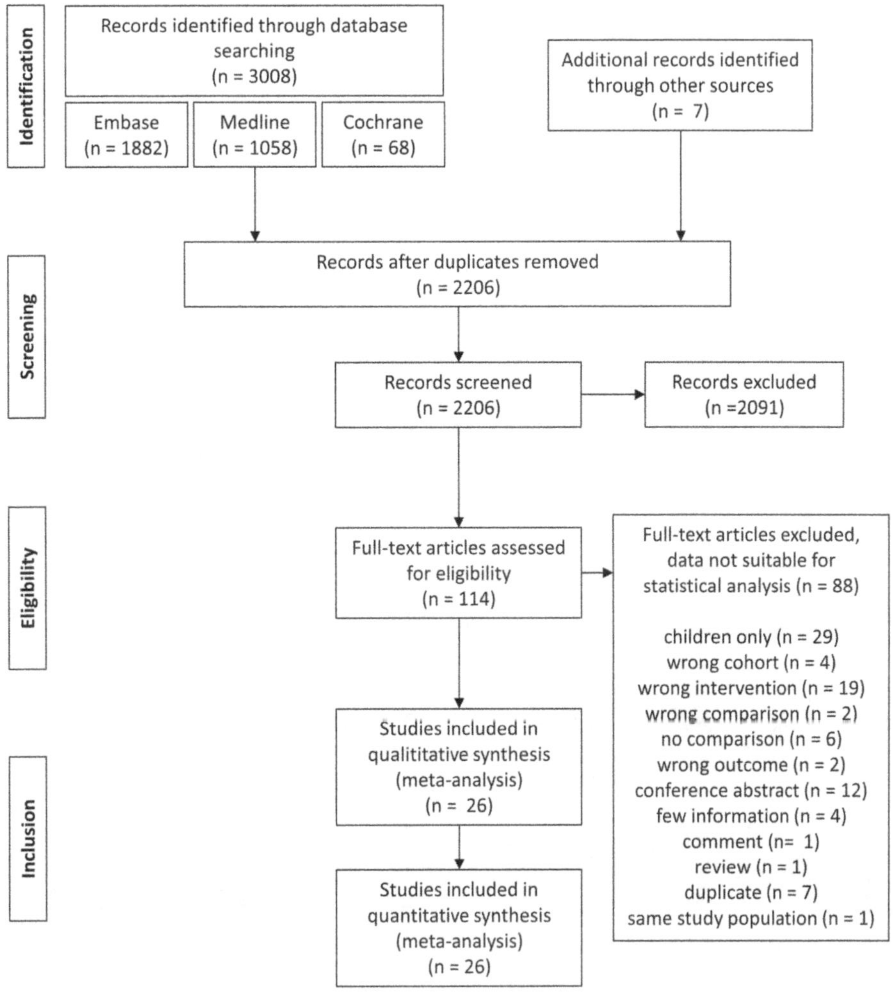

Fig. 1 Flow diagram of study inclusion process

Study quality

The median study quality was 14 points (range from 6 to 25 points). Reasons for the moderate quality were missing randomization, allocation concealment and blinding as well insufficient confounder adjustment and loss to follow-up in almost all studies. Nevertheless, many studies clearly described study hypothesis, main outcomes and findings as well as patient characteristics and selected participants representative for the source population. Table 2 details the study quality separately for the most important endpoints success and complications. Comparable results were obtained using the Newcastle Ottawa scale (Additional file 1: Table S3).

Network meta-analyses for different outcomes

Network meta-analysis of operative success

The analysis of operative success included 34 pairwise comparisons from 24 studies. Compared with RP, EP and LP showed lower success rates with OR = 0.09 (95%CI 0.05–0.19; $p < 0.001$) for EP and OR = 0.51 (95%CI0.31–0.84; $p = 0.008$) for LP. No statistically significant difference was evident comparing OP and RP (OR = 0.69, 95%CI 0.34–1.4; $p = 0.306$). Table 3 depicts all pairwise comparisons in a league table. Associated p-scores are presented in Table 4. There was no evidence of study heterogeneity ($I^2 = 0\%$, $p = 0.9041$). Neither Cochran's Q (Q = 1.98; $p = 0.9213$) nor the net heat plot depicted inconsistencies. Comparisons for OP, RP, LP, and EP as forest-plot are shown in Fig. 3a. Upon sensitivity analyses including only those studies with at least 12 months follow-up time ($n = 13$), comparable results were obtained (Additional file 1: Table S1). A total of 15 studies provided information on primary versus secondary UPJO [14, 16, 21, 22, 25, 27–29, 35–37, 39–41, 44]. Of these, only 9 studies explicitly included secondary UPJO [16, 21, 22, 25, 27, 28, 35, 37, 44]: Only 2 studies compared operative success between primary and secondary UPJO [25, 30]. Baldwin et al. stated, that for LP operative success was higher in the group with secondary UPJO (100% vs 89%). But for EP operative success

Table 1 Study characteristics of included studies

Author	Publication year	Design	Operative approaches	End points	Study size	Secondary UPJO	Uro-lithiasis	Country	Population	Mean age [years]	Percent female	Follow up [monts]
Baldwin et al. [25]	2003	retrospective	EP, LP, OP	operative success, operating time, estimated blood loss, transfusion, complications, length of stay, analgesia requirement	32	LP 44%, EP 33%, OP 43%	NA	USA	adult	44,4 and 37 and 42	NA	11,0 and 9,9 and 5,4
Bernie et al. [26]	2005	retrospective	LP, RP	operative success, operating time, estimated blood loss, complications, urinary leakage, length of stay	14	NA	NA	USA	adult	34 and 32	NA	24 and 10
Bird et al. [27]	2011	prospective	LP, RP	operative success, operating time, suturing time, estimated blood loss, conversion, complications, length of stay	172	13% overall	LP 16%, RP 30%	USA	adult	39,7+/−14,6	53	NA
Brooks et al. [28]	1995	retrospective	EP, LP, OP	operative success, operating time, transfusion, re-operation, complications, length of stay, time to return to normal activity, analgesia requirement	45	EP 23%, LP 8%, OP 18%	EP 1%, LP 0%, OP 9%	USA	adult	42 and 38,4 and 30,6	60	22,0 and 13,6 and 26,0
Calvert et al. [29]	2008	retrospective	LP, OP	operative success, operating time, conversion, complications, length of stay	100	OP 6%, LP 14%	NA	UK	adult	36,5	77	9 and 12
Chen et al. [30]	2016	retrospective	EP, LP, OP	operative success, operating time, estimated blood loss, conversion, complications, urinary leakage, length of stay	109	NA	NA	China	children and adult	32,8+/−15,6 and 30,9+/ − 12,9 and 37,5+/− 12, 0	39	51,9+/− 40,1
Danuser et al. [31]	2012	NA	LP, RP	operative success, operating time, conversion, complications, length of stay	82	NA	NA	Switzerland	NA	NA	NA	NA
Desai et al. [14]	2004	retrospective	EP, LP	operative success, operating time, re-operation, complications, length of stay	29	none	NA	USA and India	adult	38,6+/−16,1 and 38,9+/ − 17	48	31,4+/− 12,6 and 20,0+/−14,0
Fahad [32]	2017	NA	LP, OP	operative success, operating time, conversion, re-operation, complications, urinary leakage, deaths, length of stay, time to return to normal activity, analgesia requirement	40	NA	NA	Iraq	children and adult	24	35	9
Garcia-Galisteo et al. [33]	2011	retrospective	LP, RP	operative success, operating time, suturing time, estimated blood loss, transfusion, complications, deaths, length of stay	50	NA	NA	Spain	children and adult	33,9	60	20,6 and 42,5
Han et al. [22]	2008	retrospective	EP, LP	operative success, operating time, transfusion, complications, length of stay, renal function	45	EP 31%, LP 13%	NA	Korea	adult	45,22 and 49,5 ± 13,6	47	15,2 and 14,3
Hanske et al. [20]	2015	retrospective	LP, OP	transfusion, re-operation, complications, deaths	593	NA	NA	USA	adult	median 48	57	1
Hemal et al. [34]	2010	retrospective	LP, RP	operative success, operating time, suturing time, estimated blood loss, conversion, re-operation, complications, length of stay, time to return to normal activity, analgesia requirement	60	NA	NA	India	children and adult	24,9 and 28,1	32	18

Table 1 Study characteristics of included studies *(Continued)*

Author	Publication year	Design	Operative approaches	End points	Study size	Secondary UPJO	Uro-lithiasis	Country	Population	Mean age [years]	Percent female	Follow up [monts]
Klingler et al. [35]	2003	retrospective	LP, OP	operative success, re-operation, complications, pain, analgesia requirement	55	LF 8%, OP 0%	NA	Switzerland	adult	35,9+/−21,1 and 41,0+/−27,9	60	19,4+/−9,1 and 17,9+/−8,8
Link et al. [36]	2006	prospective	LP, RP	operating time, complications, urinary leakage	20	none	NA	USA	adult	46,5 and 38,0	65	5,6
Lucas et al. [16]	2012	retrospective	LP, RP	operative success, operating time, estimated blood loss, complications, urinary leakage	759	RP 27%, LP 24%	RP 18%, LP 12%	North America	NA	35	NA	11+/−13 and 15+/− 16
Memon et al. [37]	2016	retrospective	LP, OP	operative success, operating time, estimated blood loss, complications, length of stay	73	none	NA	Pakistan	adult	28 and 30	59	2,7+/−1,2
Mohammed [38]	2017	prospective	LP, OP	operative success, operating time, estimated blood loss, re-operation, length of stay	55	NA	NA	Germany	obese, NA	NA	NA	> 12
Olweny et al. [39]	2012	retrospective	LP, RP	operative success, operating time, estimated blood loss, conversion, complications, length of stay, analgesia requirement	20	none	NA	USA	adult	40,3 and 35,8	57	2,8 and 9,2
Pahwa et al. [40]	2014	pro- and retrospective	LP, OP, RP	operative success, operating time, estimated blood loss, complications, length of stay	90	none	NA	India	adult	31,4 and 34,4 and 32	33	32,0 and 18,0 and 13,5
Rivas et al. [15]	2015	retrospective	LP, OP	operative success, conversion, complications, deaths, length of stay	92	NA	LP 19%, OP 20%	Spain	adult	44,5 and 38,5	NA	45
Simforoosh et al. [41]	2004	prospective	LP, OP	operative success, operating time, transfusion, re-operation, complications, urinary leakage, length of stay	69	none	NA	Iran	children and adult	18,2 and 23,1	38	16,5 and 11,4
Umari et al. [42]	2011	retrospective	LP, OP	operative success, operating time, conversion, complications, length of stay	49	NA	LP 17%, OP 32%	Italy	children and adult	42	51	72,3 and 40,9
Wang et al. [43]	2013	retrospective	LP, OP	operative success, operating time, estimated blood loss, complications, urinary leakage, length of stay, analgesia requirement	172	NA	NA	China	children and adult	21 AND 25 years	34	32,7 AND 38,4 months
Weise and Winfield [44]	2006	prospective	LP, RP	operative success, operating time, estimated blood loss, transfusion, complications, length of stay	45	LP 7%, RP 0%	NA	USA	children and adult	26 and 24,5	59	6 and 10
Yanke et al. [21]	2008	retrospective	EP, LP, RP	operative success	273	EP 29%; LP 23%, RP 31%	NA	USA	adult	NA	61	20 and 20 and 19

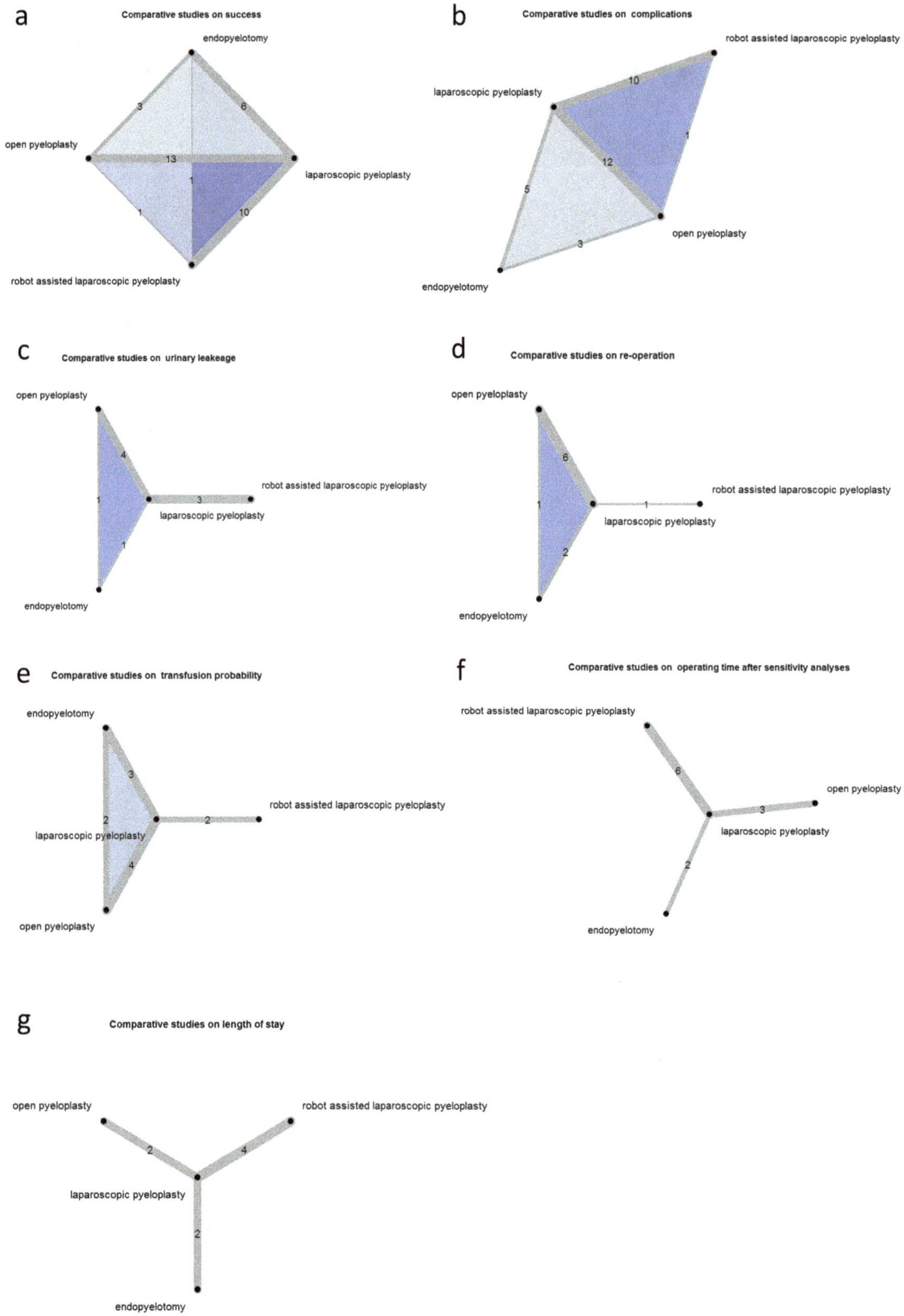

Fig. 2 Number of comparisons for each end point. **a**) Comparative studies on success. **b**) Comparative studies on complications. **c**) Comparative studies on urinary leakeage. **d**) Comparative studies on re-operation. **e**) Comparative studies on transfusion probability. **f**) Comparative studies on operating time after sensitivity analyses. **g**) Comparative studies on length of stay

Table 2 study quality according to the Downs and Black instrument for success and complications

	Baldwin et al. [25]	Bernie et al. [26]	Bird et al. [27]	Brooks et al. [28]	Calvert et al. [29]	Chen et al. [30]	Danuser et al. [31]	Desai et al. [14]	Fahad [32]	Garcia-Galisteo et al. [33]	Han et al. [22]	Hanske et al. [20]	Hemal et al. [34]
Success													
Hypothesis/aim/objective clearly described	1	1	1	1	1	1	1	0	1	1	1	NA	1
Main outcomes in Introduction or Methods	0	0	1	1	1	1	0	1	0	0	1	NA	0
Patient characteristics clearly described	0	0	1	1	1	1	0	1	0	1	1	NA	1
Interventions of interest clearly described	1	0	1	0	0	1	0	1	1	1	1	NA	1
Principal confounders clearly described	0	0	1	0	0	0	0	0	0	0	0	NA	0
Main findings clearly described	1	0	1	1	1	1	1	1	1	1	1	NA	0
Estimates of random variability provided for main outcomes	0	0	1	0	1	1	1	1	0	0	1	NA	1
All adverse events of intervention reported	1	0	1	1	0	1	0	1	1	1	0	NA	1
Characteristics of patients lost to follow-up described	0	0	0	0	0	0	0	0	0	0	0	NA	0
Probability values reported for main outcomes	1	1	1	1	0	0	0	0	0	0	0	NA	0
Subjects asked to participate were representative of source population	0	0	0	0	0	1	0	0	1	1	0	NA	1
Subjects prepared to participate were representative of source population	0	0	0	0	1	1	0	0	1	1	0	NA	1
Location and delivery of study treatment was representative of source population	1	1	1	1	1	1	1	0	1	1	1	NA	1
Study participants blinded to treatment	0	0	0	0	0	0	0	0	0	0	0	NA	0
Blinded outcome assessment	0	0	0	0	0	0	0	0	0	0	0	NA	0
Any data dredging clearly described	0	0	0	0	0	0	0	0	0	0	0	NA	0
Analyses adjust for differing lengths of follow-up	0	0	0	0	0	0	0	0	0	0	0	NA	0
Appropriate statistical tests performed	1	0	1	0	1	0	0	1	0	1	1	NA	0
Compliance with interventions was reliable	0	0	0	0	0	0	0	0	0	0	0	NA	1
Outcome measures were reliable and valid	1	0	1	0	1	0	0	0	0	1	1	NA	0
All participants recruited from the same source population	1	1	1	1	0	1	1	0	1	1	1	NA	1
All participants recruited over the same time period	1	1	1	1	0	0	0	0	1	0	1	NA	0
Participants randomized to treatment(s)	0	0	0	0	0	0	0	0	0	0	0	NA	0
Allocation of treatment concealed from investigators and participants	0	0	0	0	0	0	0	0	0	0	0	NA	0
Adequate adjustment for confounding	0	0	0	0	0	0	0	0	0	0	0	NA	0

Table 2 study quality according to the Downs and Black instrument for success and complications *(Continued)*

	Baldwin et al. [25]	Bernie et al. [26]	Bird et al. [27]	Brooks et al. [28]	Calvert et al. [29]	Chen et al. [30]	Danuser et al. [31]	Desai et al. [14]	Fahad [32]	Garcia-Galisteo et al. [33]	Han et al. [22]	Hanske et al. [20]	Hemal et al. [34]
Losses to follow-up taken into account	0	0	0	0	0	0	0	0	0	0	0	NA	0
Study power	2	1	5	3	4	5	4	2	2	3	3	NA	4
Sum	12	6	19	12	13	16	9	9	11	14	14	NA	14
Complications													
Hypothesis/aim/objective clearly described	1	1	1	1	1	1	1	0	1	1	1	1	1
Main outcomes in Introduction or Methods	0	0	1	1	1	1	0	1	0	0	1	1	0
Patient characteristics clearly described	0	0	1	1	1	1	0	1	0	1	1	1	1
Interventions of interest clearly described	1	0	1	0	0	1	0	1	1	1	1	0	1
Principal confounders clearly described	0	0	1	0	0	0	0	0	0	0	0	2	0
Main findings clearly described	1	0	1	1	1	1	1	1	1	1	1	1	0
Estimates of random variability provided for main outcomes	0	0	1	0	1	1	1	1	0	0	1	1	1
All adverse events of intervention reported	1	0	1	1	0	1	0	1	1	1	0	1	1
Characteristics of patients lost to follow-up described	0	0	0	0	0	0	0	0	0	0	0	0	0
Probability values reported for main outcomes	1	1	1	1	0	0	0	0	0	0	0	1	0
Subjects asked to participate were representative of source population	0	0	0	0	0	1	0	0	1	1	0	1	1
Subjects prepared to participate were representative of source population	0	0	0	0	1	1	0	0	1	1	0	1	1
Location and delivery of study treatment was representative of source population	1	1	1	1	1	1	1	0	1	1	1	1	1
Study participants blinded to treatment	0	0	0	0	0	0	0	0	0	0	0	0	0
Blinded outcome assessment	0	0	0	0	0	0	0	0	0	0	0	0	0
Any data dredging clearly described	0	0	0	0	0	0	0	0	0	0	0	0	0
Analyses adjust for differing lengths of follow-up	0	0	0	0	0	0	0	0	0	0	0	0	0
Appropriate statistical tests performed	1	0	1	0	1	0	0	1	0	1	1	1	0
Compliance with interventions was reliable	0	0	0	0	0	0	0	0	0	0	0	1	1
Outcome measures were reliable and valid	1	0	1	0	1	0	0	0	0	1	1	1	0
All participants recruited from the same source population	1	1	1	1	0	1	1	0	1	1	1	1	1
All participants recruited over the same time period	1	1	1	1	0	0	0	0	1	0	1	1	0

Table 2 study quality according to the Downs and Black instrument for success and complications *(Continued)*

	Baldwin et al. [25]	Bernie et al. [26]	Bird et al. [27]	Brooks et al. [28]	Calvert et al. [29]	Chen et al. [30]	Danuser et al. [31]	Desai et al. [14]	Fahad [32]	Garcia-Galisteo et al. [33]	Han et al. [22]	Hanske et al. [20]	Hemal et al. [34]
Participants randomized to treatment(s)	0	0	0	0	0	0	0	0	0	0	0	0	0
Allocation of treatment concealed from investigators and participants	0	0	0	0	0	0	0	0	0	0	0	0	0
Adequate adjustment for confounding	0	0	0	0	0	0	0	0	0	0	0	1	0
Losses to follow-up taken into account	0	0	0	0	0	0	0	0	0	0	0	0	0
Study power	2	1	5	3	4	5	4	2	2	3	3	5	4
Sum	12	6	19	12	13	16	9	9	11	14	14	23	14

NA **not applicable**

Table 2 study quality according to the Downs and Black instrument for success and complications *(Continued)*

	Klingler et al. [35]	Link et al. [36]	Lucas et al. [16]	Memon et al. [37]	Mohammed [38]	Olweny et al. [39]	Pahwa et al. [40]	Rivas et al. [15]	Simforoosh et al. [41]	Umari et al. [42]	Wang et al. [43]	Weise and Winfield [44]	Yanke et al. [21]
Success													
Hypothesis/aim/objective clearly described	1	NA	1	1	1	1	1	0	1	1	1	1	1
Main outcomes in Introduction or Methods	1	NA	1	1	1	1	1	1	1	1	1	1	1
Patient characteristics clearly described	1	NA	0	1	0	1	0	1	0	1	1	1	1
Interventions of interest clearly described	1	NA	1	0	0	1	0	1	0	0	0	1	1
Principal confounders clearly described	0	NA	1	1	0	0	0	1	0	1	0	1	2
Main findings clearly described	0	NA	1	1	1	1	1	1	1	1	1	1	1
Estimates of random variability provided for main outcomes	1	NA	1	0	1	1	0	1	0	0	1	0	1
All adverse events of intervention reported	1	NA	0	1	0	0	1	1	1	1	0	1	0
Characteristics of patients lost to follow-up described	0	NA	1	0	0	0	0	0	0	1	1	0	0
Probability values reported for main outcomes	0	NA	1	0	0	0	0	0	0	0	1	0	1
Subjects asked to participate were representative of source population	1	NA	1	1	0	1	1	1	0	1	0	1	1
Subjects prepared to participate were representative of source population	1	NA	1	0	0	1	1	1	1	1	1	1	1
Location and delivery of study treatment was representative of source population	1	NA	1	1	1	1	1	1	1	1	1	1	1
Study participants blinded to treatment	0	NA	0	0	0	0	0	0	0	0	0	0	0
Blinded outcome assessment	0	NA	0	0	0	0	0	0	0	0	0	0	0
Any data dredging clearly described	0	NA	1	0	0	0	0	1	0	0	0	0	0
Analyses adjust for differing lengths of follow-up	0	NA	1	0	1	0	0	0	0	0	0	0	1
Appropriate statistical tests performed	0	NA	1	0	0	1	0	1	1	0	1	1	1
Compliance with interventions was reliable	1	NA	1	1	1	1	1	1	1	1	1	1	1
Outcome measures were reliable and valid	0	NA	1	1	0	1	0	1	0	1	1	1	1
All participants recruited from the same source population	1	NA	1	1	1	1	1	1	0	1	1	1	1
All participants recruited over the same time period	1	NA	0	1	1	0	0	0	1	1	1	0	1
Participants randomized to treatment(s)	0	NA	0	0	1	0	0	0	0	0	0	0	0
Allocation of treatment concealed from investigators and participants	0	NA	0	0	0	0	0	1	0	0	0	0	0

Table 2 study quality according to the Downs and Black instrument for success and complications *(Continued)*

	Klingler et al. [35]	Link et al. [36]	Lucas et al. [16]	Memon et al. [37]	Mohammed [38]	Olweny et al. [39]	Pahwa et al. [40]	Rivas et al. [15]	Simforoosh et al. [41]	Umari et al. [42]	Wang et al. [43]	Weise and Winfield [44]	Yanke et al. [21]
Adequate adjustment for confounding	0	NA	0	0	0	0	0	0	0	0	0	0	1
Losses to follow-up taken into account	0	NA	1	0	0	0	0	0	0	0	0	0	1
Study power	3	NA	5	4	3	2	4	4	4	3	5	3	5
Sum	15	NA	23	16	13	15	13	20	13	17	19	17	25
Complications													
Hypothesis/aim/objective clearly described	1	1	1	1	NA	1	1	0	1	1	1	1	1
Main outcomes in Introduction or Methods	1	0	1	1	NA	1	1	1	1	1	1	1	1
Patient characteristics clearly described	1	1	0	1	NA	1	0	1	0	1	1	1	1
Interventions of interest clearly described	1	0	1	0	NA	1	0	1	0	0	0	1	1
Principal confounders clearly described	0	1	1	1	NA	0	0	1	0	1	0	1	2
Main findings clearly described	0	1	1	1	NA	1	1	1	1	1	1	1	1
Estimates of random variability provided for main outcomes	1	1	1	0	NA	1	0	1	0	0	1	0	1
All adverse events of intervention reported	1	0	0	1	NA	0	1	1	1	1	0	1	0
Characteristics of patients lost to follow-up described	0	0	1	0	NA	0	0	0	0	1	1	0	0
Probability values reported for main outcomes	0	0	1	0	NA	0	0	0	0	0	1	0	1
Subjects asked to participate were representative of source population	1	1	1	1	NA	1	1	1	0	1	0	1	1
Subjects prepared to participate were representative of source population	1	1	1	0	NA	1	1	1	1	1	1	1	1
Location and delivery of study treatment was representative of source population	1	0	1	1	NA	1	1	1	1	1	1	1	1
Study participants blinded to treatment	0	0	0	0	NA	0	0	0	0	0	0	0	0
Blinded outcome assessment	0	0	0	0	NA	0	0	0	0	0	0	0	0
Any data dredging clearly described	0	0	1	0	NA	0	0	1	0	0	0	0	0
Analyses adjust for differing lengths of follow-up	0	0	1	0	NA	0	0	0	0	0	0	0	1
Appropriate statistical tests performed	0	0	1	0	NA	1	0	1	1	0	1	1	1
Compliance with interventions was reliable	1	1	1	1	NA	1	1	1	1	1	1	1	1
Outcome measures were reliable and valid	0	1	1	1	NA	1	0	1	0	1	1	1	1
All participants recruited from the same source population	1	1	1	1	NA	1	1	1	0	1	1	1	1

Table 2 study quality according to the Downs and Black instrument for success and complications *(Continued)*

	Klingler et al. [35]	Link et al. [36]	Lucas et al. [16]	Memon et al. [37]	Mohammed [38]	Olweny et al. [39]	Pahwa et al. [40]	Rivas et al. [15]	Simforoosh et al. [41]	Umari et al. [42]	Wang et al. [43]	Weise and Winfield [44]	Yanke et al. [21]
All participants recruited over the same time period	1	1	0	1	NA	0	0	0	1	1	1	0	1
Participants randomized to treatment(s)	0	0	0	0	NA	0	0	0	0	0	0	0	0
Allocation of treatment concealed from investigators and participants	0	0	0	0	NA	0	0	1	0	0	0	0	0
Adequate adjustment for confounding	0	0	0	0	NA	0	0	0	0	0	0	0	1
Losses to follow-up taken into account	0	0	1	0	NA	0	0	0	0	0	0	0	1
Study power	3	1	5	4	NA	2	4	4	4	3	5	3	5
Sum	15	12	23	16	NA	15	13	20	13	17	19	17	25

Table 3 League table showing pairwise comparisons for all surgical approaches and end points included in the quantitative network meta-analysis

End point		Endopyelotomy (reference)	Laparoscopic pyeloplasty (reference)	Open pyeloplasty (reference)	Robot assisted laparoscopic pyeloplasty (reference)
operative success (OR)	EP (comparator)	1 (1–1), p = NA	**0.18 (0.11–0.31), p = < 0.001**	**0.14 (0.07–0.27), p = < 0.001**	**0.09 (0.05–0.19), p = < 0.001**
	LP (comparator)	**5.44 (3.26–9.08), p = < 0.001**	1 (1–1), p = NA	0.74 (0.44–1.26), p = 0.27	**0.51 (0.31–0.84), p = 0.008**
	OP (comparator)	**7.31 (3.72–14.39), p = < 0.001**	1.34 (0.8–2.27), p = 0.27	1 (1–1), p = NA	0.69 (0.34–1.4), p = 0.306
	RP (comparator)	**10.59 (5.25–21.37), p = < 0.001**	**1.94 (1.19–3.19), p = 0.008**	1.45 (0.71–2.94), p = 0.306	1 (1–1), p = NA
		EP (reference)	LP (reference)	OP (reference)	RP (reference)
overall complications (OR)	EP (comparator)	1 (1–1), p = NA	0.95 (0.41–2.18), p = 0.898	0.59 (0.25–1.39), p = 0.226	1.43 (0.54–3.78), p = 0.474
	LP (comparator)	1.06 (0.46–2.43), p = 0.898	1 (1–1), p = NA	**0.62 (0.41–0.95), p = 0.027**	1.51 (0.91–2.51), p = 0.115
	OP (comparator)	1.7 (0.72–4.01), p = 0.226	**1.61 (1.05–2.45), p = 0.027**	1 (1–1), p = NA	**2.42 (1.27–4.63), p = 0.007**
	RP (comparator)	0.7 (0.26–1.85), p = 0.474	0.66 (0.4–1.1), p = 0.115	**0.41 (0.22–0.79), p = 0.007**	1 (1–1), p = NA
		EP (reference)	LP (reference)	OP (reference)	RP (reference)
urinary leakage (OR)	EP (comparator)	1 (1–1), p = NA	0.14 (0.01–3.01), p = 0.211	0.17 (0.01–3.41), p = 0.247	0.25 (0.01–5.95), p = 0.392
	LP (comparator)	6.98 (0.33–146.48), p = 0.211	1 (1–1), p = NA	1.19 (0.39–3.62), p = 0.761	1.75 (0.74–4.17), p = 0.206
	OP (comparator)	5.87 (0.29–117.38), p = 0.247	0.84 (0.28–2.56), p = 0.761	1 (1–1), p = NA	1.47 (0.36–6.05), p = 0.591
	RP (comparator)	3.99 (0.17–94.46), p = 0.392	0.57 (0.24–1.36), p = 0.206	0.68 (0.17–2.79), p = 0.591	1 (1–1), p = NA
		EP (reference)	LP (reference)	OP (reference)	RP (reference)
re-operation (OR)	EP (comparator)	1 (1–1), p = NA	6.18 (0.97–39.29), p = 0.053	4.75 (0.7–32.39), p = 0.112	19.18 (0.46–800.12), p = 0.121
	LP (comparator)	0.16 (0.03–1.03), p = 0.053	1 (1–1), p = NA	0.77 (0.32–1.85), p = 0.557	3.1 (0.12–79.23), p = 0.494
	OP (comparator)	0.21 (0.03–1.43), p = 0.112	1.3 (0.54–3.14), p = 0.557	1 (1–1), p = NA	4.04 (0.14–116), p = 0.415
	RP (comparator)	0.05 (0–2.17), p = 0.121	0.32 (0.01–8.24), p = 0.494	0.25 (0.01–7.11), p = 0.415	1 (1–1), p = NA
		EP (reference)	LP (reference)	OP (reference)	RP (reference)
transfusion rate (OR)	EP (comparator)	1 (1–1), p = NA	2.74 (0.33–22.72), p = 0.35	0.78 (0.07–9.02), p = 0.844	6.17 (0.14–273.11), p = 0.347

Table 3 League table showing pairwise comparisons for all surgical approaches and end points included in the quantitative network meta-analysis *(Continued)*

End point		Endopyelotomy (reference)	Laparoscopic pyeloplasty (reference)	Open pyeloplasty (reference)	Robot assisted laparoscopic pyeloplasty (reference)
	LP (comparator)	0.36 (0.04–3.03), $p = 0.35$	1 (1–1), $p = NA$	0.29 (0.04–2.16), $p = 0.225$	2.25 (0.1–52.29), $p = 0.613$
	OP (comparator)	1.28 (0.11–14.72), $p = 0.844$	3.5 (0.46–26.44), $p = 0.225$	1 (1–1), $p = NA$	7.88 (0.19–331.49), $p = 0.279$
	RP (comparator)	0.16 (0–7.18), $p = 0.347$	0.44 (0.02–10.32), $p = 0.613$	0.13 (0–5.34), $p = 0.279$	1 (1–1), $p = NA$
		EP (reference)	LP (reference)	OP (reference)	RP (reference)
operating time (mean minutes and SD) after sensitivity analyses	EP (comparator)	0 (0–0), $p = NA$	**−127.51 (−179.83–-75.19), $p = < 0.001$**	**−76.16 (− 142.85–-9.47), $p = 0.025$**	**−115.39 (− 175.19–-55.58), $p = < 0.001$**
	LP (comparator)	**127.51 (75.19–179.83), $p = < 0.001$**	0 (0–0), $p = NA$	**51.35 (10–92.7), $p = 0.015$**	12.12 (− 16.84–41.08), $p = 0.412$
	OP (comparator)	**76.16 (9.47–142.85), $p = 0.025$**	**−51.35 (−92.7–-10), $p = 0.015$**	0 (0–0), $p = NA$	−39.22 (−89.71–11.26), $p = 0.128$
	RP (comparator)	**115.39 (55.58–175.19), $p = < 0.001$**	−12.12 (−41.08–16.84), $p = 0.412$	39.22 (− 11.26–89.71), $p = 0.128$	0 (0–0), $p = NA$
		EP (reference)	LP (reference)	OP (reference)	RP (reference)
length of stay (mean days and SD)	EP (comparator)	0 (0–0), $p = NA$	0.32 (−2.55–3.18), $p = 0.827$	−0.69 (−4.76–3.37), $p = 0.739$	1.19 (− 2.52–4.9), $p = 0.53$
	LP (comparator)	−0.32 (−3.18–2.55), $p = 0.827$	0 (0–0), $p = NA$	−1.01 (− 3.89–1.87), $p = 0.492$	0.87 (− 1.49–3.23), $p = 0.471$
	OP (comparator)	0.69 (− 3.37–4.76), $p = 0.739$	1.01 (− 1.87–3.89), $p = 0.492$	0 (0–0), $p = NA$	1.88 (− 1.85–5.61), $p = 0.323$
	RP (comparator)	−1.19 (− 4.9–2.52), $p = 0.53$	−0.87 (− 3.23–1.49), $p = 0.471$	−1.88 (− 5.61–1.85), $p = 0.323$	0 (0–0), $p = NA$

Estimates with corresponding statistically significant p-values ($p < 0.05$) are written in boldface

Table 4 P-scores ranking the surgical approaches for every outcome based on the amount of certainty that a single treatment outperforms the average of competing interventions. The p-score ranges from 0 to 1, the latter indicating the highest certainty possible

	Endopyelotomy	Laparoscopic pyeloplasty	Open pyeloplasty	Robot assisted laparoscopic pyeloplasty
Operative success	0.0000	0.3797	0.6727	0.9476
Few overall complications	0.5583	0.4975	0.0435	0.9007
Few cases of urinary leakage	0.8584	0.1963	0.3462	0.5991
Low re-operation rate	0.0476	0.6472	0.4768	0.8284
Low transfusion rate	0.3089	0.6730	0.2247	0.7934
Short operating time after sensitivity analyses	0.9958	0.0712	0.6471	0.2860
Short length of stay	0.4365	0.5252	0.2589	0.7794

was higher among patients with primary UPJO [25]. Calvert et al. reported higher success rates among patients with primary UPJO for LP (98% vs. 57%) and OP (96% vs 67%) [29].

Network meta-analysis of overall complications

The network meta-analysis of overall complications included 31 pairwise comparisons from 23 studies. Compared with OP, LP (OR = 0.62; 95%CI 0.41–0.95; p = 0.027) as well as RP (OR = 0.41; 95%CI 0.22–0.79; p = 0.007) had a statistically lower risk for complications. No statistically significant difference was detected comparing EP and OP. All pairwise comparisons are depicted in Table 3. Associated p-scores are presented in Table 4. The study heterogeneity was potentially irrelevant (I^2 = 13.7%, p = 0.1416). Neither Cochran's Q (Q = 1.02; p = 0.9064) nor the net heat plot depicted inconsistencies. Figure 3b depicts comparisons for OP, RP, LP, and EP.

Network meta-analysis of urinary leakage

The network meta-analysis of urinary leakage included 9 pairwise comparisons from 7 different studies. Compared with RP none of the other surgical treatment options had a statistically significant higher or lower risk for urinary leakage. Table 3 summarizes these findings, and Table 4 depicts the associated p-scores. There was no evidence of study heterogeneity (I^2 = 0%, p = 0.5161). No inconsistencies were depicted by Cochran's Q (Q = 0,58; p = 0.4471) or the net heat plot. Comparisons for OP, RP, LP, and EP as forest-plot are shown in Fig. 3c.

Network meta-analysis of re-operation

The analysis of re-operation was based on 10 pairwise comparisons from 8 studies. Compared with RP, none of the other surgical treatment options had a statistically significant higher or lower risk for re-operation. All pairwise comparisons are depicted in Table 3. Associated p-scores are presented in Table 4. There was no evidence of study heterogeneity (I^2 = 0%, p = 0.3001). Neither Cochran's Q (Q = 0.02; p = 0.9897) nor the net heat plot revealed inconsistencies. Figure 3d depicts comparisons for OP, RP, LP, and EP. Upon sensitivity analyses including only those studies with at least 12 months follow-up time (n = 13), comparable results were obtained and are depicted in Additional file 1: Table S2 [8, 14, 15, 21, 22, 28, 30, 33–35, 38, 40, 42]. Five studies stated, whether concomitant stones were present at the time of pyeloplasty but only 2 studies evaluated any effect on one of the outcomes [15, 16, 27, 28, 42]. Lucas et al. reported that presence of urolithiasis did not affect the rate of secondary interventions [16].

Network meta-analysis of transfusion rate

The analysis of transfusion rates included 11 pairwise comparisons from 7 studies. Compared with RP none of the other surgical treatment strategies reached a statistically significant difference in transfusion rates as presented in Table 3. Associated p-scores are depicted by Table 4. The study heterogeneity was "moderate" but not statistically significant (I^2 = 42.3.7%, p = 0.4396). There were statistically significant inconsistencies (Cochran's Q = 6.64, p = 0.0361) for which the sources were not identifiable by visual assessment of the net heat plot. Therefore, no sensitivity analyses excluding any studies were possible. Comparisons for OP, RP, LP and EP are depicted by Fig. 3e.

Network meta-analysis of operating time

A total of 14 pairwise comparisons from 12 studies were included in the analysis of operating time. Compared with EP, RP had a statistically significant longer operating time: mean = 102.87 min (95%CI 41.79 min–163.95 min, p = < 0.001). Further statistically significant differences in operating times were detected when comparing LP to EP with mean = 115.13 min (95%CI 65.63 min–164.63 min, p = < 0.001) and OP to EP with mean = 91.96 min (95%CI 32.33 min–151.58 min, p = 0.003). No statistically significant differences resulted from comparisons of the operative techniques against each other. The study heterogeneity was "considerable" and statistically significant (I^2 = 95.2%, p < 0.001). The net heat plot suggested that the study design comparing EP, LP, and OP

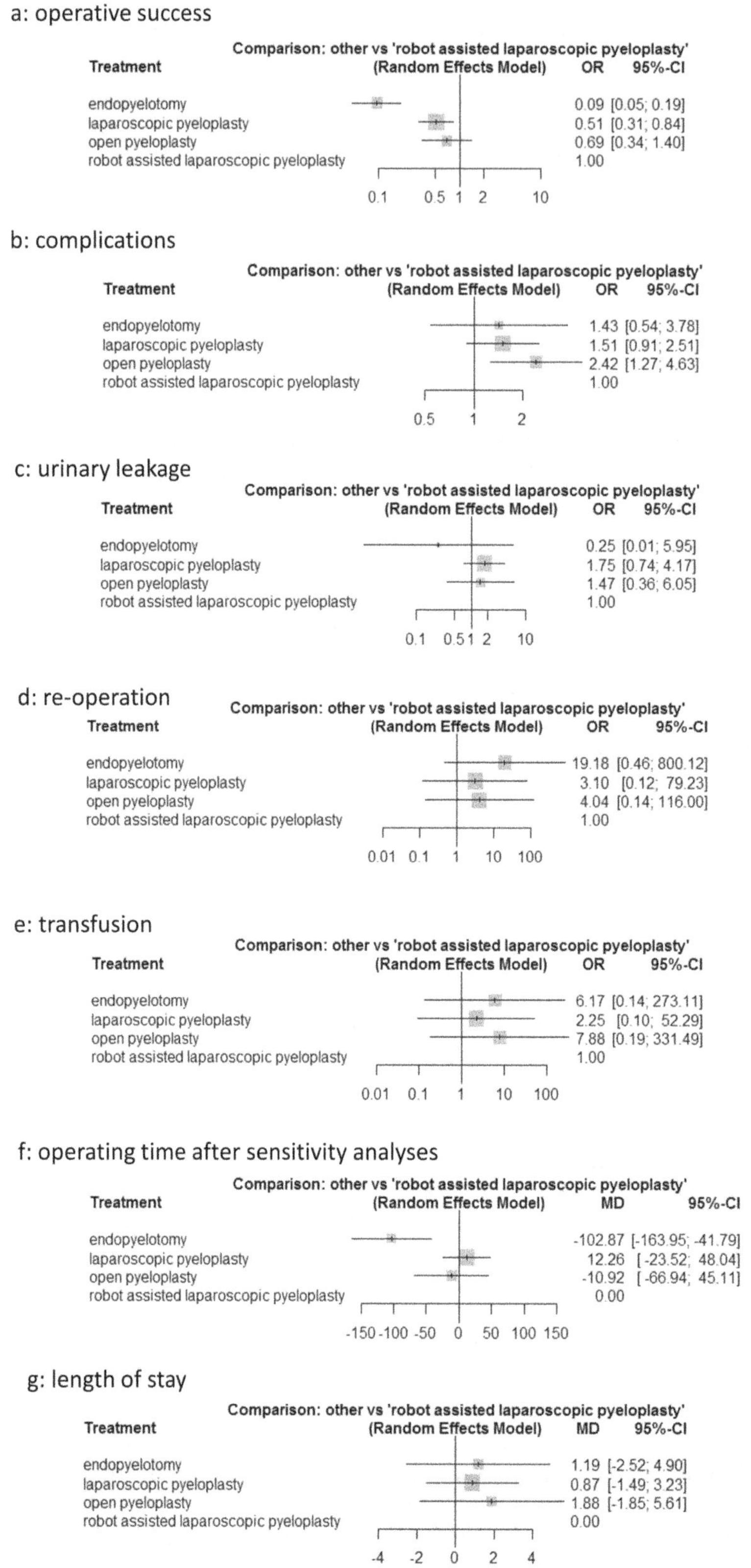

Fig. 3 Pooled estimates for each endpoint. **a**) operative success. **b**) complications. **c**) urinary leakeage. **d**) re-operation. **e**) transfusion. **f**) operating time after sensitivity analyses. **g**) length of stay

contributed most to network inconsistencies (Q = 101.59, $p < 0.001$). In consequence, sensitivity analyses excluding the study of Chen et al. were conducted. This resulted in 11 pairwise comparisons from 11 studies. Again, RP had a statistically significant longer operating time when compared to EP mean = 115.39 min (95%CI 55.58 min–175.19 min, $p = < 0.001$). This was also true for comparisons of LP or OP to EP. For LP to EP with mean = 127.51 min (95%CI 75.19 min - 179.83 min, $p = < 0.001$) and for OP to EP mean 76.16 min (95%CI 9.47 min–142.85 min, $p = 0.025$). In addition, statistically significant longer operating times resulted from a comparison of LP to OP with mean = 51.35 min (95%CI 10 min–92.7 min, $p = 0.015$). Table 3 depicts all pairwise comparisons of the reduced analysis. Associated p-scores of the reduced model are detailed in Table 4. The aforementioned "considerable" heterogeneity remained (I^2 = 92.4%, $p < 0.001$) which was not explored further in order to maintain adequate numbers of comparisons. As only direct comparisons remained in the reduced analysis, no evaluation of inconsistencies was reasonable. Bird et al. reported that concurrent treatment of nephrolithiasis did not affect operating time [27]. Figure 3f depicts comparisons for OP, RP, LP, and EP after sensitivity analyses.

Network meta-analysis of length of stay

The analysis of length of stay included 8 pairwise comparisons from 8 studies. Compared with RP none of the surgical treatment options had a statistically significant shorter or longer length of stay. All pairwise comparisons are depicted in Table 3 whereas Table 4 shows the associated p-scores. Analyses of heterogeneity revealed an I^2 of 96.7% ($p < 0.001$). Due to the available study designs with direct comparisons only, no evaluation of inconsistency was warranted. Again, no further subgroup analyses were performed because of low numbers of comparisons. Comparisons for OP, RP, LP, and EP as forest-plot are shown in Fig. 3g.

Publication bias

Assessment of publication bias was possible for operative success and complications with the interventions LP versus OP and LP versus RP each. On visual assessment, slight asymmetry was evident for operative success with the comparison of LP versus OP. Less studies reported on ORs < 0.74. Statistical evaluation did not reveal significant publication bias ($p = 0.9118$). Visual assessment of publication bias for operative success with RP compared to LP showed slight publication bias as well. Less studies reported on ORs > 1.94. Again, statistical evaluation did not reveal significant publication bias ($p = 0.1519$). Moreover, visual assessment comparing LP versus OP with respect to complications also resulted in the impression of slight publication bias which was not statistically significant: $p = 0.365$. Fewer studies reported on ORs < 0.62.Visual assessment and statistical evaluation of the comparison of LP and RP yielded no publication bias ($p = 0.4808$). Figure S1 in the Additional file 1 illustrates the funnel plots.

Narrative meta-analysis of other outcomes

Only three studies reported on suturing time for RP versus LP [27, 33, 34]. In all cases, suturing time was shorter for RP. Estimated blood loss was reported by 13 studies of which only 4 studies provided estimates of dispersion which did not allow for meta-analyses. In most studies, EP had the lowest blood loss, followed by LP and RP. The highest blood loss was reported for OP in all studies. Due to the nature of the intervention, conversion rates were only reported for RP and LP: Low event rates did not allow for any reliable pooling which applied to death rates as well. Analgesia requirement was reported by 7 studies with different medication such as morphine equivalents, diclophenac, pethidine or tramadol and most of the time without measure of dispersion. Overall, the studies reported EP to have the lowest analgesic requirement, followed by LP and OP. Only one study compared RP and LP and described lower need for analgesic medication for RP. For time to return to normal activity, renal function, and costs only 1 to 3 studies reported estimates with heterogeneous outcome definitions. Therefore, no meta-analysis was possible in these cases.

Discussion

Several surgical techniques have been developed for treatment of UPJO, each yielding unique advantages and potential limitations. Although RP and LP are allegedly superior, these claims are based on pairwise meta-analyses that failed to evaluate all available techniques at once. In contrast, our study provides a comprehensive overview on OP, EP, LP and RP, comparing their performance with respect to crucial clinical outcomes. Our results indicate that RP is the technique with highest rates of operative success, lowest overall complication rates, shortest hospital stay as well as lowest re-operation rates and transfusion rates. On the other hand, EP yields lowest rates of urinary leakage and shortest operating times. Robot assisted surgery is known for its minimally invasive nature which goes along with less postoperative pain and earlier recovery, which probably causes shorter hospital stays. In addition, robot assisted surgery allows for high precision movements with articulated arms and provides magnified 3-D vision for the surgeon [45]. This might explain high operative success rates of RP. Low transfusion rates of RP are the consequence of the minimally invasive nature of robotic surgery which allows immediate and precise reaction to local bleeding [46]. The reason for short operating time in EP probably is that the kidney access requires more time during abdominal surgery than this endoscopic procedure. In addition, EP is less complex, even though the percutaneous approach involves a short flank incision and sewing techniques which are both of low complexity [47, 48]. Another advantage of EP are low rates of urinary leakage, which might be due to the small extent of manipulation compared to pyeloplasty approaches. However, the reduced invasiveness of EP is on the cost of high recidive rates. Urothelial scarring probably explains these differences since EO only involves an urothelial incision as opposed to surgical approaches where strictured tissue is resected [49, 50]. When evaluating different treatment approaches, costs have to be taken into account as well. Only one of the included studies evaluated treatment costs [36]: Link et al. reported 2.7 times higher costs for RP ($5323.80) compared to LP ($1989.87). More literature is available comparing LP, RP and OP: Yu et al. found RP to be associated with the highest median costs ($11,829), followed by OP ($9520) and LP ($8291) [51]. Gettmann et al. published costs for EP ranging between $3842 and $5297 compared to higher costs for LP ($7026) and OP ($7119) [52]. No decision tree analyses have been published to evaluate whether the differences in these expenditures outbalance the benefits of the approaches. Overall study quality was moderate due to limitations in study design such as randomization, concealment of treatment allocation, blinding and omission of multivariable analyses. Still, the nature of interventions and outcomes assessed in this meta-analysis questions, whether higher quality trials would yield relevant changes in the observed effects. Our study is not devoid of limitations, which are mainly inherent to the published trials as its data source: most publications did not adjust for confounding and only one randomized controlled trial could be included. Therefore, the pooled estimates might slightly vary from the true effects. Visual assessment of publication bias yielded minor asymmetries for some the funnel plots. Nevertheless, statistical tests did not return statistically significant evidence for publication bias, which does not completely exclude such bias but suggests low impact. The network meta-analyses of operating time and length of stay yielded statistically significant heterogeneity which could not be bypassed by subgroup analyses in order to maintain adequate numbers of comparisons. Therefore, the pooled estimates might not be generalizable to specific patient subpopulations. Finally, results on the inferiority of EP might be due to differing failure patterns, which is mainly due to missed diagnosis of crossing vessels in EP, and due to inadequate spatulation or incomplete excision of the diseased segment in RP, LP and OP. Still, EP studies were included since they contributed indirect evidence for comparison of other surgical approaches as well. Still, our findings are based on a total of 26 included studies which is the largest meta-analysis published so far and the first comparing more than two interventions simultaneously. The novel network meta-analyses approach further allows for combination of direct and indirect evidence to enhance comparisons of formerly underpowered treatment approaches [53–55].

Conclusions

Comparing OP, EP, LP and RP for UPJO in a comprehensive network meta-analysis approach, our study found that RP has the highest rates of operative success and as well as LP lower complication rates than OP. Operating time is shortest for EP, followed by OP, RP, and LP. Surgeons should consider these findings when selecting the optimal treatment method for individual UPJO patients. Further research should aim for improvement of study quality and decision tree analyses based on associated costs.

Supplementary information

Additional file 1: Figure S1. Funnel plots for operative success and complications with different comparisons **Table S1.** Operative success based on studies with at least 12 months follow-up (n = 13) **Table S2.** Probability of re-operation based on studies with at least 12 months follow-up (n = 13). **Table S3.** Study quality according to the Newcastle Ottawa Scale.

Abbreviations

EP: Endopyelotomy; IVU: Intravenous urography; LP: Laparoscopic pyeloplasty; OP: Open pyeloplasty; RP: Robotic assisted pyeloplasty; UPJO: Ureteropelvic junction obstruction

Acknowledgements

Parts of this paper have been presented as poster presentation at the 2019 European Association of Urology (EAU) conference in Barcelona (poster 1085).

Authors' contributions

The prespecified title and abstract screening of the EMBASE, MEDLINE and COCHRANE libraries as well as full text assessment were performed by AU, JU, AvH and AS. All other authors performed additional literature screening e.g. of publication lists of reviews and included articles as well as conference proceedings. Data extraction and assessment was performed by all authors. AU and JU performed all statistical analyses, data interpretation and drafted the manuscript. AS and AvH contributed technical knowledge with respect to different surgical techniques. LT and MH supervised the study. Data interpretation and drafting of the manuscript were performed by all authors. All authors read and approved the final manuscript.

Author details

[1]Department of Urology, University Medical Center Goettingen, Goettingen, Germany. [2]Department of Diagnostic and Interventional Radiology, University Medical Center Goettingen, Goettingen, Germany. [3]Division of Interventional Radiology, Department of Radiology and Biomedical Imaging, Yale School of Medicine, New Haven, CT, USA. [4]Department of Thoracic and Cardiovascular Surgery, University Medical Center Goettingen, Goettingen, Germany.

References

1. Gettman MT, Neururer R, Bartsch G, Peschel R. Anderson-Hynes dismembered pyeloplasty performed using the da Vinci robotic system. Urology. 2002;60:509–13.
2. Schuessler WW, Grune MT, Tecuanhuey LV, Preminger GM. Laparoscopic dismembered pyeloplasty. J Urol. 1993;150(6):1795–9.
3. Mei H, Pu J, Yang C, Zhang H, Zheng L, Tong Q. Laparoscopic versus open pyeloplasty for ureteropelvic junction obstruction in children: a systematic review and meta-analysis. J Endourol. 2011;25(5):727–36.
4. Huang Y, Wu Y, Shan W, Zeng L, Huang L. An updated meta-analysis of laparoscopic versus open pyeloplasty for ureteropelvic junction obstruction in children. Int J Clin Exp Med. 2015;8(4):4922–31.
5. Bansal P, Gupta A, Mongha R, Narayan S, Kundu AK, Chakraborty SC, et al. Laparoscopic versus open pyeloplasty: comparison of two surgical approaches -- a single Centre experience of three years. J Minim Access Surg. 2008;4(3):76–9.
6. Jacobs BL, Kaufman SR, Morgenstern H, Hollenbeck BK, Wolf JS Jr, Hollingsworth JM. Trends in the treatment of adults with ureteropelvic junction obstruction. J Endourol. 2013;27(3):355–60.
7. Khan F, Ahmed K, Lee N, Challacombe B, Khan MS, Dasgupta P. Management of ureteropelvic junction obstruction in adults. Nat Rev Urol. 2014;11(11):629–38.
8. Wang FX, Xu Y, Zhong H. Robot-assisted versus laparoscopic pyeloplasty for patients with ureteropelvic junction obstruction: an updated systematic review and meta-analysis (Provisional abstract). Scand J Urol. 2013;47(4):251–64 Available from: http://onlinelibrary.wiley.com/o/cochrane/cldare/articles/DARE-12013047147/frame.html.
9. Light A, Karthikeyan S, Maruthan S, Elhage O, Danuser H, Dasgupta P. Peri-operative outcomes and complications after laparoscopic vs robot-assisted dismembered pyeloplasty: a systematic review and meta-analysis. BJU Int. 2018,122(2).181–94.
10. Cundy TH, Harling L, Hughes-Hallett A, Mayer EK, Najmaldin AS, Athanasiou T, Yang GZ, Darzi A. Meta-analysis of robot-assisted vs conventional laparoscopic and open pyeloplasty in children (Provisional abstract). Database Abstr Rev Eff. 2014;2:582–94 Available from: http://onlinelibrary.wiley.com/o/cochrane/cldare/articles/DARE-12014066171/frame.html.
11. Autorino R, Eden C, El-Ghoneimi A, Guazzoni G, Buffi N, Peters CA, et al. Robot-assisted and laparoscopic repair of ureteropelvic junction obstruction: a systematic review and meta-analysis. Eur Urol. 2014;65(2):430–52.
12. Corbett HJ, Mullassery D. Outcomes of endopyelotomy for pelviureteric junction obstruction in the paediatric population: A systematic review. J Pediatr Urol. 2015;11(6):328–36.
13. Samarasekera D, Chew BH. Endopyelotomy still has an important role in the management of ureteropelvic junction obstruction. Can Urol Assoc J. 2011; 5(2):134–6.
14. Desai MM, Desai MR, Gill IS. Endopyeloplasty versus endopyelotomy versus laparoscopic pyeloplasty for primary ureteropelvic junction obstruction. Urology. 2004;64(1):16–21 discussion.
15. Rivas JG, Gregorio SA, Sanchez LC, Portella PF, Gomez AT, Ledo JC, et al. Evolution in the treatment of the ureteropelvic junction obstruction syndrome. Laparoscopic versus open pyeloplasty. Cent European J Urol. 2015;68(3):384–8.
16. Lucas SM, Sundaram CP, Wolf JS Jr, Leveillee RJ, Bird VG, Aziz M, Pautler SE, Luke P, Erdeljan P, Baldwin DD, Ebrahimi K, Nadler RB, Rebuck D, Thomas R, Lee BR, Boylu U, Figenshau RS, Munver R, Averch TD, Gayed B, Shalhav AL, Gundeti MS, Castle EP, Anderson JK, Duffey BG, Landman J, Okhunov Z, Wong C, Strom KH. Factors That Impact the Outcome of Minimally Invasive Pyeloplasty: Results of the Multi-Institutional Laparoscopic and Robotic Pyeloplasty Collaborative Group. J Urol. 2012;187:522–7.
17. Rothman KJ, Greenland S, Lash TL. Modern epidemiology, vol. x. 3rd ed. Philadelphia: Wolters Kluwer Health/Lippincott Williams & Wilkins; 2008. p. 758.
18. Downs SH, Black N. The feasibility of creating a checklist for the assessment of the methodological quality both of randomised and non-randomised studies of health care interventions. J Epidemiol Community Health. 1998; 52(6):377–84.
19. Higgins JPT, Green S (editors). Cochrane Handbook for Systematic Reviews of Interventions Version 5.1.0 [updated March 2011]. The Cochrane Collaboration, 2011. Available from www.handbook.cochrane.org.
20. Hanske J, Sanchez A, Schmid M, Meyer CP, Abdollah F, Roghmann F, et al. Comparison of 30-day perioperative outcomes in adults undergoing open versus minimally invasive pyeloplasty for ureteropelvic junction obstruction: analysis of 593 patients in a prospective national database. World J Urol. 2015;33(12):2107–13.
21. Yanke BV, Lallas CD, Pagnani C, McGinnis DE, Bagley DH. The minimally invasive treatment of ureteropelvic junction obstruction: a review of our experience during the last decade. J Urol. 2008;180:1397–402.
22. Han DY, Park KS, Seo IL, Rim JS. A comparison of minimally invasive surgical techniques for ureteropelvic junction obstructions: Endopyelotomy, acucise endopyelotomy, and laparoscopic pyeloplasty. Korean J Urol. 2008;49:592–7.
23. Rucker G, Schwarzer G. Ranking treatments in frequentist network meta-analysis works without resampling methods. BMC Med Res Methodol. 2015;15:58.
24. Egger M, Davey Smith G, Schneider M, Minder C. Bias in meta-analysis detected by a simple, graphical test. BMJ. 1997;315(7109):629–34.
25. Baldwin DD, Dunbar JA, Wells N, McDougall EM. Single-center comparison of laparoscopic pyeloplasty, Acucise endopyelotomy, and open pyeloplasty (Structured abstract). J Endourol. 2003;17(3):155–60 Available from: http://onlinelibrary.wiley.com/o/cochrane/cleed/articles/NHSEED-22003000812/frame.html.
26. Bernie JE, Venkatesh R, Brown J, Gardner TA, Sundaram CP. Comparison of laparoscopic pyeloplasty with and without robotic assistance; 2005.
27. Bird VG, Leveillee RJ, Eldefrawy A, Bracho J, Aziz MS. Comparison of robot-assisted versus conventional laparoscopic transperitoneal pyeloplasty for patients with ureteropelvic junction obstruction: a single-center study. Urology. 2011;77(3):730–4.
28. Brooks JD, Kavoussi LR, Preminger GM, Schuessler WW, Moore RG. Comparison of open and endourologic approaches to the obstructed ureteropelvic junction. Urology. 1995;46(6):791–5.
29. Calvert RC, Morsy MM, Zelhof B, Rhodes M, Burgess NA. Comparison of laparoscopic and open pyeloplasty in 100 patients with pelvi-ureteric junction obstruction. Surg Endosc. 2008;22(2):411–4.
30. Chen WN, Ye XJ, Liu SJ, Xiong LL, Huang XB, Xu T, Wang XF. Comparison of three surgical methods of ureteropelvic junction obstruction in therapeutic effect and complication. Beijing Da Xue Xue Bao Yi Xue Ban. 2016;48(5):817–21.
31. Danuser H, Stucki P, Pierro GBd, Mattei A. 7 Are there differences in outcome of laparoscopic and robot assisted pyeloplasties and how long is stenting of the anastomosis necessary? J Urol. 2012;187(4S):e3-e.
32. Fahad AH. A comparative study between open and laparoscopic pyeloplasty. J Pharm Sci Res. 2017;9:1961-5.
33. Garcia-Galisteo E, Emmanuel-Tejero E, Navarro Vilchez P, Garcia-Galisteo J, Baena-Gonzalez V. Comparison of the operation time and complications between conventional and robotic-assisted laparoscopic pyeloplasty. Actas Urol Esp. 2011;35(9):523–8.
34. Hemal AK, Mukherjee S, Singh K. Laparoscopic pyeloplasty versus robotic pyeloplasty for ureteropelvic junction obstruction: a series of 60 cases performed by a single surgeon. Can J Urol. 2010;17(1):5012–6.
35. Klingler HC, Remzi M, Janetschek G, Kratzik C, Marberger MJ. Comparison of open versus laparoscopic pyeloplasty techniques in treatment of uretero-pelvic junction obstruction. Eur Urol. 2003;44(3):340–5.
36. Link RE, Bhayani SB, Kavoussi LR. A prospective comparison of robotic and laparoscopic pyeloplasty. Ann Surg. 2006;243:486–91.
37. Memon MA, Biyabani SR, Ghirano R, Aziz W, Siddiqui KM. Is laparoscopic pyeloplasty a comparable option to treat ureteropelvic junction obstruction (UPJO)? A comparative study. J Pak Med Assoc. 2016;66(3):324–7.
38. Mohammed N, Zarzour M, Gadelmoula M, Muhlstadt S, Kawan F, Schumman A, Gollert C, Fornara P. Laparoscopic versus open pyeloplasty in overweight and obese patients. European Urology Supplements. 2017;16(3):e803.
39. Olweny EO, Park SK, Tan YK, Gurbuz C, Cadeddu JA, Best SL. Perioperative comparison of robotic assisted laparoendoscopic single-site (LESS) pyeloplasty versus conventional LESS pyeloplasty. Eur Urol. 2012;61(2):410–4.
40. Pahwa M, Pahwa AR, Girotra M, Abrahm RR, Kathuria S, Sharma A. Defining the pros and cons of open, conventional laparoscopy, and robot-assisted pyeloplasty in a developing nation. Adv Urol. 2014;2014:850156.
41. Simforoosh N, Basiri A, Tabibi A, Danesh AK, Sharifi-Aghdas F, Ziaee SA, Nooralizadeh A, Hosseini-Moghaddam SM. A comparison between laparoscopic and open pyeloplasty in patients with ureteropelvic junction obstruction. Urol J. 2004;1(3):165–9.
42. Umari P, Lissiani A, Trombetta C, Belgrano E. Comparison of open and laparoscopic pyeloplasty in ureteropelvic junction obstruction surgery: report of 49 cases. Arch Ital Urol Androl. 2011;83(4):169–74.
43. Wang X, Zhang Z, Peng N, Liu C. Retroperitoneal laparoscopic versus open dismembered pyeloplasty for ureteropelvic junction obstruction. J Xray Sci Technol. 2013;21(3):429–39.

44. Weise ES, Winfield HN. Robotic computer-assisted pyeloplasty versus conventional laparoscopic pyeloplasty. J Endourol. 2006;20(10):813–9.
45. Kim KC. Ohio library and information network. Robotics in general surgery. Online Resource. 2014;xvii:511. https://www.amazon.com/Robotics-General-Surgery-Keith-Chae-ebook/dp/B00GL0NSF2.
46. Farnham SB, Webster TM, Herrell SD, Smith JA. Intraoperative blood loss and transfusion requirements for robotic-assisted radical prostatectomy versus radical retropubic prostatectomy. Urology. 2006;67(2):360–3.
47. Novick AC, Gill IS, Klein EA, Rackley R, Ross JH. Operative Urology: Springer Science & Business Media; 2007.
48. Hofmann R. Endoskopische Urologie: Springer; 2005.
49. Hashim H, Woodhouse CRJ. Ureteropelvic junction obstruction. Eur Urol Suppl. 2012;11(2):25–32.
50. Rohrmann D, Snyder HM, Duckett JW, Canning DA, Zderic SA. The operative Management of Recurrent Ureteropelvic Junction Obstruction. J Urol. 1997; 158(3):1257–9.
51. Yu HY, Hevelone ND, Lipsitz SR, Kowalczyk KJ, Hu JC. Use, costs and comparative effectiveness of robotic assisted, laparoscopic and open urological surgery. J Urol. 2012;187(4):1392–8.
52. Gettman M, Lotan Y, Roerhborn CG, Cadeddu JA, Pearle MS. Cost-effective treatment for ureteropelvic junction obstruction: a decision tree analysis. J Urol. 2003;169(1):228–32.
53. Rucker G. Network meta-analysis, electrical networks and graph theory. Res Synth Methods. 2012;3(4):312–24.
54. Caldwell DM, Ades AE, Higgins JP. Simultaneous comparison of multiple treatments: combining direct and indirect evidence. BMJ. 2005;331(7521): 897–900.
55. Mills EJ, Thorlund K, Ioannidis JP. Demystifying trial networks and network meta-analysis. BMJ. 2013;346:f2914.

8

Definitive external-beam radiotherapy versus radical prostatectomy in clinically localized high-risk prostate cancer: A retrospective study

Fundagul Andic[1,6*], Volkan Izol[2], Serkan Gokcay[3], Hasan Suat Arslantas[1], Yildirim Bayazit[2], Hatice Coskun[4], Mustafa Zuhtu Tansug[2] and Yasar Sertdemir[5]

Abstract

Background: Optimal treatment of high-risk prostate cancer remains controversial. We aimed to compare treatment outcomes of prostate cancer patients treated with definitive external-beam radiotherapy (ExRT) or radical prostatectomy (RP).

Methods: The records of 120 high-risk clinical stage T2b-T4 N0 M0 prostate cancer patients treated with definitive ExRT or RP were reviewed. Patients with pretreatment prostate-specific antigen (PSA) levels ≥20 ng/mL or clinical ≥T3 stage or Gleason score (GS) ≥8 were included in the study. Biochemical failure free survival (BFFS), distant metastasis free survival (DMFS), cancer-specific survival (CSS) and overall survival (OS) were analyzed. Cox regression analysis was performed to determine predictors of BF.

Results: Seventy-two patients received definitive ExRT with androgen-deprivation therapy in 95.8% and 48 patients underwent RP with pelvic lymph node dissection. Mean age (67.7 ± 6.6 vs 64.5 ± 7.6 year, $p = 0.017$) and the rate of patients with PSA levels ≥20 ng/mL (69.4% vs 47.9%, $p = 0.022$) were higher in the definitive ExRT group than the RP group. Distributions of GS and clinical T stage were similar. Mean follow-up was 60.2 ± 30.3 months in the definitive ExRT group and 41.3 ± 21.5 months in the RP group ($p < 0.001$). Twenty-five % of the RP group received adjuvant ExRT and 41.7% received salvage ExRT. Biochemical failure was significantly higher (52.1% vs 21.4%, $p < 0.001$) and the mean BFFS was significantly lesser (34.4 ± 3.9 vs 97.8 ± 5.9 months, $p < 0.001$) in the RP group than the definitive ExRT group. However, DMFS, CSS and OS were similar in both groups. In multivariate analysis, being in the RP group significantly increased the risk of BF ($p < 0.001$). Furthermore, not receiving pelvic lymphatic irradiation in the definitive ExRT group ($p = 0.048$) and having positive surgical margin in the RP group ($p = 0.050$) increased the risk of BF.

Conclusions: BF was significantly higher and the mean BFFS was significantly lesser in high-risk prostate cancer patients undergoing RP than definitive ExRT while DMFS, CSS and OS were similar in both treatment groups.

Keywords: High-risk prostate cancer, Radiotherapy, Radical prostatectomy, Treatment outcomes

* Correspondence: fgandic@gmail.com
[1]Faculty of Medicine, Department of Radiation Oncology, Cukurova University, Adana, Turkey
[6]Balcali Hastanesi, Radyasyon Onkolojisi AD, Cukurova Universitesi, 01330 Sarıcam, Adana, Turkey
Full list of author information is available at the end of the article

Background

High-risk disease accounts approximately 30% of prostate cancer (PCa) [1, 2]. However, the current definitions of high-risk PCa include a heterogeneous group of patients with a range of prognoses and the optimal management of the subgroups is under debate [3–7].

Local treatment of high-risk PCa provides local control and also prevents further seeding of distant metastatic sites. Conventionally, high-risk PCa patients are treated with a combination of definitive external-beam radiotherapy (ExRT) and androgen-deprivation therapy (ADT) [8–10]. However, recent published data suggests that radical prostatectomy (RP) shows excellent local tumor control and similar oncological results in high-risk PCa patients, especially in combination with multimodal treatments involving ADT and radiotherapy [11–14]. Consequently, the American Urological Association (AUA) and European Association of Urology (EAU) support RP with extended pelvic lymph node dissection (PLND) as an optional treatment for a selective group of patients in the context of multimodal treatment [3, 4].

While outcomes for definitive ExRT and RP have been published independently these treatments have not been compared prospectively and the optimal management of high-risk PCa is still controversial. However, side effect profiles of definitive ExRT and RP might play a role in the decision of treatment. Treatment specific quality of life studies in clinically localized PCa demonstrate that sexual function and urinary control are better after ExRT than RP and gastro-intestinal side effects are more common after ExRT [15, 16]. Furthermore, adverse events due to combination of radiotherapy with long-term ADT, such as heart failure, arrhythmia, liver dysfunction, glucose intolerance, hot flush and diabetes may pose additional problems [17, 18].

In this single-institution retrospective study, we aimed to analyze the treatment outcomes of high-risk PCa patients either treated with definitive ExRT or RP as first-line treatment of the disease.

Methods

This study is approved by the Institutional Ethics Review Board.

The records of 120 patients with clinical stage T2b-T4 N0 M0 high-risk PCa who were treated with definitive ExRT or RP with PLND and/or followed at the Departments of Radiation Oncology and Urology between August 2007 and March 2018 were analyzed retrospectively. Patients were staged according to the seventh edition of the American Joint Committee on Cancer Classification and Staging of Tumors [19].

Eligibility criteria included: untreated, high-risk, clinical node negative, none-metastatic, histologically confirmed adenocarcinoma of the prostate. Patients at least having one of the following factors at pretreatment diagnostic evaluation: prostate-specific antigen (PSA) level ≥ 20 ng/mL, clinical ≥T3 stage and Gleason score (GS) ≥8 were accepted as high-risk PCa as defined in the AUA guideline [3].

All patients were evaluated with complete history, physical examination and blood PSA counts. Pelvic computed tomography (CT) and or magnetic resonance imaging, and bone scan were used for staging. Additionally, positron emission tomography (PET)/CT scan or prostate-specific membrane antigen PET /CT were applied in some patients as a part of their workup.

Follow-up of asymptomatic patients included disease specific history and blood PSA measurement at least 3 times (at three, six and twelve months) in the first year after treatment, then every six months until three years, and then annually. Restaging work-up was done if necessary. Examination intervals were adjusted individually at biochemical and clinical progression. Patient follow-up was completed through the review of medical records and phone calls from the patients.

In patients who underwent RP, a detectable or rising PSA value after surgery that is ≥0.2 ng/ml with a second confirmatory level is accepted as biochemical failure (BF) and the date of BF is accepted as the first rise (≥0.2 ng/mL) in PSA [20]. In patients receiving definitive ExRT, a PSA rise of ≥2 ng/mL above the nadir PSA after radiotherapy is accepted as BF and the date of BF is defined by the time the rise in PSA (≥2 ng/mL above the nadir) [21].

Postoperative ExRT was accepted as adjuvant if ExRT was started before BF without local and distant metastatic disease within 6 months after RP and accepted as salvage if ExRT was started after local and/or BF without distant metastatic disease. The decision of adjuvant or salvage ExRT and/or ADT were made by an urologist in cooperation with a radiation oncologist. The patients with positive surgical margins and positive lymph nodes were mostly treated with adjuvant ExRT. However, the patients with negative surgical margins and negative lymph nodes were most regularly followed-up and were further treated if they concluded with clinical failure.

Following definitive treatment, patients who have only BF with or without local recurrence are assessed for salvage local therapy often combined with ADT and patients who have subsequent metastatic disease received docetaxel or abiraterone acetate in combination with ADT.

Upgrading and downgrading of GS were defined as an increase or decrease, respectively, from one prognostic risk group to another, similar to upstaging and downstaging of T stage. Based on the AUA guideline, prognostic risk groups for GS were defined as follows: GS ≤6 (low risk), GS 7 (intermediate risk), and GS ≥8 (high risk) and prognostic risk groups for T stage were defined as follows: ≤T2a (low risk), T2b-T2c (intermediate risk) and ≥ T3 stage (high risk) [3].

End points

Mean follow-up was 60.2 ± 30.3 months in the definitive ExRT group and 41.3 ± 21.5 in the RP group. The primary end point was the rate of BF and BF free survival (BFFS). Additionally, distant metastases free survival (DMFS), cancer-specific survival (CSS) and overall survival (OS) were analyzed.

Possible predictive risk factors for BF were defined as age, pretreatment PSA level ≥ 20 ng/mL, GS ≥8 at biopsy and RP specimen, clinical and pathological ≥T3 tumor, pathological N1 stage, positive surgical margins, pelvic lymphatic irradiation (PLI) and short term (< 2 year) ADT use.

In the definitive ExRT group, in order to analyze whether duration of ADT may predict BF or not, ADT duration was calculated from the day of initiation of ADT to the last day of ADT effectiveness in cases without BF and to the day of BF in cases with BF.

Statistical analysis

All analyses were performed using IBM SPSS Statistics for Windows Version 19.0 statistical software package (Armonk, NY: IBM Corp). Categorical variables were expressed as numbers and percentages, whereas continuous variables were summarized as mean and standard deviation and as median and minimum-maximum where appropriate. Chi-square/Fisher Exact test was used to compare categorical variables between groups. For comparison of continuous variables between two groups, the Student's t-test or Mann-Whitney U test was used depending on whether the statistical hypotheses were fulfilled or not. Kaplan-Meier method and log rank test was performed for survival analysis. Cox regression analysis was performed to determine significant predictors of BF. Results of univariate and multivariate Cox regression analysis are given with odds ratio and 95% confidence interval. The statistical level of significance for all tests was considered to be 0.05.

Results

Seventy-two (60%) patients underwent definitive ExRT and 48 (40%) patients underwent RP with PLND as first-line therapy of high-risk PCa. The characteristics of high-risk PCa patients are shown in Table 1. No difference with regard to pretreatment clinical T stage and GS was found between the treatment groups. However, pretreatment mean PSA levels ($p = 0.049$) and the rate of patients with pretreatment PSA levels ≥20 ng/mL ($p = 0.022$) were significantly higher in the definitive ExRT group than the RP group.

Sixty-nine (95.8%) of the patients receiving definitive ExRT also received ADT in combination with ExRT as first-line treatment. ADT was not prescribed in three patients because of their cardiovascular comorbidities. While 65.3% ($n = 47$) of the patients receiving definitive ExRT received ADT ≥2-years, 25% ($n = 18$) of them received ≥1-year to < 2-year and 5.6% ($n = 4$) of them received less than < 1-year.

All patients had RP with extended PLND. However, 3 patients underwent surgery at an outside facility. Pathological characteristics of RP are given in Table 2. Forty-four out of 48 (91.7%) patients who underwent RP had adverse pathological risk factors (≥T3 tumor and/or positive surgical margins and/or positive lymph nodes and or GS ≥8).

Characteristics of definitive, adjuvant and salvage ExRT are given in Table 3. Three-dimensional conformal

Table 1 Characteristics of patients

	ExRT ($n = 72$)	RP ($n = 48$)	p
Age (years)	67.7 ± 6.6 67.2 (43.9–80.1)	64.5 ± 7.6 65.3 (47.3–79.9)	0.017
Follow-up (months)	60.2 ± 30.3 53.7 (10.3–125.8)	41.3 ± 21.5 37.8 (9.6–128.9)	< 0.001
Pretreatment PSA (ng/mL)	34.6 ± 30.7 25.4 (3.4–172)	27.2 ± 26.3 17 (3.2–138.7)	0.049
Pretreatment PSA ≥20 ng/mL n (%)	50 (69.4)	23 (47.9)	0.022
Clinical T stage n (%)			
T2	46 (63.9)	35 (72.9)	0.474
T3	22 (30.6)	12 (25.0)	
T4	4 (5.6)	1 (2.1)	
Gleason score (biopsy) n (%)			
6	17 (23.6)	8 (16.7)	0.636
7	15 (20.8)	10 (20.8)	
> 8	40 (55.6)	30 (62.5)	

ExRT, external-beam radiotherapy; *RP*, radical prostatectomy; *PSA*, prostate-specific antigen

Table 2 Pathological characteristics of radical prostatectomy

Extended PLND n (%)	48 (100)
Removed LN	13.3 ± 7.4 12 (5–38)
N1 stage n (%)	16 (33.3)
Positive surgical margin n (%)	28 (58.3)
Gleason score n (%)	
6	2 (4.2)
7	19 (39.6)
≥ 8	27 (56.3)
Gleason score upgrading n (%)	8 (16.7)
Gleason score downgrading n (%)	7 (14.6)
T stage n (%)	
T2	9 (18.8)
T3	38 (79.2)
T4	1 (2.1)
T stage upgrading n (%)	25 (52.1)
T stage downgrading n (%)	0 (0)

PLND: pelvic lymph node dissection; *LN*: lymph nodes

radiation therapy (3D-CRT) or intensity modulated radiation therapy (IMRT) techniques were used in all 104 patients receiving ExRT. However, 11.5% of the patients (5 in definitive ExRT group, 4 in adjuvant ExRT group and 3 in salvage ExRT group) received their ExRT at an outside facility.

In the RP group, 12 (25%) patients received adjuvant ExRT and 20 (41.7%) patients received salvage ExRT for local and/or BF. Furthermore, 9 of the patient in adjuvant ExRT group and 12 of the patients in salvage ExRT group also received ADT in combination with ExRT.

Prior to salvage ExRT, median PSA level of totally 20 patients was 1.09 (0.25–43.5). Salvage ExRT was administered at a PSA level of < 0.5 ng/mL in 3 (15%) patients, at a PSA level of 0.5 to1.5 in 10 (50%) patients and > 1.5 ng/mL in 7 (35%) patients.

Table 3 Characteristics of external-beam radiotherapy

	Definitive ExRT (n = 72)	Adjuvant ExRT (n = 12)	Salvage ExRT (n = 20)
Volume	P + SV +/− PLI	Operation bed +/− PLI	Operation bed +/− PLI
Dose*	74 Gy (70–76)	66 Gy (60–70.2)	66 Gy (60–74)
PLI n (%)	18 (25.0)	3 (33.3)	8 (40)
Technique n (%)			
3D-CRT	65 (90.3)	10 (83.3)	18 (90)
IMRT	7 (9.7)	2 (16.7)	2 (10)

ExRT, external-beam radiotherapy; *P*, prostate; *SV*, seminal vesicle; *PLI*, pelvic lymphatic irradiation; *3D-CRT*, three-dimensional conformal radiotherapy; *IMRT*, intensity modulated radiotherapy
*, radiotherapy was given with 1.8–2 Gy daily fraction dose

Risk groups of GS were confirmed on RP specimen in 33 (68.8%) out of 48 patients who underwent RP. Eight patients (16.7%) had upgrading on RP specimen: 4 patients upgraded from a low risk GS 6 to an intermediate risk GS 7, 2 patients from a low risk GS 6 to a high risk GS 9 and 2 patients from an intermediate risk GS 7 to a high risk GS 8. Furthermore, 7 (14.6%) patients had downgrading on RP specimen from a high risk GS 8 to an intermediate risk GS 7.

Risk groups of clinical T stages were confirmed on RP specimen in 23 (47.9%) out of 48 patients. However, 25 (52.1%) patients had upstaging on RP specimen from a T2b-T2c stage to a T3 stage in 24 patients and from a T2c to a T4 stage in 1 patient.

Treatment outcomes according to the treatment groups are given in Figs. 1, 2, 3 and 4 and Table 4. BF was significantly higher (52.1% vs 21.4%, $p < 0.001$) and the mean BFFS was significantly lesser (34.4 ± 3.9 vs 97.8 ± 5.9 months, p < 0.001) in the RP group than the definitive ExRT group. However, distant metastasis, cancer-specific mortality, all-cause mortality, DMFS, CSS and OS were similar in both groups.

Results of the univariate Cox regression analyses for potential predictors of BF are given in Table 5. When all patients were included, univariate analysis showed that being in the treatment group RP was the only significant (p < 0.001) predictor of BF while age was borderline significant ($p = 0.066$) and multivariate analysis showed that being in the treatment group RP was still the only significant ($p < 0.001$) predictor of BF and pretreatment PSA level ≥ 20 ng/mL was borderline significant ($p = 0.069$). When only definitive

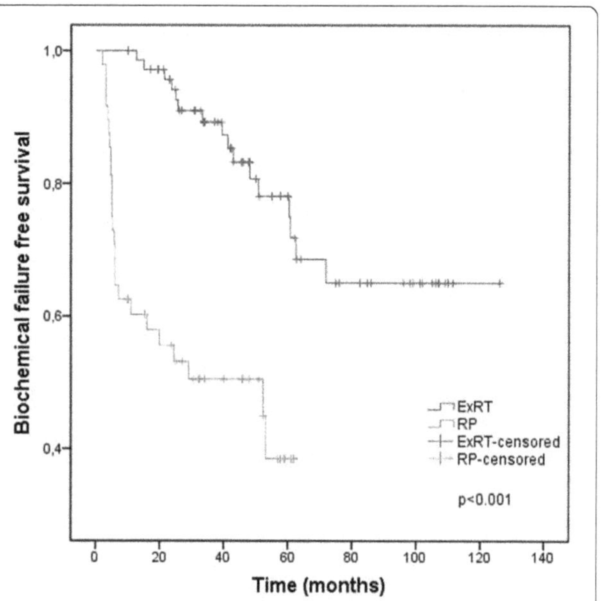

Fig. 1 Biochemical failure free survival. ExRT, external-beam radiotherapy; RP, radical prostatectomy

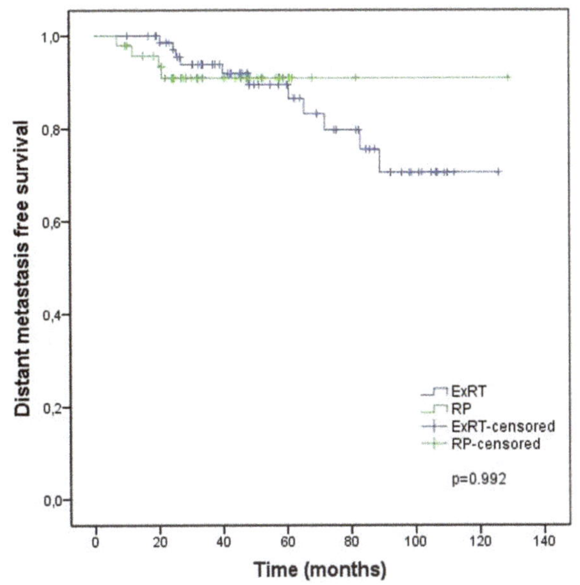

Fig. 2 Distant metastasis free survival. ExRT, external-beam radiotherapy; RP, radical prostatectomy

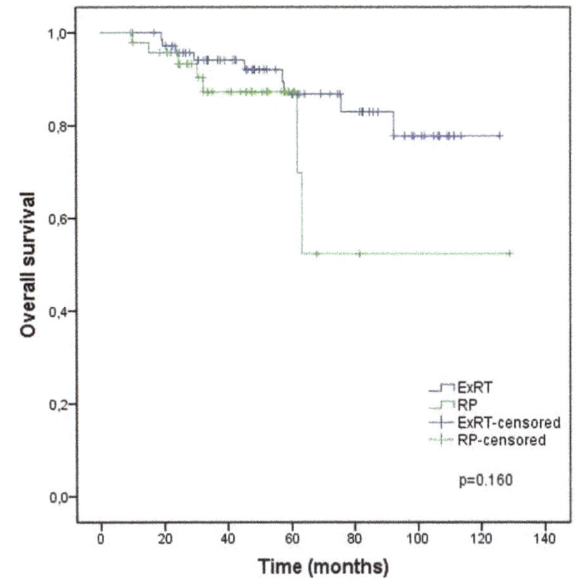

Fig. 4 Overall survival. ExRT, external-beam radiotherapy; RP, radical prostatectomy

ExRT treatment group was included, univariate analysis showed that not receiving PLI was borderline significant ($p = 0.071$) to predict BF and multivariate analysis showed that after risk adjustment according to ≥2-year ADT use, BF risk was significantly higher in patients who did not receive PLI ($p = 0.048$) than patients who received. When only RP treatment group was included, both univariate and multivariate analysis showed that positive surgical margin was the only significant ($p = 0.050$) predictor of BF.

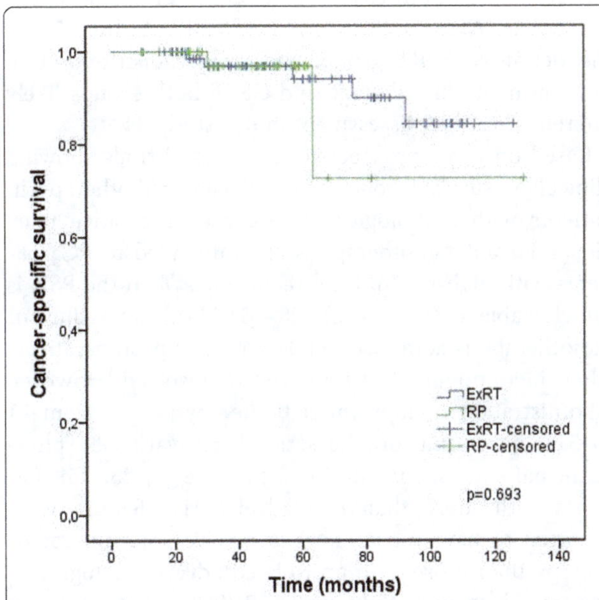

Fig. 3 Cancer-specific survival. ExRT, external-beam radiotherapy; RP, radical prostatectomy

Discussion

There is no consensus on the best treatment for high-risk PCa patients. Options include definitive ExRT with ADT or RP with PLND followed by adjuvant radiotherapy in cases with unfavorable pathological features. The results of this study showed that the rate of BF was significantly higher (52.1% vs 21.4%, $p < 0.001$) and the mean BFFS was significantly lesser (34.4 ± 3.9 vs 97.8 ± 5.9 months, $p < 0.001$) in the RP group than the definitive ExRT group. Five-year BFFS was 38.5 and 78.1% in the RP and the definitive ExRT group, respectively. Furthermore, 5-year DMFS, CSS and OS were similar in both groups. In multivariate analysis, when all patients were included, being in the treatment group RP significantly increased the risk of BF (p < 0.001) and pretreatment PSA levels ≥20 ng/mL was borderline significant ($p = 0.069$); when only definitive ExRT group was included, after risk adjustment according to ≥2-year ADT use, not receiving PLI significantly increased the risk of BF ($p = 0.048$); and when only RP group was included, positive surgical margin was the only significant ($p = 0.050$) predictor of BF.

Suggestion of RP as a first-line treatment option in high-risk PCa patients is based on several large published retrospective series demonstrating favorable 10-year CSS rates ranging around 90 to 80% and 5-year BFFS rates ranging around 70 to 50% [12, 22–24]. However, such high survival rates and high BFFS rates may be associated with the definitions of high-risk disease and thus capturing the patients with more favorable high-risk disease. In our study, 5-year CSS rate was 96.9% and 5-year BFFS was 38.5% in the RP group.

Table 4 Outcomes of treatment groups

Treatment Outcomes	Definitive ExRT (*n* = 72)	RP (*n* = 48)	p
BF n (%)	16 (21.4)	25 (52.1)	< 0.001
Mean BFFS (months)	97.8 ± 5.9	34.4 ± 3.9	< 0.001
3 year BFFS (%) (95% CI)	89.3 (95 81.7–96.9)	50.6 (36.1–65.1)	
5 year BFFS (%) (95% CI)	78.1 (66.7–89.5)	38.5 (20.1–56.9)	
DM n (%)	11 (15.3)	4 (8.3)	0.399
Mean DMFS (months)	106.6 ± 5.1	118.5 ± 4.9	0.992
3-year DMFS (%) (95% CI)	93.8 (87.9–99.7)	90.9 (82.4–99.4)	
5-year DMFS (%) (95% CI)	89.5 (81.4–97.6)	90.9 (82.4–99.4)	
Cancer-specific mortality n (%)	5 (6.9)	2 (4.2)	0.701
Mean CSS (months)	116.9 ± 5.1	109.9 ± 14.0	0.693
3 year CSS (%)	96.8 (92.5–100.0)	96.9 (90.8–100.0)	
5 year CSS (%)	94.1 (87.2–100.0)	96.9 (90.8–100.0)	
All-cause mortality n (%)	9 (12.5)	7 (14.6)	0.788
Mean OS (months)	110.9 ± 4.6	92.3 ± 13.4	0.160
3 year OS (%) (95% CI)	94.1 (88.4–99.7)	87.2 (76.6–97.9)	
5 year OS (%) (95% CI)	86.8 (77.2–96.3)	87.2 (76.6–97.9)	

ExRT, external-beam radiotherapy; *RP*, radical prostatectomy; *BF*, biochemical failure; *BFFS*, biochemical failure free survival; *DM*, distant metastasis; *DMFS*, distant metastasis free survival; *CSS*, cancer-specific survival; *OS*, overall survival

Furthermore, several studies have retrospectively compared RP with ExRT in high-risk PCa patients. In a combined analysis including 1238 patients undergoing RP and 609 patients undergoing ExRT with or without ADT, 10-year CCS rates were 92, 92, and 88% for patients receiving RP, ExRT with ADT, and ExRT alone, respectively ($p = 0.06$) [25]. After multivariable risk adjustment, there was no significant difference in DMFS or CSS. However, the risk of all-cause mortality was greater after ExRT with ADT when compared to RP which could be explained by selection bias and contribution of potential adverse cardiovascular effects of ADT [25]. In our study 5-year DMFS and 5-year CCS was similar (89.5% vs 90.9 and 94.1% vs 96.9%) in the definitive ExRT and the RP groups, respectively, as well as the rate of all-cause mortality (86.8% vs 87.2%).

In a retrospective study from Italy reported outcomes of 288 patients with high-risk PCa either underwent ExRT ($n = 162$) in combination with nine months of ADT or underwent ($n = 122$) RP with pelvic lymph node sampling. Three-year BFFS favored ExRT targeted to prostate and seminal vesicle without PLI (86.8% vs 69.8%, $p = 0.001$) [26]. However, ADT duration was none-optimal and follow-up period was relatively short. In our study, 95.8% ($n = 69$) of the patients receiving definitive ExRT also received ADT in combination with ExRT as initial treatment. Furthermore, ADT duration was ≥2-years in 65.3% ($n = 47$) of the patients and ≥ 1-year to < 2-year in 25% ($n = 18$) of them.

Another retrospective study reported 7.8% absolute benefit in 8-year metastatic progression with RP compared to ExRT in a high-risk cohort of PCa patients [27]. However, omission of PLI and short term (3 to 6 months) ADT use in combination with ExRT and higher pretreatment risk factors (PSA, clinical stage, and GS) in the ExRT group than the RP group were the major limitations of the study [27]. In our study, 5-year DMFS were similar in both treatment groups. Furthermore, use of ≥2-years ADT in 65.3% and performing PLI in 25% of the definitive ExRT group, and similar distribution of pretreatment clinical stage and GS in both groups likely offered a healthier assessment in our study.

Based on three prospective randomized trials showing clinical or survival benefit for adjuvant radiotherapy in patients with pathological T3 disease or positive margins, adjuvant radiotherapy is recommended to PCa patients with high-risk of local recurrence when the PSA is undetectable (< 0.2 ng/mL) [28–31]. Typically, adjuvant radiotherapy is administered 3–6 months postoperatively when incontinence has stabilized or resolved. However, administration of adjuvant radiotherapy ranged from 11 to 51% depending on the series likely varied by physician, patient, and institutional practice [7, 23, 25]. Patients with more than one adverse risk feature were reported to have more likely to receive adjuvant radiotherapy than those with an isolated adverse or high-risk feature [7]. In our study, while 12 (25%) of the patients in the RP group received adjuvant ExRT, 9 of them also received ADT in combination with adjuvant ExRT.

Table 5 Possible predictive factors in univariate and multivariate analysis

	OR	95% CI	p
All patients-univariate			
Age	0.96	0.92–1.00	0.066+
PSA ≥20 ng/mL	1.26	0.66–2.41	0.480
Clinical ≥T3 stage	0.70	0.35–1.41	0.319
GS ≥8 at biopsy	1.29	0.69–2.42	0.430
Treatment group RP	4.61	2.36–9.00	< 0.001*
All patients-multivariate			
PSA ≥20 ng/mL	1.85	0.95–3.59	0.069+
Treatment group RP	5.35	2.69–10.61	< 0.001*
ExRT group-univariate			
ADT use < 2-year	1.98	0.72–5.49	0.188
No PLI	2.53	0.93–6.91	0.071+
ExRT group-multivariate			
ADT use < 2-year	2.42	0.85–6.89	0.098
No PLI	2.87	1.01–8.16	0.048*
RP group-univariate			
Positive surgical margin	2.41	1.00–5.78	0.050*
Pathological N1 stage	1.97	0.87–4.46	0.105
Pathological ≥T3 stage	2.17	0.65–7.32	0.210
GS ≥8 at RP specimen	1.83	0.80–4.18	0.154
RP group-multivariate			
Positive surgical margin#	2.41	1.00–5.78	0.050*

OR, Odds ratio; *CI*, confidence Interval; *PSA*, prostate specific antigen; *GS*, Gleason score; *RP*, radical prostatectomy; *ExRT*, external-beam radiotherapy; *ADT*, androgen deprivation treatment; *PLI*, pelvic lymphatic irradiation
*indicates statistically significant data; + indicates borderline significant data
#, for the RP group, positive surgical margin was the only significant risk factor predicting BF in multivariate analysis

Furthermore, management of local and/or BF after RP with salvage radiotherapy and ADT may permit excellent long-term outcomes comparable to definitive ExRT. In our study, while 20 (41.7%) of the patients in the RP group received salvage ExRT for local and/or BF, 12 of them received ADT in combination with salvage ExRT. In addition, the effectiveness of radiotherapy for PSA failure is greatest when given at lower levels of PSA [20]. In our study, salvage ExRT was administered at a PSA level of ≤1.5 ng/mL in 65% of the patients.

RP may reveal ascertainment errors particularly in patients who are characterized as high-risk by biopsy alone and may represent the sole, initial definitive therapy in some high-risk PCa patients with specimen-confined disease. A recent study of 1424 PCa who underwent open or robotic-assisted RP found that 61.5% (91/148) of patients with clinical GS 8 disease on prostate biopsy were downgraded on RP [32]. In our study 7 (14.6%) patients were downgraded on RP specimen from a high risk GS 8 to an intermediate risk GS 7. However, 5 of them had T3 disease with or without positive lymph node(s) on RP and the rest 2 patients had no other pathological or clinical high-risk factor except the initial GS 8 at biopsy.

Since high-risk PCa patients have high frequency of nodal spread, RP with PLND provides accurate staging to estimate prognosis and to inform the need for subsequent therapy [33]. In two systematic reviews, extended PLND had been suggested to increase the detection of positive nodes, with an associated improvement in survival [34, 35]. The observed survival benefit was attributed to the elimination of micro metastatic disease. In our study, all patients underwent RP with extended PLND and the median number of removed lymph nodes was 12 (5–38).

Radiotherapy dose escalation may provide better biochemical control in patients with high-risk disease [36–38]. Additionally, a better local control and improvement in distant metastases and disease-specific survival with higher doses of radiation are reported previously [36, 39]. However, an improvement in OS has not been demonstrated up to date. Thus, it brings to mind the question of whether the addition of long-term ADT to radiotherapy may be more important than dose escalation; most likely related to the effect of ADT on micro metastatic disease [40]. In our study, median definitive ExRT dose was 74 Gy (70–76) and 90.3% of the definitive ExRT group used ADT more than one year.

The limitations of this study are being a retrospective study, having a relatively short observation period and the use of BF as a primary endpoint since the definitions of BF are different after radiotherapy and after surgery. Furthermore, we recognize that our study is also limited by the imbalanced distributions of PSA levels and age, and the differed follow-up period between the treatment groups which could have impacted our long-term comparisons. Higher pretreatment PSA levels and older age in the definitive ExRT group than the RP group could be explained by the referral of these patients considerably to radiotherapy rather than surgery and shorter follow-up period in the RP group than the definitive ExRT group could be explained by the recently recognition of RP as an optional treatment in the context of multimodal treatment [3, 4] in high-risk PCa patients.

The strength of this study is using 3D-CRT or IMRT in all patients receiving ExRT and administration of long term ADT in most of the patients receiving definitive ExRT, and having extended PLND in all patents who underwent RP.

In high-risk PCa patients, RP as a component of multimodal therapy including radiotherapy and ADT may provide excellent oncological outcomes comparable to definitive radiotherapy. In our study, 66.7% of the patients in the RP group received either adjuvant or salvage ExRT with or without ADT and both treatment groups had similar mortality rates though the BF rate was higher in the RP group.

Conclusion

This study showed that while the rate of BF was significantly higher and the mean BFFS was significantly lesser in high-risk PCa patients undergoing RP than definitive ExRT; 5-year DMFS, CSS and OS were similar in both treatment groups. However, further randomized trials investigating optimal management of high-risk PCa and the sub-groups are needed.

Abbreviations

3D-CRT: Three dimensional conformal radiation therapy; ADT: Androgen-deprivation therapy; AUA: American urological association; BF: Biochemical failure; BFFS: Biochemical failure free survival; CSS: Cancer-specific survival; CT: Computed tomography; DMFS: Distant metastasis free survival; EAU: European association of urology; ExRT: External-beam radiotherapy; GS: Gleason score; IMRT: Intensity modulated radiation therapy; OS: Overall survival; PCa: Prostate cancer; PET: Positron emission tomography; PLI: Pelvic lymphatic irradiation; PLND: Pelvic lymph node dissection; PSA: Prostate-specific antigen; RP: Radical prostatectomy

Acknowledgements

Not applicable.

Authors' contributions

FA made substantial contributions to conception and design of the study; acquisition, analysis and interpretation of data; and drafted and revised the manuscript. VI and YB contributed to conception and design of the study; acquisition, analysis and interpretation of data; and assisted with drafting and revising the manuscript. SG, HSA, HC, MZT contributed to conception and design of the study and acquisition of data; and revised the manuscript critically for important intellectual content. YS contributed to conception and design of the study; analysis and interpretation of data; and revised the manuscript critically for important intellectual content. Furthermore, all authors approved the final version of the manuscript to be published; agreed to be accountable for all aspects of the work in ensuring that questions related to the accuracy or integrity of any part of the work are appropriately investigated and resolved.

Author details

[1]Faculty of Medicine, Department of Radiation Oncology, Cukurova University, Adana, Turkey. [2]Faculty of Medicine, Department of Urology, Cukurova University, Adana, Turkey. [3]Department of Medical Oncology, Mehmet Akif Inan Training and Research Hospital, Sanliurfa, Turkey. [4]Faculty of Medicine, Department of Radiation Oncology, Gaziantep University, Gaziantep, Turkey. [5]Faculty of Medicine, Department of Biostatistics, Cukurova University, Adana, Turkey. [6]Balcali Hastanesi, Radyasyon Onkolojisi AD, Cukurova Universitesi, 01330 Sarıcam, Adana, Turkey.

References

1. Cooperberg MR, Cowan J, Broering JM, Carroll PR. High-risk prostate cancer in the United States, 1990-2007. World J Urol. 2008;26:211–8.
2. Abdollah F, Sun M, Thuret R, Jeldres C, Tian Z, Briganti A, et al. A competing-risks analysis of survival after alternative treatment modalities for prostate cancer patients:1988–2006. Eur Urol. 2011;59:88–95.
3. Sanda MG, Cadeddu JA, Kirkby E, Chen RC, Crispino T, Fontanarosa J, et al. Clinically Localized Prostate Cancer: AUA/ASTRO/SUO Guideline. Part I: Risk Stratification, Shared Decision Making, and Care Options. J Urol. 2017; doi: https://doi.org/10.1016/j.juro.2017.11.095
4. Mottet N, Bellmunt J, Bolla M, Briers E, Cumberbatch MG, De Santis M, et al. EAU-ESTRO-SIOG guidelines on prostate cancer. Part 1: screening, diagnosis, and local treatment with curative intent. Eur Urol. 2017;71:618–29.
5. Briganti A, Joniau S, Gontero P, Abdollah F, Passoni NM, Tombal B, et al. Identifying the best candidate for radical prostatectomy among patients with high-risk prostate cancer. Eur Urol. 2012;61:584–92.
6. Yossepowitch O, Eggener SE, Serio AM, Carver BS, Bianco FJ Jr, Scardino PT, et al. Secondary therapy, metastatic progression, and cancer-specific mortality in men with clinically high-risk prostate cancer treated with radical prostatectomy. Eur Urol. 2008;53:950–9.
7. Spahn M, Joniau S, Gontero P, Fieuws S, Marchioro G, Tombal B, et al. Outcome predictors of radical prostatectomy in patients with prostate-specific antigen greater than 20 ng/ml: a European multi-institutional study of 712 patients. Eur Urol. 2010;58:1–7.
8. Bolla M, Collette L, Blank L, Warde P, Dubois JB, Mirimanoff RO, et al. Longterm results with immediate androgen suppression an external irradiation in patients with locally advanced prostate cancer (an EORTC study): a phase III randomised trial. Lancet. 2002;360:103–6.
9. Bolla M, Van Tienhoven G, Warde P, Dubois JB, Mirimanoff RO, Storme G, et al. External irradiation with or without longterm androgen suppression for prostate cancer with high metastatic risk: 10-year results of an EORTC randomised study. Lancet Oncol. 2010;11:1066–73.
10. Horwitz EM, Bae K, Hanks GE, Porter A, Grignon DJ, Brereton HD, et al. Ten-year follow-up of radiation therapy oncology group protocol 92-02: a phase III trial of the duration of elective androgen deprivation in locally advanced prostate cancer. J Clin Oncol. 2008;26:2497–504.
11. Johnstone PA, Ward KC, Goodman M, Assikis V, Petros JA. Radical prostatectomy for clinical T4 prostate cancer. Cancer. 2006;106:2603–9.
12. Spahn M, Weiss C, Bader P, Ströbel P, Gerharz EW, Kneitz B, et al. Longterm outcome of patients with highrisk prostate cancer following radical prostatectomy and stage-dependent adjuvant androgen deprivation. Urol Int. 2010;84:164–73.
13. Steuber T, Budäus L, Walz J, Zorn KC, Schlomm T, Chun F, et al. Radical prostatectomy improves progression-free and cancer-specific survival in men with lymph node positive prostate cancer in the prostate-specific antigen era: a confirmatory study. BJU Int. 2011;107:1755–61.
14. Siddiqui SA, Boorjian SA, Blute ML, Rangel LJ, Bergstralh EJ, Karnes RJ, et al. Impact of adjuvant androgen deprivation therapy after radical prostatectomy on the survival of patients with pathological T3b prostate cancer. BJU Int. 2011;107:383–8.
15. Litwin MS, Gore JL, Kwan L, Brandeis JM, Lee SP, Withers HR, et al. Quality of life after surgery, external beam irradiation, or brachytherapy for early-s tage prostate cancer. Cancer. 2007;109:2239–47.
16. Potosky AL, Davis WW, Hoffman RM, Stanford JL, Stephenson RA, Penson DF, et al. Five-year outcomes after prostatectomy or radiotherapy for prostate cancer: the prostate cancer outcomes study. J Natl Cancer Inst. 2004;96:1358–67.
17. Keating NL, O'Malley AJ, Smith MR. Diabetes and cardiovascular disease during androgen deprivation therapy for prostate cancer. J Clin Oncol. 2006; 24:4448–56.
18. Haque R, UlcickasYood M, Xu X, Cassidy-Bushrow AE, Tsai HT, Keating NL, et al. Cardiovascular disease risk and androgen deprivation therapy in patients with localised prostate cancer: a prospective cohort study. Br J Cancer. 2017;117:1233–40.
19. Genitourinary sites: Prostate cancer. In: Edge SB, Byrd DR, Compton CC, Fritz AG, Greene FL and Trotti III A, editors. American Joint Committee on Cancer Staging Manuel Seventh Edition. New York, Dordrecht, Heidelberg, London, Springer; 2015. p. 457–68.
20. Thompson IM, Valicenti RK, Albertsen P, Davis BJ, Goldenberg SL, Hahn C, et al. Adjuvant and salvage radiotherapy after prostatectomy: AUA/ASTRO guideline. J Urol. 2013;190:441–9.
21. Roach M 3rd, Hanks G, Thames H Jr, Schellhammer P, Shipley WU, Sokol GH, et al. Defining biochemical failure following radiotherapy with or without hormonal therapy in men with clinically localized prostate cancer: recommendations of the RTOG-ASTRO Phoenix consensus conference. Int J Radiat Oncol Biol Phys. 2006;65:965–74.
22. Zwergel U, Suttmann H, Schroeder T, Siemer S, Wullich B, Kamradt J, et al. Outcome of prostate cancer patients with initial PSA> or =20 ng/ml undergoing radical prostatectomy. Eur Urol. 2007;52:1058–65.

23. Ward JF, Slezak JM, Blute ML, Bergstralh EJ, Zincke H. Radical prostatectomy for clinically advanced (cT3) prostate cancer since the advent of prostate-specific antigen testing: 15-year outcome. BJU Int. 2005;95:751–6.
24. Nagao K, Matsuyama H, Matsumoto H, Nasu T, Yamamoto M, Kamiryo Y, et al. Identification of curable high-risk prostate cancer using radical prostatectomy alone: who are the good candidates for undergoing radical prostatectomy among patients with high-risk prostate cancer? Int J Clin Oncol. https://doi.org/10.1007/s10147-018-1272-9.
25. Boorjian SA, Karnes RJ, Viterbo R, Rangel LJ, Bergstralh EJ, Horwitz EM, et al. Long-term survival after radical prostatectomy versus external-beam radiotherapy for patients with high-risk prostate cancer. Cancer. 2011;117:2883–91.
26. Arcangeli G, Strigari L, Arcangeli S, Petrongari MG, Saracino B, Gomellini S, et al. Retrospective comparison of external beam radiotherapy and radical prostatectomy in high-risk, clinically localized prostate cancer. Int J Radiat Oncol Biol Phys. 2009;75:975–82.
27. Zelefsky MJ, Eastham JA, Cronin AM, Fuks Z, Zhang Z, Yamada Y, et al. Metastasis after radical prostatectomy or external beam radiotherapy for patients with clinically localized prostate cancer: a comparison of clinical cohorts adjusted for case mix. J Clin Oncol. 2010;28:1508–13.
28. Bolla M, van Poppel H, Collette L, van Cangh P, Vekemans K, Da Pozzo L, et al. Postoperative radiotherapy after radical prostatectomy: a randomised controlled trial (EORTC trial 22911). Lancet. 2005;366:572–8.
29. Bolla M, van Poppel H, Tombal B, Vekemans K, Da Pozzo L, de Reijke TM, et al. Postoperative radiotherapy after radical prostatectomy for high-risk prostate cancer: long-term results of a randomised controlled trial (EORTC trial 22911). Lancet. 2012;380:2018–27.
30. Thompson IM, Tangen CM, Paradelo J, Lucia MS, Miller G, Troyer D, et al. Adjuvant radiotherapy for pathological T3N0M0 prostate cancer significantly reduces risk of metastases and improves survival: long-term followup of a randomized clinical trial. J Urol. 2009;181:956–62.
31. Wiegel T, Bottke D, Steiner U, Siegmann A, Golz R, Störkel S, et al. Phase III postoperative adjuvant radiotherapy after radical prostatectomy compared with radical prostatectomy alone in pT3 prostate cancer with postoperative undetectable prostate-specific antigen: ARO 96-02/AUO AP 09/95. J Clin Oncol. 2009;27:2924–30.
32. Qi R, Foo WC, Ferrandino MN, Davis LG, Sekar S, Longo TA, et al. Over half of contemporary clinical Gleason 8 on prostate biopsy are downgraded at radical prostatectomy. Can J Urol. 2017;24:8982–9.
33. Heidenreich A, Ohlmann CH, Polyakov S. Anatomical extent of pelvic lymphadenectomy in patients undergoing radical prostatectomy. Eur Urol. 2007;52:29–37.
34. Briganti A, Blute ML, Eastham JH, Graefen M, Heidenreich A, Karnes JR, et al. Pelvic lymph node dissection in prostate cancer. Eur Urol. 2009;55:1251–65.
35. Wagner M, Sokoloff M, Daneshmand S. The role of pelvic lymphadenectomy for prostate cancer--therapeutic? J Urol. 2008;179:408–13.
36. Kuban DA, Levy LB, Cheung MR, Lee AK, Choi S, Frank S, et al. Long-term failure patterns and survival in a randomized dose-escalation trial for prostate cancer. Who dies of disease? Int J Radiat Oncol Biol Phys. 2011;79:1310–7.
37. Zietman AL, Bae K, Slater JD, Shipley WU, Efstathiou JA, Coen JJ, et al. Randomized trial comparing conventional-dose with high-dose conformal radiation therapy in early-stage adenocarcinoma of the prostate: long-term results from proton radiation oncology group/american college of radiology 95-09. J Clin Oncol. 2010;28:1106–11.
38. Beckendorf V, Guerif S, Le Prisé E, Cosset JM, Bougnoux A, Chauvet B, et al. 70 Gy versus 80 Gy in localized prostate cancer: 5-year results of GETUG 06 randomized trial. Int J Radiat Oncol Biol Phys. 2011;80:1056–63.
39. Zelefsky MJ, Reuter VE, Fuks Z, Scardino P, Shippy A. Influence of local tumor control on distant metastases and cancer related mortality after external beam radiotherapy for prostate cancer. J Urol. 2008;179:1368–73.
40. Roach M 3rd. Dose escalated external beam radiotherapy versus neoadjuvant androgen deprivation therapy and conventional dose external beam radiotherapy for clinically localized prostate cancer: do we need both? Strahlenther Onkol. 2007;183:26–8.

9

Predictive factors for response to salvage stereotactic body radiotherapy in oligorecurrent prostate cancer limited to lymph nodes: A single institution experience

Christoph Oehler[1*†], Michel Zimmermann[1†], Lukas Adam[1], Juergen Curschmann[2], Marcin Sumila[2], Räto T. Strebel[3], Richard Cathomas[4], Qiyu Li[5], Uwe Schneider[2] and Daniel R. Zwahlen[1]

Abstract

Background: In patients presenting with limited nodal recurrence following radical prostatectomy (RP), stereotactic body radiotherapy (SBRT) results might improve with a better case selection.

Methods: Single-institution retrospective analysis of patients presenting with 1–3 lymph node (LN) recurrences (N1 or M1a) on 18F-Choline PET/CT. Prior therapy included radical prostatectomy (RP) ± salvage radiotherapy (RT), in absence of any systemic therapy.

Outcome parameters were biochemical response (BR), time to biochemical recurrence (TBR) and time interval between SBRT and androgen deprivation therapy start (TADT). Time to event endpoints was analysed using Kaplan-Meier method. Potential prognostic factors were examined using univariate proportional hazards regression for TADT and logistic regression for BR. The optimal cut-off point for LN size was calculated using the Contal and O'Quigley method.

Results: 25 patients fulfilling study criteria were treated with SBRT from January 2010 to January 2015 and retrospectively analysed. Median follow up was 18 months and median LN diameter 10.5 mm. SBRT was delivered to a median dose of 36 Gy in three fractions (range: 30–45 Gy). BR was reached in 52% of cases. Median TBR was 11.9 months and significantly longer in patients with larger LN (Hazard ratio [HR] = 0.87, $P = 0.03$). Using 14 mm as cut off for LN, median TBR was 10.8 months for patients with small LN (18 patients), and 21.2 months for patients with large LN (6 patients) (P unadjusted = 0.009; P adjusted = 0.099). ADT was started in 32% of patients after a median follow-up of 18 months.

Conclusions: For PCa patients with 1–3 LN recurrence after RP (± salvage RT), SBRT might result in a better biochemical control when delivered to larger sized (≥ 14 mm) LN metastases. This study is hypothesis generating and results should be tested in a larger prospective trial.

Keywords: Body radiotherapy, Stereotactic, Prostate cancer, Lymph node metastases, Salvage therapy, Recurrence

* Correspondence: christoph.oehler@ksgr.ch
Presented in part at the 59th Annual Meeting of the American Society of Radiation Oncology (ASTRO), San Diego, CA, September 24-27, 2017
†Christoph Oehler and Michel Zimmermann contributed equally to this work.
[1]Department of Radiation Oncology, Kantonsspital Graubünden, Loëstrasse 170, 7000, Chur, Switzerland
Full list of author information is available at the end of the article

Background

Prostate cancer (PCa) patients diagnosed with biochemical recurrence and limited metastatic disease are conventionally treated with androgen deprivation therapy (ADT). Recently, stereotactic body radiation therapy (SBRT) has emerged as a promising approach for oligometastatic PCa recurrence. This strategy might have the potential to defer disease progression, thereby lengthening the time till initiation of hormonal therapy, and thus improving quality of life.

Results from a recent prospective phase II study (STOMP trial) suggest that metastasis-directed therapy (surgery or SBRT) of up to three extracranial metastases (any N1 or M1) benefited patients by postponing the start of ADT when compared to surveillance (median ADT-free survival of 21 months and 13 months, respectively) [1]. In a pilot phase I/II study (POPSTAR trial), SBRT delivered to 1–3 metastatic lesions (bone or LN) resulted in a 2-year ADT-free survival rate of 48% among 22 patients who did not have ADT at the time of SBRT [2]. Results from the promising ORIOLE phase II trial (52 patients randomized 2: 1 to SBRT or observation, combined with exhaustive translational research) are not expected before 2022 [3].

Retrospective series published are quite heterogeneous regarding the location of treated metastases (including various amounts of bone, nodal or visceral locations), the irradiated volume for patients with nodal disease (involved-nodes only, or associated to a prophylactic irradiation of the pelvic lymph drainage), and the initial radical PCa treatment (mixing radical prostatectomy (RP) ± radiotherapy (RT) with "RT only" or brachytherapy cases) [4].

The aim of this single-institution study was to investigate a homogenous population of exclusively ADT-naïve prostate cancer patients following RP ± salvage RT, presenting with one to three metachronous LN metastases on 18F-Choline PET/CT (CholPET/CT) and treated by SBRT. Endpoints of interest were biochemical response (BR), time to biochemical recurrence (TBR), and time interval between SBRT and ADT start (TADT).

Methods

Design and participants

This retrospective study obtained ethical approval. Patients provided written consent for SBRT treatment and for the use of their anonymized data for research purposes (ClinicalTrial.gov Identifier NCT03604211).

Inclusion criteria were as follows: histologically proven diagnosis of PCa; prior treatment with RP and pelvic lymphadenectomy (± salvage RT limited to the prostatic bed only), followed by a PSA relapse, defined by two consecutive rising PSA values > 0.2 µg/l [5]; maximum one to three N1 or M1a lesions (CholPET/CT positive) with a controlled primary tumor (CholPET/CT negative); WHO performance status of 0–1; no prior chemotherapy or ADT for PCa (castration-naïve patients).

Exclusion criteria included a primary treatment for PCa by RT or brachytherapy to achieve a more homogeneous patient cohort. PCa patients after RP experience actually a disturbed lymph drainage, with a high occurrence of aberrant LN spread [6], which has not been described after primary RT or brachytherapy, as far as we are aware of. Furthermore, primary RT for high-risk PCa is often combined with pelvic LN irradiation, which might lead to delivering non-ablative SBRT for nodal recurrences in the obturator and iliac basins, to respect the dose constraints for organs at risk. Similarly, patients having received salvage RT of the prostatic bed combined with pelvic nodal irradiation were excluded.

Further exclusion criteria were the occurrence of > 3 LN lesions, or bone (M1b) or visceral (M1c) metastases, or any symptomatic nodal lesion.

LN were considered as positive on CholPET/CT if either their uptake was markedly increased (higher than normal liver uptake) or if their uptake was moderately increased, and their size and shape did not indicate a clear benign LN. For our study, the reference diameter was based on the long-axis of positive LN; small-axis diameters were often not mentioned in nuclear medicine records. Measurements were performed on intravenous contrast enhanced CT images collected during each CholPET/CT examination.

PSA doubling-time (PSADT) before SBRT was calculated using the natural log of 2 divided by the slope of the linear regression line of the natural log of PSA against time (months) [7]; results were stratified according to three distinct PSADT categories: < 3, 3–6 and > 6 months.

During follow-up after SBRT, patients were reviewed clinically at approximately 3 to 6 month intervals by their urologist; PSA testing and imaging frequency was left up to the discretion of the physician in charge.

For patients experiencing radiological progression after SBRT, recurrence was considered as in-field, marginal or out-of-field, if it was located inside, at the border or outside the initial planning target volume (PTV).

ADT was started after SBRT for patients with radiological progression of baseline-detected soft-tissue lesions using the Response Evaluation Criteria in Solid Tumours [8], or detection of new bone or soft tissue metastases, as long as they were not amenable to further RT. PSA progression only was generally not an indication to start ADT.

SBRT treatment

All patients were treated with SBRT delivered by CyberKnife®. Patients were immobilized using a customized external vacuum-type cast (CIVCO Medical Solutions, Kalona, IO, USA) prior to their CT planning scan (without IV contrast), acquiring images of 1.5 mm slice thickness.

Dose and fractionation were dependent on whether the patient had received previous external beam RT and normal tissue tolerances within the area to be treated. The prescribed doses ranged between 30.0 Gy and 45.0 Gy in three fractions, and were defined by the treating radiation oncologist. The prescribed dose was unrelated to LN size and increased progressively during the study period with growing experience. Treatments were designed using Multiplan software (Accuray, version 2.0.5). The planning target volume (PTV) was generated with 2–4 mm margin around the gross tumor volume (GTV).

SBRT was delivered every other day, using a non-isocentric treatment technique. Patient movement was monitored using the CyberKnife® intrafractional image guidance solution using implanted fiducial markers and relevant corrections applied.

Endpoints

Endpoints of interest were biochemical response (BR), time to biochemical recurrence (TBR), and time interval from SBRT to ADT start (TADT).

PSA reduction in percent was calculated as follows: 100 x [PSA (ug/l) at SBRT- PSA (ug/l) at nadir post-SBRT/PSA (ug/l) at SBRT].

BR was defined as a reduction in PSA level by more than 50% of the baseline value, biochemical progression as a PSA increase ≥25% and ≥ 2μg/l if baseline PSA ≥ 2 μg/l, or a PSA increase ≥2μg/l if baseline PSA < 2 μg/l [9].

BR was also defined according to Jereczek criteria, with PSA cut-offs of + 10% (progression), – 10% (minor response) and – 50% (major response) [10].

TBR was defined as the time interval between SBRT until second consecutive PSA rise above reference PSA value. For patients responding to SBRT, the reference PSA was defined as the PSA nadir after SBRT. For patients not responding to SBRT, the reference PSA was the last PSA before SBRT (baseline PSA value).

TADT was defined as the time between SBRT and the start of palliative ADT or death of any cause.

Toxicity data were not evaluated; follow-up after SBRT was mostly performed by urologists, and toxicities not systematically assessed and reported.

Statistical analysis

Descriptive statistics were used to summarize patient characteristics; results are expressed as median ± interquartile range (IQR). BR was calculated based on the maximum percentage change in PSA from baseline; it is reported for each patient using a waterfall plot. Time to event endpoints were analysed using Kaplan-Meier method. Time intervals were calculated from SBRT start to the event of interest. Censoring was at the date of last clinical follow-up in those not known to be deceased. Potential prognostic factors including age, last PSA and PSA doubling-time before SBRT, radiation dose, largest size and number of LN treated, as well as pathology results dating back to the initial prostatectomy, salvage RT after RP or not, were examined using univariate proportional hazards regression for TADT and logistic regression for BR. The optimal cut-off point for LN size was calculated using the method proposed by Contal and O'Quigley [11]; it is based on the log rank test statistic, and allows to identify a cutpoint when the outcome of interest is measured as time to event. The differences in survival between the groups were compared by the log-rank test. Statistical analyses were performed with R version 3.2.3.

Results

Patients

Thirty-eight patients treated with SBRT for oligometastatic recurrence following primary treatment of localized PCa were identified over a five-year period (January 2010 to January 2015) and entered into study. Thirteen patients did not meet all our inclusion criteria and had to be excluded. Three cases did not get RP as primary treatment [brachytherapy ($n = 1$) and external beam RT ($n = 2$)]. Six cases received ADT before SBRT, and another four were lost to follow-up (international patients residing outside the country). Twenty-five patients were included in the analysis.

Initial findings at RP are shown in Table 1. According to d'Amico classification [12], seven (28%) patients had intermediate risk disease and 18 (72%) high risk disease. The median time interval between RP and nodal SBRT was 35 months (range: 8–157). Baseline characteristics at SBRT are summarized in Table 2. Two thirds ($N = 16$, 64%) of patients had only one positive LN on CholPET/CT, with a total of 36 LNs treated for 25 patients, one third ($N = 9$, 36%) of patients had 2–3 positive LN on CholPET/CT. Location and size of involved LN are provided in Table 2 and (Additional file 1: Table S1). Median follow-up after SBRT was 18 months (IQR: 14–22). Three patients received a second SBRT treatment: one patient with infield relapse (obturator LN) and two cases of out-of-field relapse (obturator LN = > internal iliac LN; common iliac LN = > para-aortal LN; one each). Time interval between both SBRT was 8, 13 and 14 months, respectively.

Outcomes

Biochemical response (BR)

Results are provided as a waterfall plot on a per-patient basis (Fig. 1). BR was observed in 13 patients (52%),

Table 1 Patient and tumor characteristics ($n = 25$ patients)

Characteristic	Value	
Initial treatment		
RP	10	40%
RP + salvage RT	15	60%
Pre-operative PSA (μg/l)[a]		
median (IQR)	9.1	(5.4–20.4)
mean (range)	12.7	(1.8–40.5)
Gleason score		
6	1	4%
7	13	52%
8	7	28%
9	4	16%
T stage		
pT2	11	44%
pT3	14	56%
ECE		
no	13	52%
yes	12	48%
SVI		
no	19	76%
yes	6	24%
SM		
negative	13	52%
positive	12	48%

[a] one data missing ($n = 24$)

while five patients (20%) experienced biochemical progression.

According to the response criteria from Jereczek et al., 17 patients (68%) experienced a PSA drop by at least 10%, 13 patients (52%) by more than 50%. On the other hand, PSA progressed by more than 10% in six patients (24%).

Time to biochemical recurrence (TBR)

Results from the univariate Cox regression analysis of the potentially prognostic factors on time between SBRT and second PSA rise are presented in (Additional file 1: Table S2). The risk of having a second PSA rise after SBRT decreased with the size of the largest LN, with a HR of 0.87 ([95% CI: 0.77–0.99]; $P = 0.030$). In our study, a LN size of 14 mm corresponded to the optimal cut-off, based on the Contal and O'Quigley method [13]. Median TBR was 10.8 months for patients with small LN, and 21.2 months for patients with large LN (P unadjusted = 0.009; P adjusted = 0.099). Kaplan-Meier curves of TBR stratified by LN size and number of LN are provided as Figs. 2 and 3.

Table 2 Patient and SBRT treatment characteristics ($n = 25$ patients)

Characteristics	Value	
Age at SBRT (years)		
median (IQR)	68	(62–72)
mean (range)	68	(52–81)
PSA at SBRT (ug/l)		
median (IQR)	3.53	(1.48–6.86)
mean (range)	3.49	(1.02–14.54)
PSADT		
< 3 months	5	20%
3–6 months	12	48%
> 6 months	8	32%
Number of lymph nodes at SBRT		
1	16	64%
2	7	28%
3	2	8%
LN localisation ($n = 36$)		
N1	33	92%
M1a	3	8%
Largest LN diameter (mm)[a]		
median (IQR)	10.5	(8.5–13.5)
mean (range)	12.8	(5–33)
SBRT data (Gy)		
total median dose (range)	36	(30–45)
median dose per fraction (range)	12	(10–15)
SBRT regimen		
10 Gy per 3 fractions	2	8%
11 Gy per 3 fractions	1	4%
12 Gy per 3 fractions	11	44%
13 Gy per 3 fractions	7	28%
15 Gy per 3 fractions	4	16%

[a] one data missing ($n = 35$)

Time to ADT

After a median follow-up of 18 months, 68% of patients remained free of any hormone therapy; ADT was started in 8/25 cases (32%) during the follow up period.

In a further analysis, we identified T3 stage (HR 9.34 [1.12–77.73] $P = 0.039$) and extra-prostatic extension at surgery (HR 10.29 [1.25–84.78] $P = 0.030$) as risk factors for a shorter TADT (Additional file 2: Figures S1 and S2). The influences of the Gleason score and PSA doubling-time on TADT were statistically not detectable in this small retrospective cohort ($P = 0.23$ and $P = 0.47$ respectively).

Discussion

To the best of our knowledge, this is one of the largest retrospective series on LN recurrence treated with

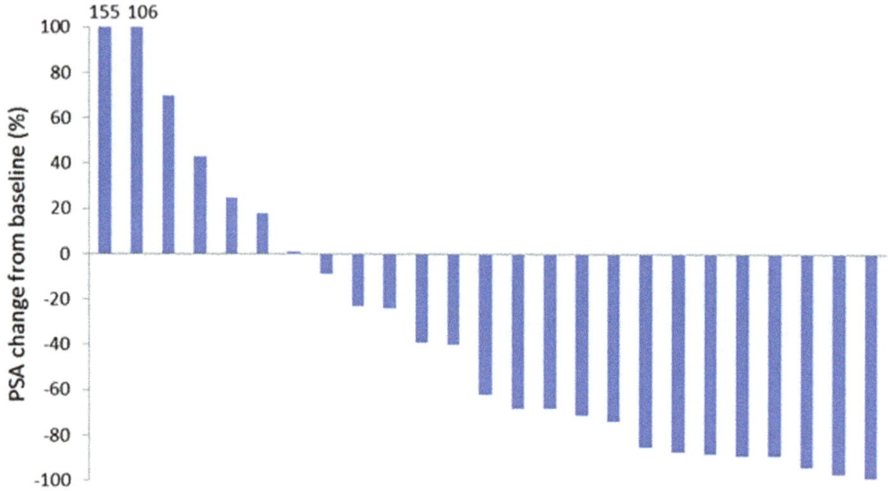

Fig. 1 Best biochemical response after SBRT

ablative SBRT exclusively in ADT-naïve prostate cancer patients. A biochemical response was observed in 52% of patients. After a median follow-up of 18 months, 68% patients were free of ADT, and only one of 36 treated LN (2.8%) required a second SBRT for in-field progression.

Jereczek-Fossa et al. recently reported on a cohort of 94 patients treated with salvage SBRT with a similar follow-up of 18.5 months [13]; initial treatment of prostate cancer was RP (42%), RP + RT (36%), RT alone (20%) and brachytherapy (2%), with or without ADT. In our series, PSA response, stabilization and progression after SBRT were observed in 68, 8 and 24% of cases, respectively. Our results replicate the 67, 16 and 18% reported by the colleagues from Milan, using similar biochemical response criteria. During the study period,

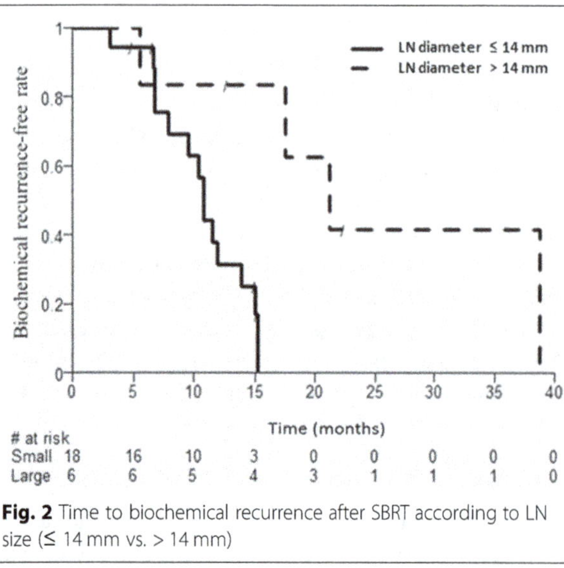

Fig. 2 Time to biochemical recurrence after SBRT according to LN size (≤ 14 mm vs. > 14 mm)

ADT was started in 32% of our patients and in 36% in Milan [13]. Interestingly, for those receiving ADT after SBRT during the study period, treatment could be deferred by at least 1 year in 63% of our cases but only in 38% by the Milan group. Potential explanations for a later ADT start in our institution might include differences in ADT prescription practices or in tumour biology (8% M1a LN against 39.5% in Milan), but might just reflect higher median dose prescriptions (3 × 12 Gy in our center versus 3 × 8 Gy in Milan), corresponding to a twice higher biological equivalent dose (BED) with an $\alpha/\beta = 2$ [14, 15] for prostate cancer (BED_2 of 252 Gy versus 120 Gy). The latter BED might not be ablative for all LN metastases, and would provide a reasonable explanation for the 10% rate of in-field progression observed by Jereczek-Fossa et al.

In prostate cancer, conventional imaging has very poor accuracy for identifying LN metastases. In a meta-analysis including 24 studies, sensitivity was 42% for CT and 39% for MRI, specificity 82% for both [16]. Integration of CholPET/CT into routine evaluation of PCa patients improved both staging accuracy and RT planning [17, 18]. The detection rate of CholPET/CT is higher in cases of high PSA velocity (> 5 µg/l/yr) and short PSA doubling time (< 2 mo or 3 mo). Detection rate falls to < 30% for PSA levels < 1 µg/l, but rises > 50% for PSA levels > 2 µg/l [19]. Kitajima et al. reported a 75% detection rate for a PSA level between 4 and 10 µg/l [20].

Prostate-specific membrane antigen (PSMA) PET was not available at the time of our study. PSMA PET outperforms CholPET/CT for the localization of disease sites at biochemical recurrence, particularly in small lymph nodes and at lower PSA levels (< 1 µg/l). [21]. Many PSMA PET positive lesions present actually without an anatomic correlation on CT or MRI, indicating

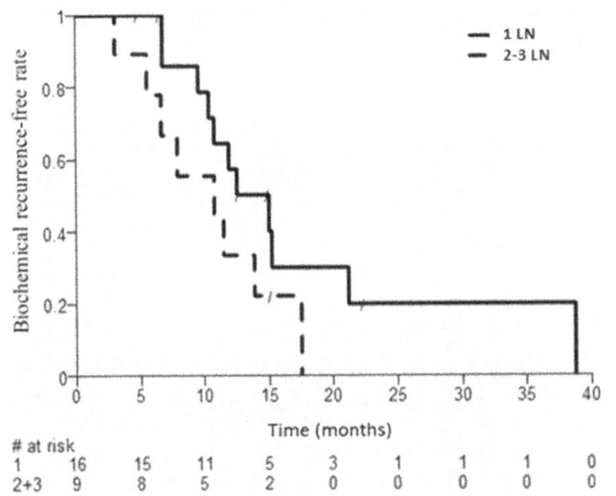

Fig. 3 Time to biochemical recurrence after SBRT according to LN number (1 vs. 2–3)

that focal treatment can be initiated at an early stage of metastatic disease [21].

It remains unclear if PSMA PET instead of CholPET/CT guided salvage treatment would have had a major impact on our results. PSA levels before SBRT were quite high in our series (median PSA: 3.53 μg/l); it is therefore likely that most positive LNs were correctly identified on CholPET/CT.

This elevated PSA before SBRT rises also the issue of delayed referral to CholPET/CT, with the advantage to better select patients with true oligo-recurrent disease for SBRT, but at the cost of exposing other patients to a higher risk of delayed treatment for more advanced progressive disease. This selection bias appears to discriminate elderly patients, as there are only two octogenerians in our series (8%). We hypothesize that 80+ year patients are mostly followed up with PSA and CT scans, and receive ADT instead of a metastasis-directed therapy at the time of nodal progression.

We found that salvage SBRT for isolated LN recurrent PCa provides a twice longer biochemical control (21.8 months vs. 10.8 months) when delivered to patients presenting with larger LN metastases (≥ 14 mm). On the other hand, the common clinico-pathological risk factors (T3, Gleason 8–10, PSA doubling time < 3 months) didn't lead to a shorter TBR (Additional file 1: Table S2). At first glance, such results appear counterintuitive, as one would expect larger LN to reflect a higher tumor burden and a more advanced stage of disease, leading to a shorter TBR. These patients with 1–3 LN macrometastases, despite high-risk features at the time of RP, exhibit a phenotype of slow lymphatic spreading, with only a few LN metastases growing up over time without developing multiple new lesions (true oligometastatic disease). Given the retrospective nature of the study design, we hypothesize that our data result from a selection bias, selecting tumors that didn't develop yet multiple mechanisms of immune evasion. Identifying the underlying gene expression pattern in such patients would allow in the future for a better selection of candidates to metastasis-directed SBRT, and for an earlier start of treatment (PSA < 1.0 μg/l and LN size < 1 cm). MicroRNA profiling shows substantial potential to be used as prognostic biomarker for individuals with oligometastatic prostate cancer [22–25].

The main strength of this study relies on quite restrictive inclusion criteria, leading to a series of 25 consecutive patients with a limited nodal recurrence (1–3 LN) after RP, in the absence of any prior or concomitant ADT. Regarding treatment, SBRT was always delivered at ablative doses (median dose: 36 Gy/ 3 fractions [range: 30–45 Gy]).

Our series has several limitations. The number of included patients was low, limiting the validity of subgroup analysis; observed results could have occurred merely by chance. Imaging and PSA levels during follow-up after SBRT were not obtained at predefined time points. We didn't stage our patients with PSMA-PET, which has been shown in multiple studies to be superior to CholPET/CT imaging in the setting of biochemical relapse [26]. Further drawbacks include the lack of confirmatory biopsy for PET-positive LN, the absence of radiological response assessment after SBRT, and the lack of a control group. Time to ADT might also have been subscriber biased due to the lack of predefined prescription criteria. Finally, our results might not apply to patients with nodal metastases occurring with concomitant local recurrence (prostate bed) and/or distant (bone) metastases, nor to patients with castrate-resistant prostate cancer presenting with oligo-progressive disease.

Last, for patients experiencing isolated metastatic LN recurrence after primary treatment, there are currently no consensus guidelines on which strategy to follow. Besides treating only positive LN with SBRT, which could be considered in one sense as "just targeting the tip of the iceberg", more comprehensive strategies might be applied as well, like salvage radiation of the whole pelvic lymph node basin combined with a simultaneous integrated boost (SIB) to PET-positive LNs, using either CholPET/CT [27] or PSMA PET/CT guided RT [28]. Extended salvage lymph node dissection (sLND) might be a valid option for selected patients, but remains technically challenging: sLND alone is usually not associated with a durable biochemical response; 50–80% of patients will receive some kind of adjuvant treatment right after sLND (ADT or RT) regardless post-operative PSA levels [29]. In an interesting retrospective analysis of 93 patients, adjuvant RT after sLND was shown to improve significantly the 5 year- relapse-free survival from 15.4%

in the surgery only group to 34.3% in the group with additional RT ($P = 0.0122$) [30]. Prospective randomized trials are warranted to confirm these encouraging results.

Conclusions

The present work underlines the possible role of ablative SBRT in the management of patients affected by LN oligo-recurrent disease. In ADT-naïve prostate cancer patients with 1–3 LN metastases after definitive RP, SBRT can offer a good control of asymptomatic disease. After a median follow-up of 18 months, 68% of patients remained free from ADT. Our study is the first to date attempting to define an optimal LN size threshold prior to SBRT. Additional studies are required before the results should be used in usual clinical settings.

Additional files

Additional file 1: Table S1. Lymph node localisation before SBRT ($n = 36$). **Table S2.** Univariable cox regression on time interval from SBRT to second PSA rise. (DOCX 16 kb)

Additional file 2: Figure S1. Time to ADT after SBRT according to initial T stage (pT2 vs. pT3). **Figure S2.** Time to ADT after SBRT according to initial presence/absence of ECE. (ZIP 106 kb)

Abbreviations

ADT: Androgen deprivation therapy; ECE: Extra-capsular extension; IQR: Interquartile range; LN: Lymph node; PSA: Prostate specific antigen; PSADT: PSA doubling time; RP: Radical prostatectomy; RT: Radiotherapy; SBRT: Stereotactic body radiation therapy; SM: Surgical margins; SVI: Seminal vesicles involvement

Acknowledgements

Not applicable.

Authors' contributions

Conception: CO, DZ, JC, US. Design: CO, MZ. Acquisition: CO. Analysis: CO, DZ, MZ, QL. Interpretation of data: CO, DZ, MZ, QL. Drafted the manuscript: CO, DZ, MZ, QL, LA, JC, MS, RS, RC, US. All authors read and approved the final manuscript.

Author details

[1]Department of Radiation Oncology, Kantonsspital Graubünden, Loëstrasse 170, 7000, Chur, Switzerland. [2]Center for Radiation Oncology, Hirslanden Klinik, Zürich, Switzerland. [3]Department of Urology, Kantonsspital Graubünden, Chur, Switzerland. [4]Division of Medical Oncology, Kantonsspital Graubünden, Chur, Switzerland. [5]Statistics Unit, SAKK Coordinating Center, Bern, Switzerland.

References

1. Ost P, Reynders D, Decaestecker K, Fonteyne V, Lumen N, De Bruycker A, et al. Surveillance or metastasis-directed therapy for Oligometastatic prostate Cancer recurrence: a prospective, randomized, multicenter phase II trial. J Clin Oncol. 2018;36:446–53. https://doi.org/10.1200/JCO.2017.75.4853.
2. Siva S, Bressel M, Murphy DG, Shaw M, Chander S, Violet J, et al. Stereotactic Ablative Body Radiotherapy (SABR) for Oligometastatic Prostate Cancer: A Prospective Clinical Trial. Eur Urol. 2018;74(4):455–62. https://doi.org/10.1016/j.eururo.2018.06.004.
3. Radwan N, Phillips R, Ross A, Rowe SP, Gorin MA, Antonarakis ES, et al. A phase II randomized trial of Observation versus stereotactic ablative Radiation for OLigometastatic prostate CancEr (ORIOLE). BMC Cancer. 2017; 17(1):453. https://doi.org/10.1186/s12885-017-3455-6.
4. Ost P, Bossi A, Decaestecker K, De Meerleer G, Giannarini G, Karnes RJ, et al. Metastasis-directed therapy of regional and distant recurrences after curative treatment of prostate cancer: a systematic review of the literature. Eur Urol. 2015;67:852–63. https://doi.org/10.1016/j.eururo.2014.09.004.
5. Amling CL, Bergstralh EJ, Blute ML, Slezak JM, Zincke H. Defining prostate specific antigen progression after radical prostatectomy: what is the most appropriate cut point? J Urol. 2001;165:1146–51.
6. Meijer HJ, van Lin EN, Debats OA, Witjes JA, Span PN, Kaanders JH, et al. High occurrence of aberrant lymph node spread on magnetic resonance lymphography in prostate cancer patients with a biochemical recurrence after radical prostatectomy. Int J Radiat Oncol Biol Phys. 2012;82(4):1405–10. https://doi.org/10.1016/j.ijrobp.2011.04.054.
7. Pound CR, Partin AW, Eisenberger MA, Chan DW, Pearson JD, Walsh PC. Natural history of progression after PSA elevation following radical prostatectomy. JAMA. 1999;281:1591–7.
8. Eisenhauer EA, Therasse P, Bogaerts J, Schwartz LH, Sargent D, Ford R, et al. New response evaluation criteria in solid tumours: revised RECIST guideline (version 1.1). EJC. 2009;45:228–47. https://doi.org/10.1016/j.ejca.2008.10.026.
9. Scher HI, Morris MJ, Stadler WM, Higano C, Basch E, Fizazi K, et al. Trial design and objectives for castration-resistant prostate Cancer: updated recommendations from the prostate Cancer clinical trials working group 3. J Clin Oncol. 2016;34:1402–18. https://doi.org/10.1200/JCO.2015.64.2702.
10. Jereczek-Fossa BA, Beltramo G, Fariselli L, Fodor C, Santoro L, Vavassori A, et al. Robotic image-guided stereotactic radiotherapy, for isolated recurrent primary, lymph node or metastatic prostate cancer. Int J Radiat Oncol Biol Phys. 2012;82:889–97. https://doi.org/10.1016/j.ijrobp.2010.11.031.
11. Contal C, O'Quigley J. An application of changepoint methods in studying the effect of age on survival in breast cancer. Comput Stat Data Anal. 1999; 30:253–70.
12. D'Amico AV, Whittington R, Malkowicz SB, Schultz D, Blank K, Broderick GA, et al. Biochemical outcome after radical prostatectomy, external beam radiation therapy, or interstitial radiation therapy for clinically localized prostate cancer. JAMA. 1998;280:969–74.
13. Jereczek-Fossa BA, Fanetti G, Fodor C, Ciardo D, Santoro L, Francia CM, et al. Salvage stereotactic body radiotherapy for isolated lymph node recurrent prostate cancer: single institution series of 94 consecutive patients and 124 lymph nodes. Clin Genitourin Cancer. 2017;15:e623–32. https://doi.org/10.1016/j.clgc.2017.01.004.
14. Vogelius IR, Bentzen SM. Meta-analysis of the alpha/beta ratio for prostate cancer in the presence of an overall time factor: bad news, good news, or no news? Int J Radiat Oncol Biol Phys. 2013;85(1):89–94. https://doi.org/10.1016/j.ijrobp.2012.03.004.
15. Miralbell R, Roberts SA, Zubizarreta E, Hendry JH. Dose-fractionation sensitivity of prostate cancer deduced from radiotherapy outcomes of 5,969 patients in seven international institutional datasets: $\alpha/\beta = 1.4$ (0.9-2.2) Gy. Int J Radiat Oncol Biol Phys. 2012;82(1):e17–24. https://doi.org/10.1016/j.ijrobp.2010.10.075.
16. Hövels AM, Heesakkers RA, Adang EM, Jager GJ, Strum S, Hoogeveen YL, et al. The diagnostic accuracy of CT and MRI in the staging of pelvic lymph nodes in patients with prostate cancer: a meta-analysis. Clin Radiol. 2008;63: 387–95. https://doi.org/10.1016/j.crad.2007.05.022.
17. Nair R, Lamb BW, Geurts N, Alghazo O, Lam W, Lawrentschuk N, et al. The role of local therapy for Oligometastatic prostate Cancer: Should We Expect a Cure? Urol Clin North Am. 2017;44:623–63. https://doi.org/10.1016/j.ucl.2017.07.013.
18. No authors listed. FDA approves 11C-choline for PET in prostate cancer. J Nucl Med. 2012;53:11N.
19. Evangelista L, Briganti A, Fanti S, Joniau S, Reske S, Schiavina R, et al. New clinical indications for (18) F/(11) C-choline, new tracers for positron emission tomography and a promising hybrid device for prostate cancer staging: a systematic review of the literature. Eur Urol. 2016;70:161–75. https://doi.org/10.1016/j.eururo.2016.01.029.
20. Kitajima K, Murphy RC, Nathan MA, Froemming AT, Hagen CE, Takahashi N, et al. Detection of recurrent prostate cancer after radical prostatectomy: comparison of 11C-choline PET/CT with pelvic multiparametric MR imaging with endorectal coil. J Nucl Med. 2014;55:223–32. https://doi.org/10.2967/jnumed.113.123018.

21. Bailey J, Piert M. Performance of 68Ga-PSMA PET/CT for prostate Cancer Management at Initial Staging and Time of biochemical recurrence. Curr Urol Rep. 2017;18:84. https://doi.org/10.1007/s11934-017-0736-1
22. Ni J, Bucci J, Chang L, Malouf D, Graham P, Li Y. Targeting microRNAs in prostate cancer radiotherapy. Theranostics. 2017;7:3243–59. https://doi.org/10.7150/thno.19934.
23. Pashaei E, Pashaei E, Ahmady M, Ozen M, Aydin N. Meta-analysis of miRNAexpression profiles for prostate cancer recurrence following radical prostatectomy. PLoS One. 2017;12:e0179543. https://doi.org/10.1371/journal.pone.0179543.
24. Kristensen H, Thomsen AR, Haldrup C, Dyrskjøt L, Høyer S, Borre M, et al. Novel diagnostic and prognostic classifiers for prostate cancer identified by genome-wide microRNA profiling. Oncotarget. 2016;7:30760–71. https://doi.org/10.18632/oncotarget.8953.
25. Bell EH, Kirste S, Fleming JL, Stegmaier P, Drendel V, Mo X, et al. A novel miRNA-based predictive model for biochemical failure following post-prostatectomy salvage radiation therapy. PLoS One. 2015;10:e0118745. https://doi.org/10.1371/journal.pone.0118745.
26. Lenzo NP, Meyrick D, Turner JH. Review of Gallium-68 PSMA PET/CT Imaging in the Management of Prostate Cancer. Diagnostics (Basel). 2018; 8(1). https://doi.org/10.3390/diagnostics8010016.
27. Supiot S, Rio E, Pacteau V, Mauboussin MH, Campion L, Pein F. OLIGOPELVIS - GETUG P07: a multicentre phase II trial of combined salvage radiotherapy and hormone therapy in oligometastatic pelvic node relapses of prostate cancer. BMC Cancer. 2015. https://doi.org/10.1186/s12885-015-1579-0.
28. Schmidt-Hegemann NS, Stief C, Kim TH, Eze C, Kirste S, Strouthos I, et al. Outcome after PSMA PET/CT based salvage radiotherapy in patients with biochemical recurrence after radical prostatectomy: a bi-institutional retrospective analysis. J Nucl Med. 2018. https://doi.org/10.2967/jnumed.118.212563.
29. Brassetti A, Proietti F, Pansadoro V. Oligometastatic prostate cancer and salvage lymph node dissection: systematic review. Minerva Chir. 2019;74(1): 97–106. https://doi.org/10.23736/S0026-4733.18.07796-9.
30. Rischke HC, Schultze-Seemann W, Wieser G, Krönig M, Drendel V, Stegmaier P, et al. Adjuvant radiotherapy after salvage lymph node dissection because of nodal relapse of prostate cancer versus salvage lymph node dissection only. Strahlenther Onkol. 2015;191(4):310–20. https://doi.org/10.1007/s00066-014-0763-5.

10

A case report of endorectal displacement of a right ureteral stent following radiochemotherapy and Bevacizumab

Alessio Tognarelli[1*], Lorenzo Faggioni[2], Francesca Manassero[1], Angiolo Gadducci[3] and Cesare Selli[1]

Abstract

Background: The angiogenesis inhibitor monoclonal antibody Bevacizumab is presently the standard treatment for numerous neoplasms but particular toxicities are emerging, such as hypertension, haemorrhage, thromboembolism, gastrointestinal perforation, fistulae, and delayed wound healing. The addition of Bevacizumab to radio and chemotherapy has improved the overall survival rate in patients with metastatic, persistent or recurrent cervical carcinoma. However an increased risk of enteric or urinary fistula formation has been documented, related to hypoxia which is induced by the inhibition of angiogenesis. Moreover, previous pelvic surgery, repeated ureteral stenting and radiation are additional risk factors.

Case presentation: We describe the remarkable case of a right ureteral stent displacement inside the rectum lumen in a patient treated with Bevacizumab for pelvic recurrence of cervical cancer. The patient was referred to our Urology Department with urinary sepsis and bilateral hydronephrosis. Right ureteral stent substitution was planned; at cystoscopy the distal loop of the stent was not visualized inside the bladder. The presence of the distal loop of the right ureteral inside the rectum was clearly demonstrated with a CT scan.

Conclusions: Since Bevacizumab is increasingly used in the treatment of gynaecological neoplasms and indwelling ureteral stents are often required to treat or prevent ureteral compressions, similar cases are likely to be diagnosed and this complication should be considered in the management of advanced pelvic cancers.

Keywords: Ureteral stent complications, Angiogenesis inhibitors, CT scan, Urinary fistula

Background

The association of monoclonal antibodies causing angiogenesis inhibition, like Bevacizumab, to radio and chemotherapy is known to increase the incidence of fistulae [1]. In particular, the final analysis of a large randomized prospective trial on the use of Bevacizumab in women with advanced cancer of the cervix, demonstrated an advantage in the overall survival rate compared to chemotherapy alone (16.8 vs 13.3 months) but also an increased risk of fistula formation (15% vs 1%) [2]. Of note, all the women with fistulae had previously been irradiated and their history of smoking was an associated risk factor. The fistulae involved the genitourinary tract in 7% of cases and the gastrointestinal [tract] in 8%.

Bevacizumab is, at present, the standard treatment for numerous neoplasms, and particular toxicities are emerging which may cause major morbidity and even mortality [3]. Ischemia and an impaired function of nitrous oxide, prostacyclins and platelets due to VEGF inhibition are the likely causes of increased fistula formation. Additional risk factors for fistulae involving the urinary tract are represented by previous pelvic surgery, repeated ureteral stenting and mostly [do you mean 'above all'/ 'most of all'?] radiation, due to its additional toxicity on microvasculature. Moreover, the positioning of ureteral stents is often required in advanced pelvic cancer to prevent or treat hydroureteronephrosis.

Herein, we report the case of a female patient with a diagnosis of cervical cancer recurrence treated with Bevacizumab, who was referred to our Urology Unit for

* Correspondence: alessio.tognarelli@gmail.com
[1]Department of Translational Research and New Technologies in Medicine and Surgery, Sections of Urology, University of Pisa, via Paradisa 2, 56126 Pisa, Italy
Full list of author information is available at the end of the article

hydronephrosis and sepsis; the patient had an indwelling right ureteral stent, whose distal loop was found dislocated in the rectal lumen at CT scan.

Case presentation

A 40-year-old woman was referred to our Urology Department with a diagnosis of urinary sepsis and bilateral hydronephrosis; radical hysterectomy, bilateral salpingectomy with ovarian preservation as well as pelvic and para-aortic lymphadenectomy for squamous cell carcinoma of the cervix had been performed 8 years earlier. The patient received adjuvant concurrent cisplatin-based chemo radiotherapy up to a total dose of 50.4 Gy; next she underwent periodical surveillance examinations which resulted negative for long term. Twenty months earlier a CT scan revealed a right-sided pelvic recurrence involving the right ureter with concurrent hydronephrosis; treatment of the recurrence required 3 further cycles of Cisplatin, Paclitaxel and Bevacizumab, obtaining a partial response at 18F-FDG PET/CT, followed by additional cycles of Bevacizumab every 3 weeks as maintenance treatment. A right ureteral stent was placed with the retrograde cystoscopic approach at the time of recurrence diagnosis to treat the associated hydronephrosis and had already been substituted twice using the same approach without problems employing hydrophilic long-permanence stents.

At time of the admission, a urinary tract infection sustained by Enterococcus was under treatment with Linezolid; abdominal sonography revealed bilateral hydronephrosis, with the presence of the curled upper extremity of the stent inside the right kidney collecting system, but the lower extremity was not detected in the bladder. Substitution of the right ureteral stent was planned to treat the sepsis.

At cystoscopy the distal end of the stent was not visible inside the bladder, while a fistula orifice covered with fibrin was evident on the right side of the bladder trigone, so the planned procedure was suspended.

A 64-detector row multiphase CT examination of the abdomen and pelvis was performed, showing a cross-over course of the ureteral stent from the right side to the left at the level of the sacrum, which was more evident with 3D rendering (Fig. 1), presence of gas inside the right pyelocalyceal system, along the side of the upper coil of the stent (Fig. 2) with displacement of the distal third of the stent and its lower loop inside the rectum, and right-sided pelvic tumor recurrence (Fig. 3). A delayed scan revealed the presence of iodinated contrast material inside the rectal lumen, consistent with urinary fistulization. Subsequent treatment consisted in bilateral percutaneous nephrostomy in the prone position to relieve hydronephrosis and digital extraction of the stent from the rectal ampulla; an indwelling bladder catheter was placed. Two days later a left excluding colostomy was performed.

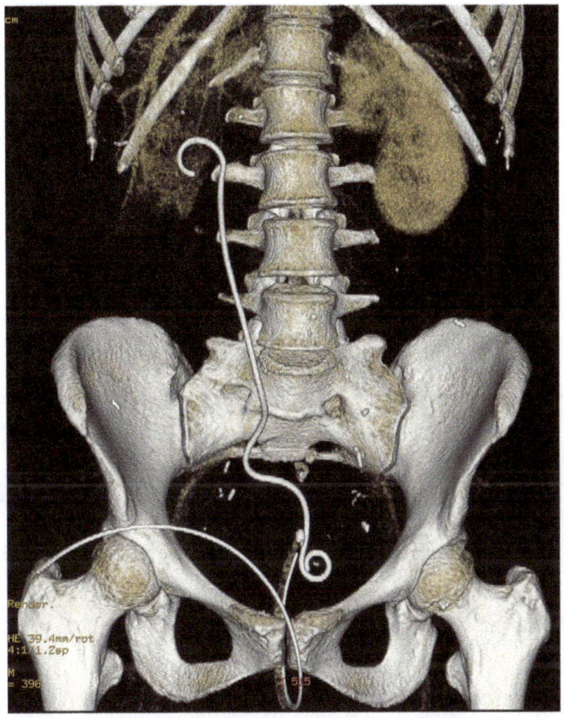

Fig. 1 3D rendering of the CT scan showing a cross-over course of the right ureteral stent at the level of mid-sacrum, while the stent distal coil is placed on the left side of the midline, defined by the presence of the bladder catheter

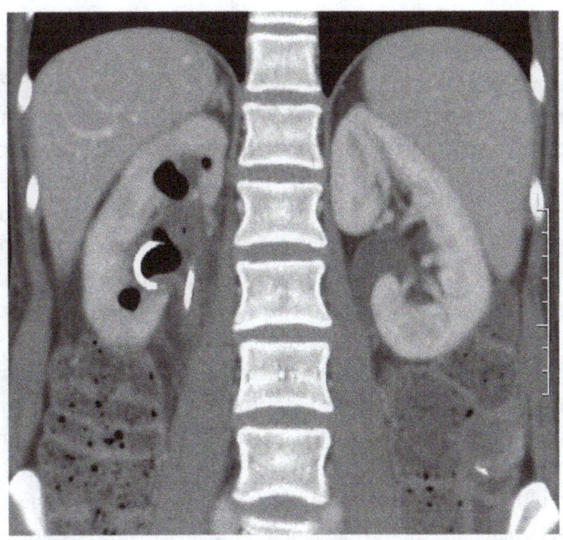

Fig. 2 Coronal section of the CT scan in a late-venous phase revealing presence of gas inside the right pyelo-calyceal system and the upper coil of the double J stent

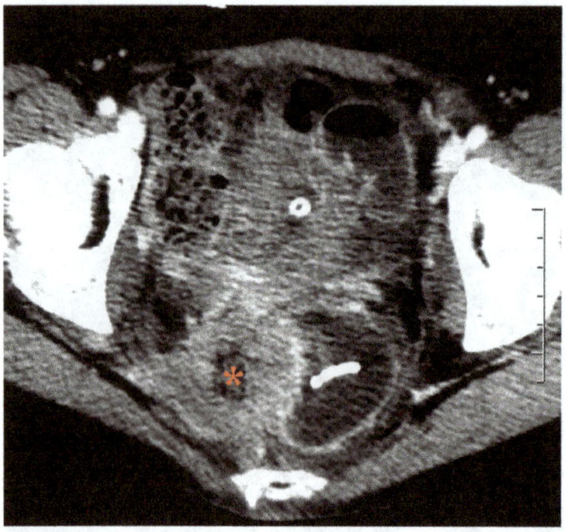

Fig. 3 Axial section of the CT scan in a venous phase demonstrating a right sided pelvic tumor recurrence with a partial central necrosis. The distal coil of the stent inside the rectal lumen and the bladder catheter are also visible

Discussion and conclusions

The present case represents, to the best of our knowledge, the first documentation with imaging techniques of the migration of a double J ureteral stent to the rectal lumen through tumor necrosis after treatment with Bevacizumab.

In the only other case of double J ureteral stent displacement inside the rectum that we are aware of, the diagnosis was made by means of colonoscopy of a woman who had been treated with radiotherapy and previous colostomy for pelvic recurrence of cervical cancer and presented with rectal bleeding [4]. Bilateral ureteral stents had been positioned 4 months earlier to relieve hydronephrosis.

Since indwelling ureteral stents are increasingly used in the management of patients with advanced gynaecological cancers where the use of Bevacizumab has become standard therapy, it is not unlikely that similar cases will be diagnosed in the future. As in our case, conventional radiology used during standard endourologic procedures is of limited help in identifying the endorectal displacement of the distal end of a double J ureteral stent, at least in the antero-posterior view. Similarly, sonography may fail to identify the absence of the distal extremity of the stent inside the bladder when it is empty or when a urinary catheter is in place. On the contrary, a CT scan provides an optimal demonstration of stent displacement and associated pelvic lesions, and gives important clues for further treatment planning. More generally, a multiphase contrast-enhanced CT allows a comprehensive assessment of the urinary tract, presence and extent of disease recurrence, and potential treatment-related complications (such as urinary fistulae) with a fast, one-stop examination. As known, the now widespread availability of CT scanners with 64 or more detector rows allows a routine acquisition of images with submillimeter spatial resolution and voxel isotropy, enabling high quality 2D and 3D image processing that yields an accurate, realistic depiction of all relevant structures under investigation [5]. Furthermore, the adoption of iterative reconstruction algorithms on modern multidetector CT equipment can significantly reduce patient exposure to ionizing radiation while maintaining the diagnostic image quality [6]. It is also worth mentioning that, in addition to mere morphological data, more advanced technological implementations of modern multidetector CT imaging (including CT perfusion and dual energy CT) and emerging applications such as CT texture analysis in oncology can provide functional information about cancer status that could help predict an early response to antiangiogenic agents and the overall patient outcome [7]. In light of this and given the increased use of Bevacizumab for the treatment of several neoplastic diseases, both clinicians and radiologists should be aware of the potential complications related to Bevacizumab treatment and so be prepared to harness the great potential of a multidetector CT to reach an accurate diagnosis, therefore possibly leading to better patient care.

Fistulization between the lower urinary tract and the rectum in the present case was, in our opinion, related to shrinkage and necrosis of the pelvic recurrence caused by angiogenesis inhibitors, which also increased wall fragility of the pelvic organs.

In order to mitigate the risk of fistulization the Urologists should try to monitor and treat concomitant urinary tract infections, use hydrophilic stents of low gauge and avoid traumatic manoeuvres during stent substitution. Advances in stent materials, such as antibacterial coating, are likely to reduce the risk of fistulization [8], while the use of metallic stents in malignant ureteral obstruction has proven to be cost-effective [9], but their increased stiffness potentially increases the risk of tissue damage.

Abbreviations

^{18}F-FDG PET/CT: fluorodeoxyglucose positron emission tomography / CT computed tomography; CT: Computed Tomography; Gy: Gray; VEGF: Vascular Endothelial Growth Factor

Acknowledgements

Not applicable.

Authors' contributions

AT: contributions to conception and design and data acquisition. LF: contributions to conception and design. FM: contributions to patient's treatment and data acquisition. AG: contributions to patient's treatment and design. CS: contributions to manuscript drafting and revising. All authors have read and approved the manuscript.

Author details
[1]Department of Translational Research and New Technologies in Medicine and Surgery, Sections of Urology, University of Pisa, via Paradisa 2, 56126 Pisa, Italy. [2]Diagnostic and Interventional Radiology, University of Pisa, Pisa, Italy. [3]Department of Clinical and Experimental Medicine, Section of Gynecologic Oncology, University of Pisa, Pisa, Italy.

References

1. Sturdza A, Hofmann S, Kranawetter, Polterauer S, Grimm C, Krainer M, Kirisitis C, Potter R, Reinthaller A, Schwameis R. Increased genitourinary fistula rate after Bevacizumab in recurrent cervical cancer patients initially treated with definitive radiochemotherapy and image-guided adaptive brachitherapy. Strahlenther Onkol. 2017;193:1056–65. https://doi.org/10.1007/s00066-017-1178-x.
2. Tewari KS, Sill MW, Penson RT, Huang H, Ramondetta LM, Landrum LM, Oaknin A, Reid TJ, Leitao MM, Michael HE, PJ DS, Copeland LJ, Creasman WT, Stehman FB, Brady MF, Burger RA, Thigpen JT, Birrer MJ, Waggoner SE, Moore DH, Look KY, Koh WJ, Monk BJ. Bevacizumab for advanced cervical cancer: final overall survival and adverse event analysis of a randomised, controlled, open-label, phase 3 trial (Gynaecologic Oncology Group 240). Lancet. 2017;390:1654–63. https://doi.org/10.1016/S0140-6736(17)31607-0.
3. Brandes AA, Bartolotti M, Tosoni A, Poggi R, Franceschi E. Practical management of Bevacizumab-related toxicities in glioblastoma. Oncologist. 2015;20:166–75. https://doi.org/10.1634/theoncologist.2014-0330.
4. Billoud E, Savoye G, Hervè S, Ramirez S, Lerebours E. Double J ureteral stent as an unusual endoscopic finding in a patient with rectal bleeding. Gastrointest Endosc. 2008;68:1239–40. https://doi.org/10.1016/j.gie.2008.02.084.
5. Dalrymple NC, Prasad SR, El-Merhi FM, Chintapalli KN. Price of isotropy in multidetector CT. Radiographics. 2007;27(1):49–62. https://doi.org/10.1148/rg.271065037.
6. Willemink MJ, Noël PB. The evolution of image reconstruction for CT-from filtered back projection to artificial intelligence. Eur Radiol. 2019;29(5):2185–95. https://doi.org/10.1007/s00330-018-5810-7.
7. García-Figueiras R, Goh VJ, Padhani AR, Baleato-González S, Garrido M, León L, Gómez-Caamaño A. CT perfusion in oncologic imaging: a useful tool? AJR Am J Roentgenol. 2013;200(1):8–19. https://doi.org/10.2214/AJR.11.8476.
8. Szell T, Dressler FF, Goelz H, Bluemel B, Miernik A, Brandstetter T, Scherag F, Schoeb DS. In vitro effects of a novel coating agent on bacterial biofilm development on ureteral stents. J Endourol. 2019;33:225–31. https://doi.org/10.1089/end.2018.0616.
9. Taylor ER, Benson AD, Schwartz BF. Cost analysis of metallic ureteral stents with 12 months of follow-up. J Endourol. 2012;26:917–21. https://doi.org/10.1089/end.2011.0481.

11

Application of hyaluronic acid/carboxymethyl cellulose membrane for early continence after nerve-sparing robot-assisted radical prostatectomy

Nobuyuki Hinata[1,2*], Yukari Bando[1], Koji Chiba[1], Junya Furukawa[1], Kenichi Harada[1], Takeshi Ishimura[1], Yuzo Nakano[1] and Masato Fujisawa[1]

Abstract

Background: To assess whether application of a hyaluronic acid-carboxymethyl cellulose membrane (HA/CMC) to the prostate bed and neurovascular plate facilitated early return of continence after nerve-sparing robot-assisted radical prostatectomy (RARP).

Methods: The subjects were 183 consecutive patients with organ-confined prostate cancer who underwent unilateral or bilateral nerve-sparing RARP. After vesicourethral anastomosis, HA/CMC was placed to cover Denonvilliers' fascia (behind the anastomotic suture) and the preserved neurovascular plate. The time until complete continence after RARP and perioperative complications were compared between patients with or without HA/CMC.

Results: HA/CMC was applied in 13/46 patients (28.3%) receiving bilateral nerve-sparing surgery and 40/137 patients (29.2%) receiving unilateral nerve-sparing surgery. After bilateral nerve-sparing RARP, the median time until continence was significantly shorter in patients with HA/CMC than in those without HA/CMC (3.2 vs. 9.3 months, respectively, $p < 0.01$). After unilateral nerve-sparing RARP, the median time until continence was also significantly shorter in patients with HA/CMC than in those without HA/CMC (3.2 vs. 12.0 months, respectively, $p < 0.01$). Multivariate Cox proportional hazards regression analysis showed that an age < 70 years (hazard ratio [HR]: 1.74, 95% confidence interval [CI]: 1.12–2.80), institutional caseload > 200, (HR: 1.64, 95%CI: 1.10–2.47), and use of HA/CMC (HR: 1.84, 95%CI: 1.22–2.76) were independent predictors of early postoperative continence. Complication rates, including urinary leakage, did not differ significantly between patients with or without HA/CMC.

Conclusion: Application of HA/CMC to the prostate bed and neurovascular plate resulted in significantly faster postoperative return of continence after both unilateral and bilateral nerve-sparing RARP.

Keywords: Prostatectomy, Surgical procedures, robotic, Sodium hyaluronate, carboxycellulose

Background

In men who undergo radical prostatectomy, urinary incontinence is one of the most unwanted postoperative complications [1], and it is well known to have multiple causes [2]. Some studies have shown that fibrosis of periurethral tissue is a risk factor for postoperative incontinence after radical prostatectomy [3, 4].

Elasticity is critical to the function of organs that undergo repeated expansion and contraction [5], and loss of elasticity due to elastic fiber damage is a major contributor to degeneration of connective tissue [6]. Hyaluronic acid (HA) is an important component of the extracellular matrix that coexists with elastic fibers and cooperates functionally with these fibers in various organs/tissues of the human body [7, 8]. HA can increase the retention of water around dehydrated elastic fibers,

* Correspondence: hinata@med.kobe-u.ac.jp
[1]Department of Urology, Kobe University Graduate School of Medicine, 7-5-1 Kusunoki-cho Chuo-ku, Kobe 650-0017, Japan
[2]Training Center for Advanced Surgery and Endoscopy, Kobe University School of Medicine, Kobe, Japan

and hydration is enhanced by self-aggregation of HA [9], leading to further accumulation of water near elastic fibers. This improves elastic fiber recoil by increasing the availability of water molecules for hydrophobic groups in the elastin polypeptide chains. These chains become more disordered with increased hydration, allowing them to store more elastic potential energy during distention [10, 11]. We previously demonstrated the coexistence of elastic fibers and HA in the urethral submucosa and smooth muscle sphincter in male human cadavers, and we also reported that HA is distributed throughout the periurethral nerves [12].

Application of a hyaluronic acid/carboxycellulose membrane (HA/CMC) has been used to prevent postoperative visceral adhesions resulting from inflammation and fibrosis [13]. Elastic fibers and HA coexist in the smooth and striated urethral sphincter muscles, which could be a target for prevention and treatment of urethral sphincter failure. Focusing on the efficacy of HA/CMC for preventing postoperative fibrosis and scarring, we hypothesized that application of HA/CMC could improve postoperative continence after radical prostatectomy. Accordingly, the aim of the present study was to investigate whether intraoperative application of HA/CMC to the prostatic bed could maintain the elasticity of periurethral connective tissue and preserve nerves after surgical invasion, thus facilitating postoperative return of continence after radical prostatectomy.

Methods

Use of an HA/CMC adhesion barrier for prevention of adhesions during abdominopelvic surgery is approved by the US Food and Drug Administration. After receiving approval from our institutional review board (approval No.170108), we conducted a retrospective study by reviewing the Kobe University Hospital database between October 2012 and June 2015. The study population was a cohort of 183 consecutive patients with a diagnosis of organ-confined prostate cancer (clinical T1c-2N0M0) who underwent robot-assisted radical prostatectomy (RARP) using unilateral or bilateral nerve-sparing techniques. Nerve-sparing surgery was defined as use of intrafascial or interfascial nerve-sparing techniques, as described previously [14]. Seprafilm® (Genzyme Corporation, Cambridge, MA) was used as HA/CMC in the present study (Fig. 1). HA/CMC turns into a gel within 24–48 h after placement and stays in place for up to 7 days. By day 7, HA/CMC is resorbed and it is excreted from the body by day 28 [15]. After the posterior reconstruction ("Rocco" stitch) [16], 6.35 cm × 7.35 cm sized HA/CMC was placed to cover Denonvilliers' fascia behind the anastomotic suture and to cover the preserved neurovascular plate. Then the vesicourethral anastomosis was performed. After the vesicourethral anastomosis, HA/CMC was placed on the ventral side of the anastomosis. The 183 patients were divided into three groups based on their treatment during the study period, since the first 42 patients underwent RARP without HA/CMC, the subsequent 53 patients underwent RARP with HA/CMC, and the final 42 patients received RARP without HA/CMC.

The four surgeons who carried out RARP in this series had all performed more than 40 RARP procedures before the study period. The nerve-sparing technique was applied if the tumor was not located ipsilaterally in the prostate on MRI. We excluded patients who had a history of urinary retention or preoperative incontinence. Demographic information was collected, including the age, body mass index, Charlson comorbidity index, pretreatment prostate specific antigen (PSA), prostate volume, hospital patient number, and clinical stage at enrollment. Perioperative and oncological outcomes were also recorded, including the console time, estimated blood loss, use of HA/CMC, perioperative complications categorized by the Clavien-Dindo classification, final pathologic diagnosis, and biochemical recurrence.

The urethral catheter was routinely removed on postoperative day 7. Continence was defined as freedom from pads and the date when each patient achieved pad-free status was determined by interview. Expanded Prostate Cancer Index Composite (EPIC) questionnaires were mailed to the patients every 3 months postoperatively. Biochemical recurrence was defined as a serum PSA level > 0.2 ng/ml on two separate occasions with an interval of at least 6 weeks.

Statistical analysis

The clinical and pathological descriptive data are presented as percentages, while continuous variables are presented as the median and interquartile range (IQR). Comparison of categorical valuables was performed by the unpaired t-test or Pearson's chi-square test, as appropriate.

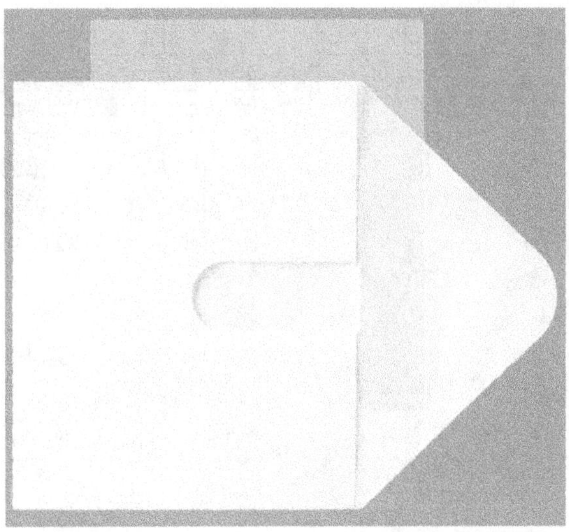

Fig. 1 A hyaluronic acid/carboxycellulose membrane (HA/CMC) used in the present study. The length of the membrane was 6.35 cm and the width was 7.35 cm

The Kaplan-Meier method was used to estimate the continence rate and curves were compared by employing the log-rank test. Cox proportional hazards regression analysis was performed to assess the prognostic significance of target covariates. All statistical analyses were done with JMP software (version 13.0; SAS Institute, Cary, NC, USA), and $P < 0.05$ was taken to indicate statistical significance.

Results

Among the 183 consecutive patients who underwent nerve-sparing RARP, none of them were excluded due to a history of urinary retention or incontinence. Consequently, all 183 patients were assessed in this study, including 46 patients who underwent bilateral nerve-sparing surgery and 137 patients who received unilateral nerve-sparing surgery. HA/CMC was used in 13/46 patients (28.3%) undergoing bilateral nerve-sparing RARP and 40/137 patients (29.2%) receiving unilateral nerve-sparing RARP.

The demographic and clinical characteristics of the bilateral and unilateral nerve-sparing RARP groups are shown in Table 1. In both groups, there were no statistically significant differences with respect to age, pretreatment PSA, prostate volume, clinical stage, Gleason score at prostate biopsy, Charlson comorbidity index, institutional caseload at surgery, and follow-up period between the patients with or without HA/CMC. Table 2 summarizes the perioperative, histological, and oncological outcomes. In both the bilateral nerve-sparing and unilateral nerve-sparing RARP groups, the operating time and complication rate did not differ significantly between patients with and without HA/CMC. There was also no significant difference of HA/CMC use between the unilateral and bilateral nerve-sparing RARP groups. Moreover, the final pathological and oncological outcomes showed no significant differences between patients with and without HA/CMC in both groups.

Among the 46 patients who received bilateral nerve-sparing RARP, the median time to achieve continence was significantly shorter in patients with HA/CMC than in those without HA/CMC (3.2 months vs. 9.3 months, respectively, $p < 0.01$) (Fig. 2a). Among the 137 patients who had unilateral nerve-sparing RARP, the median time to continence was also significantly shorter in patients with HA/CMC than in those without HA/CMC (3.2 months vs. 12.0 months, respectively, $p < 0.01$) (Fig. 2b).

Potential predictors of the time until complete postoperative continence are evaluated in Table 3. Univariate analysis showed that the age, institutional caseload, and use of HA/CMC were the predictors of achieving pad-free status. Multivariate Cox analysis indicated that an age < 70 years (hazard ratio [HR]: 1.74, 95% confidence interval [CI]: 1.12–2.80), institutional caseload > 200, (HR: 1.64, 95%CI: 1.10–2.47), and use of HA/CMC (HR: 1.84, 95%CI: 1.22–2.76) were independent predictors of the early return of continence.

Discussion

We investigated the influence of HA/CMC on early return of continence after nerve-sparing RARP and demonstrated that use of HA/CMC during nerve-sparing RARP significantly shortened the duration of postoperative incontinence. This difference was not only seen in patients undergoing bilateral nerve-sparing surgery, but also in those having unilateral nerve-sparing surgery. Multivariate analysis confirmed that use of HA/CMC was an independent predictor of postoperative recovery of continence.

Table 1 Demographic and clinical characteristics of the two groups

	Bilateral nerve-sparing RARP (*n* = 46)			Unilateral nerve-sparing RARP (*n* = 137)		
	With HA/CMC (*n* = 13)	Without HA/CMC (*n* = 33)	*P* value	With HA/CMC (*n* = 40)	Without HA/CMC (*n* = 97)	*P* value
Age	64.0 (54.1–67.2)	64.9 (59.5–71.3)	0.18	66.4 (62.5–70.7)	66.0 (63.0–71.0)	0.99
BMI	23.5 (21.3–24.4)	23.1 (21.5–25.5)	0.55	23.6 (21.5–25.0)	23.4 (21.6–25.1)	0.14
Pretreatment PSA	7.7 (6.0–9.2)	7.2 (5.5–11.5)	0.87	7.6 (5.2–10.1)	7.2 (5.3–9.6)	0.63
Prostate volume (cm^2)	24.5 (14–42.8)	28.0 (20.0–45.5)	0.26	28.0 (20.0–32.3)	25.0 (20.0–34.8)	0.82
Clinical stage			0.74			0.65
cT1c	6 (46.2)	16 (48.5)		8 (20.0)	18 (18.6)	
≥cT2	7 (53.8)	17 (51.5)		32 (80.0)	79 (81.4)	
Gleason sum	6 (6–6.5)	7 (6–7)	0.32	7 (7–8)	7 (6.5–7)	0.13
Charlson comorbidity index, n (%)			0.68			0.43
0	3 (23.1)	9 (27.3)		11 (27.5)	32 (33.0)	
≥1	10 (76.9)	24 (72.7)		29 (72.5)	65 (67.0)	
Institutional caseload> 200, n (%)	10 (76.9)	16 (48.5)	0.08	30 (75.0)	57 (57.7)	0.06

Table 2 Perioperative, pathological, and oncological outcomes

	Bilateral nerve-sparing RARP ($n = 46$)			Unilateral nerve-sparing RARP ($n = 137$)		
	With HA/CMC ($n = 13$)	Without HA/CMC ($n = 33$)	P value	With HA/CMC ($n = 40$)	Without HA/CMC ($n = 97$)	P value
Follow-up period, months: median (IQR)	20.7 (16.3–27.0)	20.1 (14.9–29.4)	0.83	21.6 (16.7–27.0)	20.3 (13.3–28.5)	0.79
Operating time, min: median (IQR)	207 (178–223)	215 (189–249)	0.10	210 (176–234)	233 (203–275)	0.09
Estimated blood loss, mL: median (IQR)	10 (2.5–125)	20 (5–125)	0.09	19 (0–88)	70 (0–105)	0.07
Complications ≥ Clavien G3, n (%)	1 (7.7)	3 (9.1)	0.32	1 (2.5)	2 (2.1)	0.87
Urine leakage at cystography, n (%)	1 (7.7)	3 (9.1)	0.81	4 (10.0)	10 (10.3)	0.96
pT, n (%)			0.81			0.38
pT2	12 (92.3)	28 (84.8)		29 (72.5)	77 (79.4)	
≥ pT3	1 (7.7)	5 (15.2)		11 (27.5)	20 (20.6)	
Gleason sum, n (%)			0.48			0.50
6	4 (30.8)	7 (21.2)		1 (2.5)	3 (3.1)	
7	7 (53.8)	23 (30.4)		31 (77.5)	85 (87.6)	
≥8	2 (15.4)	3 (9.1)		8 (20.0)	9 (9.3)	
Positive surgical margin, n (%)	2 (15.4)	3 (9.1)	0.54	5 (12.5)	15 (15.5)	0.37
Biochemical failure, n (%)	0 (0)	0 (0)	–	2 (5.0)	6 (6.2)	0.79

Periurethral fibrosis and scarring have been reported as factors that predict postoperative incontinence after radical prostatectomy [3, 4]. Technical factors such as the amount of postoperative oozing or a prolonged operating time might contribute to fibrotic change. These factors can be improved by increasing the surgeon's or institution's experience, but complete prevention of inflammation or fibrosis after surgical invasion is theoretically impossible, and no method of preventing fibrosis or scarring after radical prostatectomy has been reported to our knowledge.

One of the main causes of postoperative incontinence after radical prostatectomy could be periurethral scarring, which can lead to chronic compression and ischemia of the periurethral tissues as well as sphincteric nerves. HA is a major component of the extracellular matrix and it plays an important role in early wound healing together with fibrin [17]. HA stimulates the production of interleukin-1 (IL-1) and IL-1 promotes fibroblast proliferation and collagenase production [18]. HA is also involved in regulating leukocyte motility, adhesion, and phagocytosis, and it acts to suppress scar formation caused by infiltration of inflammatory cells into damaged tissues [19]. HA/CMC is a surgical material with a 66.6% content of HA that is widely been used to prevent visceral adhesion by inhibiting postoperative local inflammation and fibrosis [20]. The improvement of early postoperative continence after RARP observed in the present study could have been due to suppression of periurethral scarring by intraoperative application of HA/CMC. Because HA/CMC is available worldwide, easy to use, and low cost, it seems to be a reasonable option for prevention of scarring of the urethral sphincter and periurethral tissue after radical prostatectomy.

HA also has an important role in maintaining tissue elasticity. HA increases hydration of the extracellular matrix and traps water molecules around elastic fibers, thus improving their function. Elastic fibers are a major insoluble component of the extracellular matrix that permit deformation and passive recoil of organs or tissues [9, 10]. We previously demonstrated co-localization of elastic fibers and HA in the submucosa and smooth muscle of the membranous urethra [12]. Surgical invasion can reduce tissue elasticity derived from water captured by a matrix of HA and elastic fibers, so the elasticity of periurethral tissue could be impaired after radical prostatectomy. Loss of elasticity was reported to lead to the degeneration of connective tissue [6]. In the present study, faster recovery of continence after RARP was confirmed in patients with HA/CMC than in those without it. Although direct measurement of the urethral elasticity is impossible, this difference might have been related to maintenance of urethral elasticity by application of HA/CMC.

HA can also prevent cicatrization of peripheral nerves and promote nerve regeneration. For example, rats showed faster functional recovery after sciatic nerve dissection when HA was applied to the dissected nerve [21]. Furthermore, HA creates a hydrated open lattice in the extracellular matrix that facilitates migration of regenerating axons [22]. We previously reported that peripheral nerves running through the hiatus between the bilateral levator ani slings were positive for HA in human male cadavers [12]. An association between sparing the cavernous nerves and early postoperative return of urinary

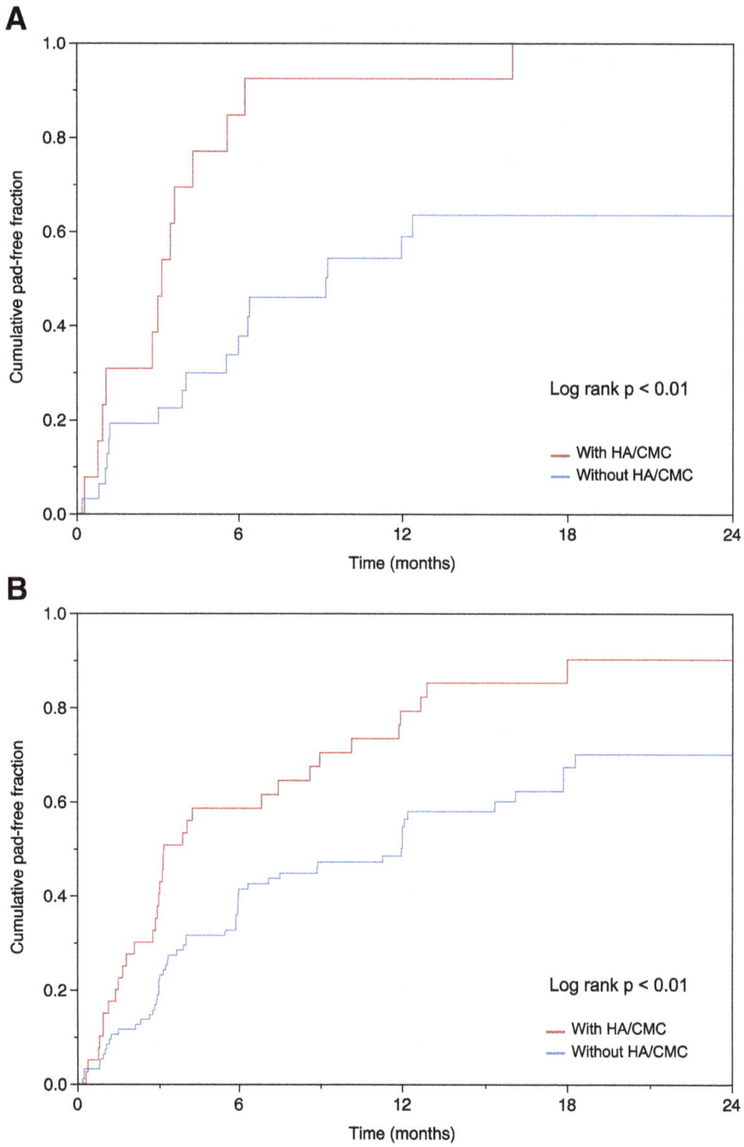

Fig. 2 Pad-free status of patients who underwent bilateral nerve-sparing RARP (*n* = 46) (**a**) and unilateral nerve-sparing RARP (*n* = 137) (**b**)

continence has already been described [23]. Repeated injection of HA into nerve conduits was reported to enhance regeneration of sciatic nerve defects in rats [22]. In another study, HA reduced perineural adhesions at 4 weeks and 12 weeks after neurorrhaphy, and also enhanced peripheral nerve regeneration at 12 weeks postoperatively [21]. Furthermore, HA/CMC has been reported to reduce extraneural adhesions and promote nerve regeneration at 3 months after sciatic nerve repair in rabbits [24]. In the present study, early return of continence after application of HA/CMC to the

Table 3 Univariate and multivariate Cox regression analysis of factors influencing achievement of pad-free status

	Univariate analysis			Multivariate analysis		
	HR	95% CI	*P* value	HR	95%CI	*P* value
Age ≤ 70 years	1.67	1.08–2.68	0.02	1.74	1.12–2.80	0.01
BMI ≤24	1.11	0.76–1.66	0.61			
Nerve-sparing (bilateral vs. unilateral)	1.24	0.80–1.87	0.33			
Institutional caseload > 200	1.86	1.28–2.71	<0.01	1.64	1.10–2.47	0.02
Use of HA/CMC	2.26	1.54–3.30	<0.01	1.84	1.22–2.76	<0.01

nerve-sparing side may have been related to enhanced regeneration of axons in the cavernous nerves. Figure 3 outlines how application of HA/CMC could prevent three potential causes of postoperative loss of tissue elasticity due to surgical invasion.

A retrospective study showed that wrapping HA/CMC around the suture line led to a higher frequency of sequelae associated with intestinal anastomotic leakage after abdominopelvic surgery [25]. However, covering the prostate bed with HA/CMC did not increase including postoperative urine leakage or other complications in the present study, even though RP involves vesicourethral anastomosis. Joung et al. reported earlier recovery of erectile function when the neurovascular bundle was coated with HA/CMC gel during RARP than in the control group [26]. They also reported that complication rates did not differ between the two groups, a similar finding to the results of the present study. It is possible that precise suturing with robotic assistance [27] could contribute to reducing urine leakage and prevent migration of dissolved HA/CMC after radical prostatectomy. Excellent hemostasis of the prostatic bed achieved with RARP could also have enabled safe application of HA/CMC.

Several limitations of this study should be considered. First, the retrospective design and small number of patients limit the conclusions that can be drawn. Second, reasons of the rather low continence outcomes of the non-HA/CMC groups in the present study might be ascribed to the strict continence definition used and the fact that not all the four surgeons were experts. Third, the treatment protocol was not randomized, so results might have been influenced by the learning curve effect. Thompson et al. reported that RARP had a long learning curve with inferior early results that progressively transform to superior functional and oncological outcomes [28]. Although patients receiving HA/CMC were assigned according to institutional policy, the caseload was still an independent predictor of postoperative continence by Cox proportional hazards analysis in the present study. However, use of HA/CMC was also an independent predictor of the earlier achievement of pad-free status by Cox analysis. Thus, intraoperative application of HA/CMC to the prostate bed during nerve-sparing RARP improved postoperative continence.

Conclusions

This study demonstrated that application of HA/CMC to the prostate bed and neurovascular plate significantly shortened the duration of postoperative incontinence after both unilateral and bilateral nerve-sparing RARP. Further researches on this working mechanism and a prospective randomized controlled trial of HA/CMC in patients undergoing RARP seems to be warranted.

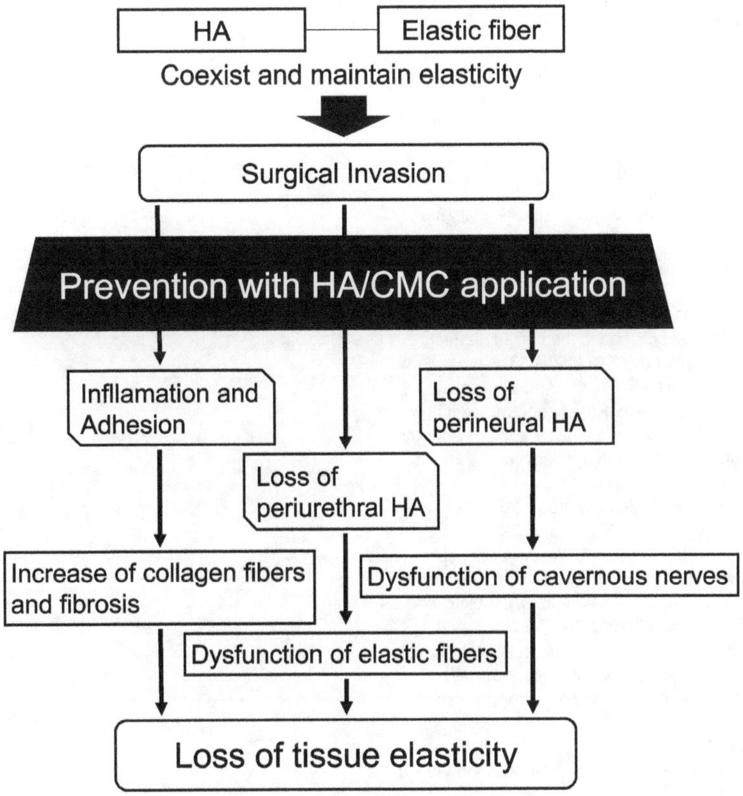

Fig. 3 Mechanism by which application of HA/CMC may prevent three possible causes of the postoperative loss of tissue elasticity due to surgical invasion

Abbreviations

HA: hyaluronic acid; HA/CMC: hyaluronic acid-carboxymethyl cellulose membrane; RARP: robot-assisted radical prostatectomy

Acknowledgements

Not applicable.

Authors' contributions

Conception and design: NH, MF, Data acquisition: NH, YB, KC, JF, KH, TI, Data analysis and interpretation: KC, Drafting the manuscript: YB, NH, MF, Critical revision of the manuscript for scientific and factual content: NH, Statistical Analysis: YB, NH Supervision: MF. All authors read and approved the final manuscript.

References

1. Ficarra V, Novara G, Rosen RC, Artibani W, Carroll PR, Costello A, et al. Systematic review and meta-analysis of studies reporting urinary continence recovery after robot-assisted radical prostatectomy. Eur Urol. 2012;62(3):405–17.
2. Heesakkers J, Farag F, Bauer RM, Sandhu J, De Ridder D, Stenzl A. Pathophysiology and contributing factors in Postprostatectomy incontinence: a review. Eur Urol. 2017;71(6):936–44.
3. Tuygun C, Imamoglu A, Keyik B, Alisir I, Yorubulut M. Significance of fibrosis around and/or at external urinary sphincter on pelvic magnetic resonance imaging in patients with postprostatectomy incontinence. Urology. 2006;68(6):1308–12.
4. Paparel P, Akin O, Sandhu JS, Otero JR, Serio AM, Scardino PT, et al. Recovery of urinary continence after radical prostatectomy: association with urethral length and urethral fibrosis measured by preoperative and postoperative endorectal magnetic resonance imaging. Eur Urol. 2009;55(3):629–37.
5. Kielty CM, Sherratt MJ, Shuttleworth CA. Elastic fibres. J Cell Sci. 2002;115(Pt 14):2817–28.
6. Watson RE, Griffiths CE, Craven NM, Shuttleworth CA, Kielty CM. Fibrillin-rich microfibrils are reduced in photoaged skin. Distribution at the dermal-epidermal junction. J Invest Dermatol. 1999;112(5):782–7.
7. Korn GP, Martins JR, Park SW, Mendes A, Kobayashi EY, Nader HB, et al. Concentration of hyaluronic acid in human vocal folds in young and old subjects. Otolaryngol Head Neck Surg. 2011;145(6):981–6.
8. Kawase T, Shibata S, Katori Y, Ohtsuka A, Murakami G, Fujimiya M. Elastic fiber-mediated enthesis in the human middle ear. J Anat. 2012;221(4):331–40.
9. Scott JE, Cummings C, Brass A, Chen Y. Secondary and tertiary structures of hyaluronan in aqueous solution, investigated by rotary shadowing-electron microscopy and computer simulation. Hyaluronan is a very efficient network-forming polymer. Biochem J. 1991;274(Pt 3):699–705.
10. Rosenbloom J, Abrams WR, Mecham R. Extracellular matrix 4: the elastic fiber. FASEB J. 1993;7(13):1208–18.
11. Kendall K. Molecular adhesion and its applications: the sticky universe: Springer; 2001.
12. Hinata N, Murakami G, Abe S, Shibata S, Morizane S, Honda M, et al. Coexistence of elastic fibers with hyaluronic acid in the human urethral sphincter complex: a histological study. J Urol. 2013;190(4):1313–9.
13. Di Saverio S, Coccolini F, Galati M, Smerieri N, Biffl WL, Ansaloni L, et al. Bologna guidelines for diagnosis and management of adhesive small bowel obstruction (ASBO): 2013 update of the evidence-based guidelines from the world society of emergency surgery ASBO working group. World J Emerg Surg. 2013;8(1):42.
14. Hinata N, Sejima T, Takenaka A. Progress in pelvic anatomy from the viewpoint of radical prostatectomy. Int J Urol. 2013;20(3):260–70.
15. Becker JM, Dayton MT, Fazio VW, Beck DE, Stryker SJ, Wexner SD, et al. Prevention of postoperative abdominal adhesions by a sodium hyaluronate-based bioresorbable membrane: a prospective, randomized, double-blind multicenter study. J Am Coll Surg. 1996;183(4):297–306.
16. Joshi N, de Blok W, van Muilekom E, van der Poel H. Impact of posterior musculofascial reconstruction on early continence after robot-assisted laparoscopic radical prostatectomy: results of a prospective parallel group trial. Eur Urol. 2010;58(1):84 9.
17. Weigel PH, Fuller GM, LeBoeuf RD. A model for the role of hyaluronic acid and fibrin in the early events during the inflammatory response and wound healing. J Theor Biol. 1986;119(2):219–34.
18. Hiro D, Ito A, Matsuta K, Mori Y. Hyaluronic acid is an endogenous inducer of interleukin-1 production by human monocytes and rabbit macrophages. Biochem Biophys Res Commun. 1986;140(2):715 22.
19. Goldberg RL, Toole BP. Hyaluronate inhibition of cell proliferation. Arthritis Rheum. 1987;30(7):769–78.
20. Kumar S, Wong PF, Leaper DJ. Intra-peritoneal prophylactic agents for preventing adhesions and adhesive intestinal obstruction after non-gynaecological abdominal surgery. Cochrane Database Syst Rev. 2009;1:CD005080.
21. Ozgenel GY. Effects of hyaluronic acid on peripheral nerve scarring and regeneration in rats. Microsurgery. 2003;23(6):575–81.
22. Wang KK, Nemeth IR, Seckel BR, Chakalis-Haley DP, Swann DA, Kuo JW, et al. Hyaluronic acid enhances peripheral nerve regeneration in vivo. Microsurgery. 1998;18(4):270–5.
23. Reeves F, Preece P, Kapoor J, Everaerts W, Murphy DG, Corcoran NM, et al. Preservation of the neurovascular bundles is associated with improved time to continence after radical prostatectomy but not long-term continence rates: results of a systematic review and meta-analysis. Eur Urol. 2015;68(4):692–704.
24. Adanali G, Verdi M, Tuncel A, Erdogan B, Kargi E. Effects of hyaluronic acid-carboxymethylcellulose membrane on extraneural adhesion formation and peripheral nerve regeneration. J Reconstr Microsurg. 2003;19(1):29–36.
25. Beck DE, Cohen Z, Fleshman JW, Kaufman HS, van Goor H, Wolff BG. A prospective, randomized, multicenter, controlled study of the safety of Seprafilm adhesion barrier in abdominopelvic surgery of the intestine. Dis Colon Rectum. 2003;46(10):1310–9.
26. Joung JY, Ha YS, Singer EA, Ercolani MC, Favaretto RL, Lee DH, et al. Use of a hyaluronic acid-carboxymethylcellulose adhesion barrier on the neurovascular bundle and prostatic bed to facilitate earlier recovery of erectile function after robot-assisted prostatectomy: an initial experience. J Endourol. 2013;27(10):1230–5.
27. Ploussard G, de la Taille A, Moulin M, Vordos D, Hoznek A, Abbou CC, et al. Comparisons of the perioperative, functional, and oncologic outcomes after robot-assisted versus pure extraperitoneal laparoscopic radical prostatectomy. Eur Urol. 2014;65(3):610–9.
28. Thompson JE, Egger S, Bohm M, Haynes AM, Matthews J, Rasiah K, et al. Superior quality of life and improved surgical margins are achievable with robotic radical prostatectomy after a long learning curve: a prospective single-surgeon study of 1552 consecutive cases. Eur Urol. 2014;65(3):521–31.

12

Agreement between patient reported outcomes and clinical reports after radical prostatectomy - A prospective longitudinal study

David Bock[1,2*], Eva Angenete[1], Anders Bjartell[3], Jonas Hugosson[4], Gunnar Steineck[5], Sofie Walming[1], Peter Wiklund[6] and Eva Haglind[1]

Abstract

Background: In clinical research information can be retrieved through various sources. The aim is to evaluate the agreement between answers in patient questionnaires and clinical reports in a study of patients after radical prostatectomy and patient characteristics associated with agreement between these two data sources.

Methods: In the prospective non-randomized longitudinal trial LAParoscopic Prostatectomy Robot Open (LAPPRO) 4003 patients undergoing radical prostatectomy at 14 centers in Sweden were followed. Analysis of agreement is made using a variety of methods, including the recently proposed Gwet's AC1, which enables us to handle the limitations of Cohen's Kappa where agreement depends on the underlying prevalence.

Results: The incidence of postoperative events was consistently reported higher by the patient compared with the clinical reports for all outcomes. Agreement regarding the absence of events (negative agreement) was consistently higher than agreement regarding events (positive agreement) for all outcome variables. Overall impression of agreement depends on which measure used for the assessment. The previously reported desirable properties of Gwet's AC1 as well as the patient characteristics associated with agreement were confirmed.

Conclusion: The differences in incidence and agreement across the different variables and time points highlight the importance of carefully assessing which source of information to use in clinical research.

Keywords: Agreement, Questionnaire, Prostate cancer, Prostatectomy, Case-report form

Background

In clinical research information can be retrieved through various sources. Three commonly used sources of information are the patient themselves (self-reported), professional caregivers (clinical reports) and medical records. The preferred source depends on the specific research objective and the kind of information retrieved from the different sources. However, there may be different sources of information to choose from for several types of data such as morbidity, symptoms and health care utilization [1].

Medical conditions are commonly assessed retrospectively through patient interviews or patient charts [2–7]. When assessing outcomes after cancer surgery, documenting patient's comorbidity is crucial as it may influence outcomes [8], such as recurrence [9], symptoms, complications [10] and bodily dysfunctions [11]. Another aim is documentation of health care utilization [12, 13]. Whereas studies comparing self-reported questionnaires with medical records are common [3, 6, 14–17], evaluation of clinical reports has received less attention [2, 6, 8].

* Correspondence: david.bock@gu.se
[1]Department of Surgery, Institute of Clinical Sciences, Sahlgrenska Academy, University of Gothenburg, SSORG (Scandinavian Surgical Outcomes Research Group), Sahlgrenska University Hospital/Östra, 416 85 Gothenburg, Sweden
[2]Health Metrics Unit, Sahlgrenska Academy, University of Gothenburg, Gothenburg, Sweden
Full list of author information is available at the end of the article

Knowledge of quality characteristics such as agreement and reliability of different sources of information is important. Evaluating agreement between different sources contributes to the choice of source for information in clinical research. The focus in this study is on the agreement between patient questionnaires and case report form in a study of patients after radical prostatectomy. Assessing agreement by a single measure is often insufficient [18]. The use of measures of agreement for continuous outcomes was explored in a systematic review [19]. For categorical outcomes where data is classified according to concordant (positive/positive or negative/negative) and discordant (positive/negative or negative/positive) pairs, any recent systematic review is to our knowledge currently not available. However, according to Wongpakaran [20] and by our current review of the literature, many studies only report Cohen's Kappa [21], sometimes combined with positive and negative agreement [18]. Kappa is a measure of the level of agreement in excess of chance, expressed as the relative difference in proportions of concordant pairs between observed and what would have occurred by chance. Positive and negative agreement estimates the conditional probability that, given that one of randomly selected rater makes a positive and negative rating, respectively, the other rater will also do so. A limitation with kappa is its dependence on the underlying prevalence, giving rise to for example low kappa values despite high percentage of agreement [18, 22]. This originates from how chance agreement is computed [23]. Gwet [24] proposed a statistic, named AC1, which is similar to kappa but use an estimator of chance agreement that is less dependent on the prevalence [20]. In the correction for chance agreement of kappa, it is assumed that all observed ratings may potentially agree by pure chance. In Gwet's AC1, the likelihood of chance agreement is instead related to the proportion of ratings that may lead to an agreement. This portion does in turn depend on the observed marginal prevalence's. This enables Gwet's AC1 to avoid the problem of over or under correction that Kappa suffer from.

Agreement can be analyzed by generalized linear models for contingency tables [25]. Log-linear models are a class of models which to enable to quantify the contribution of row, column and diagonal effects as well as covariates on the outcome. The quasi-independence model [26] enables a greater degree flexibility and a more in-depth study of the structure of agreement than simple summary measures. For the situation where a source provides the true conditions (positive/negative), referred to as gold standard, the sensitivity and specificity of the different sources can be evaluated. Sensitivity and specificity measures the rate of cases being correctly classified as positive and negative, respectively.

The aim of this study was to evaluate the agreement between patient questionnaires and clinical reports in a study of patients after radical prostatectomy and to study patient characteristics associated with agreement between these two data sources.

Methods

Laparoscopic Prostatectomy Robot Open (LAPPRO) is an ongoing open, controlled and non-randomized prospective longitudinal trial comparing open retropubic and robot-assisted laparoscopic radical prostatectomy for localized prostate cancer at 14 centers in Sweden. The trial has been previously described in detail [27]. Patient scheduled for prostatectomy at the participating centers fulfilling the inclusion criteria (informed consent, age < 75 yr., ability to read and write Swedish, tumour stage cT1, cT2, or cT3 (TNM Classification of Malignant Tumors, [28]) with no signs of distant metastases, and a prostate-specific antigen level of < 20 ng/ml) were included.

Information was collected at 6–12 weeks, 12 and 24 months postoperatively both from case report forms by study personnel (either the operating urologist or clinical nurses) and from questionnaires filled out by the patients with regard to the following five outcomes: 1. swelling of groin or lower extremities, 2. complications and re-admissions, 3. re-operations, 4. added pharmacological therapy after surgery or due to local or distant recurrence and 5. local recurrence and metastases, see Fig. 1.

The questionnaires were based on concepts introduced in previous research projects [11, 29] and were content validated by experts in the field of urology and then face validated face with patients with prostate cancer. The case report forms were face validated with professional caregivers. The case report forms and questionnaires were further tested in a pilot study, after which final revisions were made [27]. The different questions in the case report forms and the questionnaires are presented in Supplement 1.

Definition of outcomes and predictors

In the derivation of the outcome variables a broad approach was used with binary outcomes where the presence (positive) or absence (negative) of at least one occurrence of interest, for example a readmission, was required to be reported in both sources (case report form and questionnaire) to reach agreement. A higher level of similarity, for example the exact number of readmissions, was not required. The reason is that the recall of the patient and the case report form may not refer to exactly the same time period. The derived outcomes can hence be grouped according to concordant (positive/

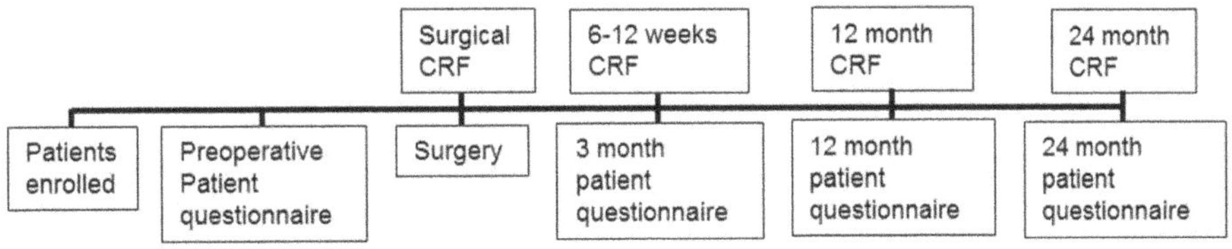

Fig. 1 Flow chart of study procedures

positive or negative/negative) and discordant (positive/negative or negative/positive) pairs.

When the recall of the patient and the case report form refer to the same time period a higher agreement is more likely compared to when there is no defined time period. However, in the study the personnel did to some extent complete the clinical record form retrospectively by investigating medical records. Therefore the time period cannot be accurately assed and is not used in the analysis. Lastly, the events studied here were anticipated to have relatively low incidence.

Swelling of groin or lower extremities

At 6–12 weeks follow-up the case report form addressed signs of swelling (lymph oedema) in groin (left or right side) and lower extremities (left or right) with response categories *"Yes"*/*"No"*. At 3 months the questionnaire addressed feeling of swelling and heaviness in (left or right) groin or leg and heaviness in legs. A positive outcome was defined as *"Yes"* on at least one of the questions. A negative outcome was defined as responding *No* on all the questions. Otherwise the outcome was set to missing.

Complications, readmissions and reoperations

The case report form collected information on complications related to surgery, complications occurring after 6–12 weeks, and if the patient had been re-admitted to hospital for other reasons than cancer treatment later than the 12 month follow-up. At 3, 12 and 24 months the questionnaire included a question on whether the patient had contacted healthcare for a specified list of reasons. If any reason included pain from the surgical wound, lower or upper part of abdomen, bleeding from surgical wound, urinary tract or catheter it was defined as an event. There was also a question on whether that patient had been readmitted to hospital. For the questionnaire, a positive outcome was defined as responding *"Yes"* on any of the questions. For the case report form positive and negative outcome was defined as responding *"Yes"* and *"No"*, respectively. Responding *"No information"* and a non-response outcome were defined as missing.

At 12 and 24 months the case report form addressed whether the patients had been re-operated after 6–12 weeks and 12 months follow-up, respectively. The questionnaire addressed if the patient had been operation during the last 12 months. For both the case report form and the questionnaire a positive and negative outcome was defined by responding *"Yes"* and *"No"*, respectively. A non-response outcome was defined as missing.

For a yet unpublished report, [30] data on all readmissions within 3 months of surgery were collected from the Patient registry, Swedish Board of Health and Welfare. These data will be compared with the questionnaire and the CRF at 3 months.

Adjuvant therapy and local recurrence and metastases

Signs of local recurrence and detection of distant metastases were assessed in the case report form at 12 and 24 months and at the same follow-up times the patients were also asked about these matters. For both the case report form and the questionnaire a positive and negative outcome was defined by responding *"Yes"* and *"No"*, respectively. For a non-response the outcome was defined as missing.

Predictor variables

Patient characteristics and demography were collected through the questionnaires preoperatively and throughout the study. Preoperatively, information on age, education, occupation and marital status was collected and evaluated with regard to association with agreement [7, 13, 16]. In addition, use of medication, alcohol consumption, quality of life, depressed mood and presence of negative intrusive thoughts were also evaluated. Use of medication was defined as use of sleeping pills or tranquilizers. Self-assessed quality of life, negative intrusive thoughts and alcohol consumption were characterized in the same way as in an earlier analysis [31]. Depressive mood was defined as either responding 'Yes' to the question 'Would you call yourself depressed?' [32] or use of anti-depressive medication.

Sensitivity and specificity

Sensitivity and specificity will be evaluated for two scenarios with regard to choice of gold standard. First, the questionnaire will be considered as gold standard and the sensitivity and specificity of the clinical reports will be evaluated. Secondly, the Patient registry will be considered as standard regarding readmissions and the questionnaire and clinical report will be evaluated.

Statistical analysis

Group sizes in LAPPRO were set to evaluate urinary incontinence [27] and were judged to be sufficient to assess the current aim. Agreement was evaluated by percent of concordant pairs, positive and negative agreement and Gwet's AC1. For comparison the kappa coefficient was computed as well. Association was evaluated by the odds that the two observers agree rather than disagree using the marginal quasi-independence model. Due to the hierarchical design where the surgeons are operating on several patients, who are longitudinally followed, there are dependency structures in the data that should ideally be accounted for in the statistical model. However, due to computational difficulties a standard fixed effect model was estimated separately at each time point.

In the evaluation of factors associated with agreement (positive or negative) between the two data sources, the following were evaluated: age, education, occupation, marital status, medication (sleeping pills or tranquilizers), alcohol consumption, quality of life, depressed mood and negative intrusive thoughts. For swelling of groin or lower extremities a standard simple logistic regression was used. For the outcomes with repeated measures a random intercept logistic regression model was used and time was included as a fixed effect ([26]). Results were presented with 95% confidence intervals. In each of the analyses, for information to be evaluable, data from both sources had to be 'non-missing' according to the definitions described above. The same analyses were made for the additional comparisons with data from the Patient registry. Analyses were conducted in SAS v9.4 (SAS Institute Inc., Cary NC), the *rel* package [33] and the software described by [34].

Results

For the 3706 eligible patients, the number of patients with evaluable data from both case report forms and questionnaires varied between the different questions from 3385 (91%) for swelling of groin and lower extremities at 3 months to 1884 (51%) for complications and readmissions at 24 months (Fig. 2). Missing information was consistently higher in the case report forms and increased at later follow-up (Table 1).

Patient characteristics and demography

Patient characteristics are reported in Table 2. The median age of the patients was 63 years. Thirty-eight percent were retired and 84% were married/cohabiting.

Agreement between case report forms and patient reported data

With the exception of local recurrence and metastases, all events were reported to a higher degree by the patient reports compared with the case report form (Table 3). The incidence of swelling of groin or lower extremities was 1 and 24% as reported by the case report form and questionnaire, respectively. Gwet's AC1 was relatively stable and varied between 0.62 and 0.96 across outcomes and time points. Both kappa and the odds of agreement varied across a much wider range. Negative agreement was consistently higher than positive agreement for all the outcome variables.

There was relatively high negative agreement across all variables and time points (84–97%) which rendered high odds of agreement. However, due to the low positive agreement for most of the variables and the low incidence as reported by the case report form, the kappa values were in general low. Gwet's AC1 was less affected by the incidence. Agreement regarding additional (chemo) radiotherapy had higher agreement compared with the other variables.

Both reoperations and recurrence at 12 months had a relatively low incidence. However, despite being similar with regard to concordant pairs (91 and 95%, respectively) and negative agreement (95 and 97%, respectively), there was a large discrepancy in kappa (0.38 and 0.22) and odds of agreement (52 and 21) attributed to differences in incidence and positive agreement. Gwet's AC1 were similar, 0.90 and 0.94, respectively. A similar pattern was observed at 24 months as well as for the comparison between additional (chemo) radiotherapy after surgery or due to recurrence at 12 and 24 months.

For the scenario where the questionnaire is regarded as gold standard the sensitivity of the case report form varied considerable between variables. Specificity was more stable at a high level which means that the case report forms have a higher likelihood of identifying absence rather than presence of events (Table 4).

Agreement with patient registry data

In the comparisons of the questionnaire and CRF with Patient registry data, the estimated readmission rate was 1083 (29%), 373 (10%) and 291 (8%), respectively. The questionnaire had lower agreement with the registry compared with the CRF. The questionnaire had slightly higher sensitivity than the CRF. The CRF had higher specificity (Table 5).

Factors associated with agreement

Being retired, using sleeping pills and/or tranquilizers as well as reporting an impaired quality of life, depressed mood and negative intrusive thoughts were all associated with a lower agreement for several of the outcome

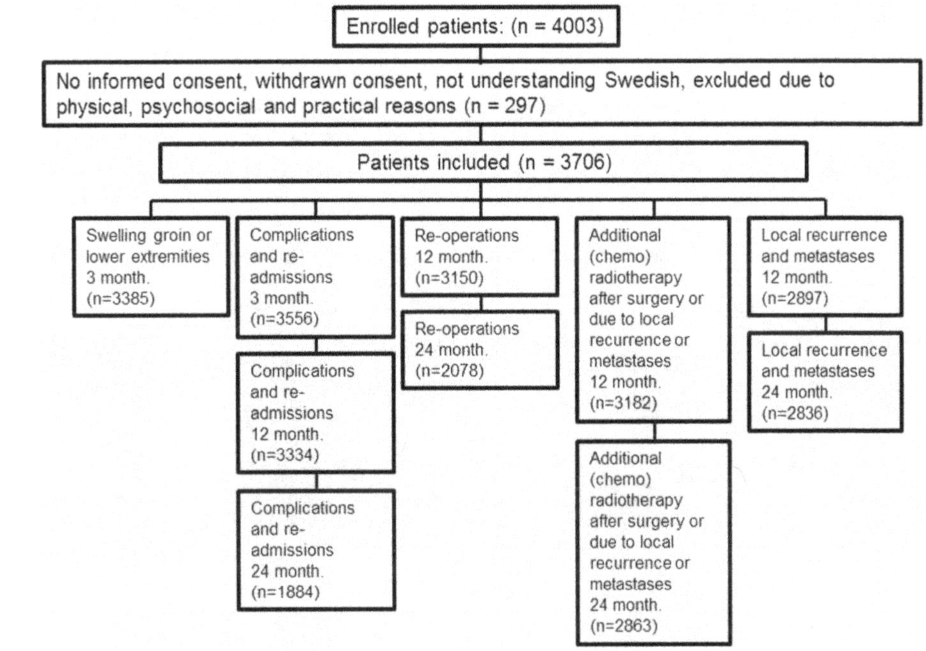

Fig. 2 Flow chart of patients included in the study

variables (Table 6). Being married/cohabiting was associated with a higher degree of agreement for swelling of the groin. Age was associated with reoperations, (chemo) radiotherapy and local recurrence and metastases with high age yielding poor agreement. No association was found for education or alcohol consumption.

Discussion

This study indicates that in a clinical trial, patients in general report a higher frequency of events than professional caregivers do. In the current study of patients after radical prostatectomy, with the exception of tumor recurrence, the incidence of various postoperative symptoms or events after radical prostatectomy for prostate cancer was consistently more frequently reported by the patients than in clinical reports. Missing information was consistently higher in the case report forms and increased at later follow-up.

Positive agreement was consistently lower than negative agreement for all the outcome variables. This is probably due to the relatively low incidence estimates and the large discrepancies in estimates between the patient and the clinical reports. Whereas both kappa and the odds of agreement varied across a wide range across

Table 1 Missing data

Assessment	Follow-up (months)	Missing data, N(%)		
		Case report form	Questionnaire	Missing on at least one
Swelling groin or lower extremities	3	163 (4%)	163 (4%)	321 (8%)
Complications and readmissions	3	150 (4%)	0	150 (4%)
	12	372 (10%)	0	372 (10%)
	24	1822 (49%)	0	1822 (49%)
Reoperations	12	300 (8%)	351 (9%)	556 (15%)
	24	1426 (38%)	356 (10%)	1628 (44%)
Additional (chemo) radiotherapy after surgery or due to local recurrence or metastases	12	251 (7%)	303 (8%)	524 (14%)
	24	555 (15%)	373 (10%)	843 (23%)
Local recurrence and metastases	12	809 (22%)	0	809 (22%)
	24	870 (23%)	0	870 (23%)

Table 2 Patient characteristics

			Not Missing / Missing
Age, median (min; max)	Years	63 (37;79)	3706/.
Education, N (%)	No higher education	1948 (60)	3236/470
	Other	55 (2)	
	University	1233 (38)	
Occupation, N(%)	Working	1759 (54)	3257/449
	Retired	1253 (38)	
	Other	245 (8)	
Marital status, N (%)	Live apart	223 (7)	3235/471
	Married/cohabiting	2731 (84)	
	No partner	281 (9)	
Medication use [a]	Yes	394 (12)	3253/453
Alcohol consumption, N (%)	High	427 (13)	3298/408
Global Quality of Life, N(%)	Low/moderate	1503 (46)	3234/467
Depression [b]	Yes	265 (8)	3257/449
Negative intrusive thoughts	At least once per week	1170 (36)	3237/469

[a]Use of use of sleeping pills or tranquilizers
[b]Depressed mood or use of anti-depressants

the different variables and time points, despite other data characteristics of agreement being relatively similar, Gwet's AC1 was relatively stable, which confirm previous findings [20, 24].

Accuracy and agreement between the different modes depends on what information is being collected [8]. For symptoms as well as events such as readmissions, an advantage with the questionnaire is that data is collected directly from the patient it concerns. However, the accuracy of recall may be questionable, especially in a retrospective setting with a long recall period [1]. Patients are more likely to recall a disease requiring a surgical or intensive pathologic/laboratory diagnostic procedure than a disease without such a procedures [14]. The time elapsed since the illness occurred and the seriousness of the disease influence agreement [3]. Diabetes has generally high agreement whereas chronic obstructive pulmonary disease and diseases with less explicit diagnostic criteria have poor agreement [6, 15]. For medical records recall bias is less of an issue as information is generally prospectively documented during a hospital admission that is data is recorded instantaneously in the course of time. A major limitation is that medical records may not cover the necessary information relevant for specific research objectives and underestimate symptoms based conditions [35]. They may also lack coverage as they miss patients not seeking health care or patients seeking health care in another county, or due to differences in reporting inpatient and outpatient visits [36]. An advantage with clinical reports is that they can be fit for purpose as opposed to medical records. A drawback is that information is filtered through the physician [11]. In the collection of signs, different types of medical examinations by an experienced clinician may be the only viable option.

The patient may be less prone to report complications when the clinical personnel asks for information compared with when he or she completes an anonymous questionnaire at home [37]. In this trial questionnaires were sent out and returned to a third party, the trial secretariat and not to the hospital/department where surgery was performed [27]. The information documented in the clinical record form was collected when clinical personnel met the patient during the follow-up meetings as well as from medical records. This probably explains the observed high agreement between the clinical record forms and the patient registry. A higher agreement between patient reports and medical records compared with patient reports versus physician reports has also been observed [8].

It has been found that patients with prostate cancer reported a higher incidence of symptoms such as fatigue compared to their physicians [38, 39]. A similar pattern was found in [40] but with a higher degree of agreement. Several study design features may contribute to these differences as discussed in [40].

Several of the studies ([5, 6, 9, 14, 16]) have used medical records as the gold standard enabling assessment of sensitivity and specificity. However, it may be an invalid assumption for other settings [35]. For the scenario where the Patient registry was regarded as the gold standard in reporting readmissions, the case report forms had a higher agreement and specificity compared

Table 3 Evaluation of agreement between case report forms and patient reported data

Assessment	Follow-up (months)	No. (%)		Concordant pairs (%)	Agreement (95% CI)		Kappa (95% CI)	Gwet's AC1 (95% CI)	Odds of agreement (95% CI)
		CRF[a]	Questionnaire		Positive	Negative			
Swelling groin or lower extremities	3	46 (1)	805 (24)	2620/3385 (77)	0.10 (0.07; 0.13)	0.87 (0.86; 0.88)	0.08 (0.06;0.10)	0.71 (0.69; 0.73)	48 (17.6;200.4)
Complications and readmissions[b]	3	373 (10)	1041 (29)	2624/3556 (74)	0.34 (0.31; 0.37)	0.84 (0.83; 0.85)	0.22 (0.19;0.25)	0.62 (0.59; 0.64)	5.4 (4.3;6.8)
	12	187 (6)	479 (14)	2884/3334 (87)	0.32 (0.28; 0.37)	0.93 (0.92; 0.93)	0.27 (0.22;0.31)	0.84 (0.82; 0.85)	10.2 (7.5;14)
	24	195 (10)	245 (13)	1554/1884 (82)	0.25 (0.20; 0.30)	0.90 (0.89; 0.91)	0.15 (0.09;0.21)	0.78 (0.75; 0.81)	3.1 (2.2;4.4)
Reoperations	12	115 (4)	348 (11)	2877/3150 (91)	0.41 (0.35; 0.47)	0.95 (0.95; 0.96)	0.38 (0.32;0.43)	0.90 (0.89; 0.91)	52 (32;88)
	24	171 (8)	264 (13)	1877/2078 (90)	0.54 (0.48; 0.60)	0.95 (0.94; 0.95)	0.49 (0.43;0.55)	0.88 (0.86; 0.90)	26 (18;38)
Additional (chemo) radiotherapy after surgery or due to local recurrence or metastases	12	212 (7)	260 (8)	3084/3182 (97)	0.79 (0.75; 0.83)	0.98 (0.98; 0.99)	0.78 (0.73;0.82)	0.96 (0.96; 0.97)	297 (187;489)
	24	207 (7)	233 (8)	2721/2863 (95)	0.68 (0.63; 0.73)	0.97 (0.97; 0.98)	0.65 (0.60;0.70)	0.94 (0.93; 0.95)	79 (55;115)
Local recurrence and metastases	12	159 (5)	49 (2)	2739/2897 (95)	0.24 (0.16; 0.32)	0.97 (0.97; 0.98)	0.22 (0.14;0.30)	0.94 (0.93; 0.95)	21 (12;38)
	24	197 (7)	44 (2)	2643/2836 (93)	0.20 (0.13; 0.27)	0.96 (0.96; 0.97)	0.18 (0.11;0.25)	0.93 (0.92; 0.94)	18 (10;34)

[a] Case Report Form
[b] Reasons: Pain in surgical wound, lower or upper part of abdomen, bleeding from surgical would, urinary tract or catheter

Table 4 Evaluation of sensitivity and specificity of case report forms

Assessment	Follow-up (months)	Sensitivity (95% CI)	Specificity (95% CI)
Swelling groin or lower extremities	3	0.05 (0.04; 0.07)	0.99 (0.99; 1.00)
Complications and readmissions*	3	0.23 (0.21; 0.26)	0.95 (0.94; 0.96)
	12	0.23 (0.19; 0.26)	0.97 (0.97; 0.98)
	24	0.22 (0.17; 0.28)	0.91 (0.90; 0.93)
Reoperations	12	0.27 (0.23; 0.32)	0.99 (0.99; 1.00)
	24	0.44 (0.38; 0.50)	0.97 (0.96; 0.98)
Additional (chemo) radiotherapy after surgery or due to local recurrence or metastases	12	0.72 (0.66; 0.77)	0.99 (0.99; 0.99)
	24	0.64 (0.58; 0.70)	0.98 (0.97; 0.98)
Local recurrence and metastases	12	0.51 (0.37; 0.65)	0.95 (0.95; 0.96)
	24	0.55 (0.40; 0.69)	0.94 (0.93; 0.95)

* Reasons: Pain in surgical wound, lower or upper part of abdomen, bleeding from surgical would, urinary tract or catheter

Table 5 Re-admission within 3 months after surgery. Evaluation of agreement and sensitivity and specificity between patient registry and case report forms and patient reported data

Assessment	Concordant pairs (%)	Positive Agreement (95%)	Negative Agreement (95% CI)	Kappa (95% CI)	Gwet's AC1 (95% CI)	Odds of agreement (95% CI)	Sensitivity (95% CI)	Specificity (95% CI)
Questionnaire	2716 (73)	0.28 (0.25; 0.31)	0.84 (0.83; 0.85)	0.18 (0.15; 0.21)	0.89 (0.88; 0.90)	5.5 (4.3; 7.1)	0.66 (0.60; 0.71)	0.74 (0.72; 0.75)
Case report forms	3228 (91)	0.50 (0.45; 0.55)	0.95 (0.94; 0.96)	0.45 (0.40; 0.50)	0.61 (0.58; 0.65)	20.2 (15.3; 26.6)	0.58 (0.52; 0.64)	0.94 (0.93; 0.95)

to the questionnaire, whereas the questionnaire had a slightly higher sensitivity.

In our study some patient characteristics were found to be associated with agreement such as age, socioeconomic factors and depressed mood, which confirmed previous results [7, 13, 16]. Younger patients, who had no self-reported impairment in quality of life, depressed mood or negative intrusive thoughts, appear to report symptoms events more in agreement with those reported by clinical personnel. However, the association with medication (sleeping pills and/or tranquilizers) has not been previously reported as far as we know.

Table 6 Evaluation of patient characteristics associated with agreement between patient self-assessed questionnaires and case report forms

Variable	Comparison	Odds ratio (95% CI) [a]				
		Swelling groin or lower extremities	Complications and readmissions[b]	Reoperations	Postoperative (chemo) radiotherapy, local recurrence or metastases	Local recurrence and metastases
Education	No higher education vs Other	1.30 (0.70; 2.42)	0.86 (0.54; 1.38)	0.71 (0.28; 1.78)	1.46 (0.58; 3.67)	0.80 (0.29; 2.22)
	No higher education vs University	0.92 (0.77; 1.10)	1.05 (0.93; 1.18)	0.92 (0.74; 1.13)	0.83 (0.61; 1.12)	1.13 (0.89; 1.43)
	Other vs University	0.71 (0.38; 1.33)	1.22 (0.76; 1.96)	1.29 (0.51; 3.25)	0.57 (0.22; 1.44)	1.40 (0.51; 3.90)
Occupation	Other vs Retired	0.78 (0.59; 1.09)	0.83 (0.67; 1.03)	1.70 (1.05; 2.73)	2.19 (1.05; 4.54)	1.23 (0.79; 1.91)
	Other vs Working	0.80 (0.58; 1.10)	0.78 (0.63; 0.96)	1.44 (0.90; 2.32)	1.57 (0.76; 3.25)	0.75 (0.48; 1.18)
	Retired vs Working	1.02 (0.85; 1.23)	0.94 (0.83; 1.06)	0.85 (0.69; 1.05)	0.72 (0.54; 0.96)	0.62 (0.49; 0.78)
Marital status	Live apart vs Married/cohabiting	0.68 (0.49; 0.93)	0.98 (0.78; 1.23)	0.90 (0.60; 1.34)	0.98 (0.56; 1.71)	1.20 (0.75; 1.94)
	Live apart vs No partner	0.79 (0.52; 1.19)	1.07 (0.80; 1.43)	0.89 (0.53; 1.50)	0.86 (0.41; 1.80)	0.72 (0.37; 1.39)
	Married/cohabiting vs No partner	1.17 (0.87; 1.57)	1.10 (0.90; 1.34)	0.99 (0.68; 1.44)	0.86 (0.51; 1.50)	0.60 (0.37; 0.97)
Medication	Medication vs No medication	0.76 (0.59; 0.97)	0.72 (0.61; 0.85)	0.80 (0.60; 1.06)	0.55 (0.38; 0.79)	0.95 (0.68; 1.33)
Alcohol consumption	Little alcohol vs Much alcohol	0.89 (0.69; 1.16)	1.29 (1.09; 1.51)	1.08 (0.81; 1.46)	0.95 (0.63; 1.43)	1.28 (0.94; 1.75)
Quality of Life	Low QoL vs High QoL	0.68 (0.57; 0.81)	0.73 (0.65; 0.82)	0.84 (0.69; 1.03)	0.86 (0.65; 1.13)	0.88 (0.70; 1.11)
Depressed mood	Depressed mood vs No depressed mood	0.66 (0.49; 0.88)	0.70 (0.58; 0.85)	1.31 (0.87; 1.98)	0.2 (0.55; 1.52)	1.06 (0.69; 1.61)
Negative intrusive thoughs	Intrusive thoughts vs No intrusive thoughts	0.65 (0.55; 0.78)	0.71 (0.63; 0.80)	0.93 (0.75; 1.14)	0.66 (0.50; 0.88)	0.69 (0.55; 0.87)
Age	Increase in age by 25 years	0.82 (0.59; 1.13)	0.86 (0.67; 1.10)	0.49 (0.32; 0.74)	0.32 (0.18; 0.58)	0.46 (0.28; 0.77)
Postoperative Time trend	24 months vs 12 months	Not applicable	0.74 (0.64; 1.15)	0.89 (0.74; 0.93)	0.61 (0.47; 1.26)	0.78 (0.63; 1.02)

[a] Ratio of odds for agreement (positive or negative) between patients (questionnaire) and clinical report (case report form)

At later follow ups (12 and 24 months) the compliance in submitting clinical record forms was significantly lower compared with compliance regarding patient reports. One reason for this could be that part of the cohort was referred for surgery to a department of urology some, or even a long, distance from their home. This would be expected to result in a lower surgeon-patient physical follow-up (out-patients visit). Other contributing explanations could be that after 12 or 24 months the follow-up was not always by the operating urologist, and thus completion of the CRF may have been missed.

This study has both strengths and limitations. Strengths include the large study cohort, the longitudinal design, a high compliance of patients and the use of validated questionnaires [27]. Limitations include a lack of information of the specific personnel who completed the case report forms at the different visits and on the specific time periods the case report forms and questionnaires covered. Difficulties in being able to account for the longitudinal structure in the statistical model must be regarded as a limitation.

Conclusions

The differences in incidence and agreement across the different variables and time points highlight the importance of carefully assessing which source of information to use in clinical research. This study confirms the importance of using several measures to assess the degree of agreement between the sources. The previously reported benefits of Gwet's AC1 are confirmed and researchers should be encouraged to consider this method. In clinical research, much effort is often devoted to increasing patient response rates. However, preventing missing data in clinical reports also needs further attention. Long-term follow-up should make use of patient reports, as clinical record forms tend to be missed by the health care. As different patient characteristics were found to increase agreement, such background information is relevant for the choice of data collection procedure.

Abbreviations

CRF: Case Report Form; LAPPRO: Laparoscopic Prostatectomy Robot Open trial

Acknowledgements

The authors gratefully acknowledge the participants in the LAPPRO trial, the members of the steering committee, the investigators at the participating hospitals and the personnel at the trial secretariat for their provision of study material and administrative support.

Assar Gabrielsson's Foundation (FB 16–24, 17–18). These funds were used in the design of the study and collection, analysis, and interpretation of data and in writing the manuscript.

Authors' contributions

Contributors to the conception and design of the study, or acquisition of data, or analysis and interpretation of data: DB, EH, GS, AB, JH and PW; drafting the article or revising it critically for important intellectual content: DB, EA, AB, JH, GS, SW, PW and EH; final approval of the version to be submitted: DB, EA, AB, JH, GS, SW, PW and EH. DB takes responsibility that this study has been reported honestly, accurately and transparently; that no important aspects of the study have been omitted; and that any discrepancies from the study as planned have been explained.

Author details

[1]Department of Surgery, Institute of Clinical Sciences, Sahlgrenska Academy, University of Gothenburg, SSORG (Scandinavian Surgical Outcomes Research Group), Sahlgrenska University Hospital/Östra, 416 85 Gothenburg, Sweden. [2]Health Metrics Unit, Sahlgrenska Academy, University of Gothenburg, Gothenburg, Sweden. [3]Department of Urology, Skåne University Hospital, Malmö, Sweden. [4]Department of Urology, Institute of Clinical Sciences, Sahlgrenska Academy, University of Gothenburg, Sahlgrenska University Hospital, Gothenburg, Sweden. [5]Division of Clinical Cancer Epidemiology, Department of Oncology, Institute of Clinical Sciences, Sahlgrenska Academy, Gothenburg, Sweden. [6]Department of Molecular Medicine and Surgery, Section of Urology, Karolinska Institutet, Stockholm, Sweden.

References

1. Harlow SD, Linet MS. Agreement between questionnaire data and medical records. The evidence for accuracy of recall. Am J Epidemiol. 1989;129(2):233–48.
2. de Groot, V., et al., How to measure comorbidity. A critical review of available methods. J Clin Epidemiol, 2003. 56(3): p. 221–9.
3. Jones MP, et al. Concordance between Sources of Morbidity Reports: Self-Reports and Medical Records. Front Pharmacol. 2011;2:16.
4. Bush TL, et al. Self-report and medical record report agreement of selected medical conditions in the elderly. Am J Public Health. 1989;79(11):1554–6.
5. Haapanen N, et al. Agreement between questionnaire data and medical records of chronic diseases in middle-aged and elderly Finnish men and women. Am J Epidemiol. 1997;145(8):762–9.
6. Merkin SS, et al. Agreement of self-reported comorbid conditions with medical and physician reports varied by disease among end-stage renal disease patients. J Clin Epidemiol. 2007;60(6):634–42.
7. Corser W, et al. Concordance between comorbidity data from patient self-report interviews and medical record documentation. BMC Health Serv Res. 2008;8:85.
8. De-loyde KJ, et al. Which information source is best? Concordance between patient report, clinician report and medical records of patient co-morbidity and adjuvant therapy health information. J Eval Clin Pract. 2015;21(2):339–46.
9. Phillips KA, et al. Agreement between self-reported breast cancer treatment and medical records in a population-based breast Cancer family registry. J Clin Oncol. 2005;23(21):4679–86.
10. Wallerstedt A, et al. Short-term results after robot-assisted laparoscopic radical prostatectomy compared to open radical prostatectomy. Eur Urol. 2015;67(4):660–70.
11. Steineck G, et al. Symptom documentation in cancer survivors as a basis for therapy modifications. Acta Oncol. 2002;41(3):244–52.
12. Wallihan DB, Stump TE, Callahan CM. Accuracy of self-reported health services use and patterns of care among urban older adults. Med Care. 1999;37(7):662–70.
13. Raina P, et al. Agreement between self-reported and routinely collected health-care utilization data among seniors. Health Serv Res. 2002;37(3):751–74.
14. Clegg LX, et al. Comparison of self-reported initial treatment with medical records: results from the prostate cancer outcomes study. Am J Epidemiol. 2001;154(6):582–7.
15. Zhu K, et al. Comparison of self-report data and medical records data: results from a case-control study on prostate cancer. Int J Epidemiol. 1999;28(3):409–17.
16. Okura Y, et al. Agreement between self-report questionnaires and medical record data was substantial for diabetes, hypertension, myocardial infarction and stroke but not for heart failure. J Clin Epidemiol. 2004;57(10):1096–103.
17. Barber J, et al. Measuring morbidity: self-report or health care records? Fam Pract. 2010;27(1):25–30.

18. Cicchetti DV, Feinstein AR. High agreement but low kappa: II. Resolving the paradoxes. J Clin Epidemiol. 1990;43(6):551–8.
19. Zaki R, et al. Statistical methods used to test for agreement of medical instruments measuring continuous variables in method comparison studies: a systematic review. PLoS One. 2012;7(5).
20. Wongpakaran N, et al. A comparison of Cohen's kappa and Gwet's AC1 when calculating inter-rater reliability coefficients: a study conducted with personality disorder samples. BMC Med Res Methodol. 2013;(13):61.
21. Cohen J. A coefficient of agreement for nominal scales. Educ Psychol Meas. 1960;20(1):37–46.
22. Feinstein AR, Cicchetti DV. High agreement but low kappa. 1. The problems of theTwo paradoxes. J Clin Epidemiol. 1990;43(6):543–9.
23. Gwet KL. Kappa statistic is not satisfactory for assessing the extent of agreement between raters. Statistical Methods for Inter-Rater Reliability Assessment. 2002;1(6):1–6.
24. Gwet KL. Handbook of inter-rater reliability. 4 ed. In: Advanced analytics; 2010.
25. Tanner MA, Young MA. Modeling Agreement Among Raters. J Am Stat Assoc. 1985;80(389):175–80.
26. Agresti A. *Categorical data analysis*. 2 ed. Wiley series in probability and mathematical statistics. Hoboken, New Jersey: Wiley-Interscience; 2002.
27. Thorsteinsdottir T, et al. LAPPRO: a prospective multicentre comparative study of robot-assisted laparoscopic and retropubic radical prostatectomy for prostate cancer. Scand J Urol Nephrol. 2011;45(2):102–12.
28. Gospodarowicz MK, Brierly JD, Wittekind C. TNM classification of malignant Tumours: Wiley-Blackwell; 2017.
29. Johansson E, et al. Long-term quality-of-life outcomes after radical prostatectomy or watchful waiting: the Scandinavian prostate Cancer Group-4 randomised trial. Lancet Oncol. 2011;12(9):891–9.
30. Wallerstedt Lantz A, et al. 90-day readmission after radical prostatectomy - a prospective comparison between robot-assisted and open surgery. Scand J Urol. 2018; to appear.
31. Bock D, et al. Habits and self-assessed quality of life, negative intrusive thoughts and depressed mood in patients with prostate cancer: a longitudinal study. Scand J Urol. 2017;51(5):353–9.
32. Skoogh J, et al. 'A no means no'--measuring depression using a single-item question versus hospital anxiety and depression scale (HADS-D). Ann Oncol. 2010;21(9):1905–9.
33. Team RC. R: a language and environment for statistical computing. R Foundation for statistical computing. Vienna, Austria; 2018.
34. Mackinnon A. A spreadsheet for the calculation of comprehensive statistics for the assessment of diagnostic tests and inter-rater agreement. Comput Biol Med. 2000;30(3):127–34.
35. Skinner KM, et al. Concordance between respondent self-reports and medical records for chronic conditions: experience from the veterans health study. J Ambul Care Manage. 2005;28(2):102–10.
36. Katz JN, et al. Can comorbidity be measured by questionnaire rather than medical record review? Med Care. 1996;34(1):73–84.
37. Mansson A, et al. Neutral third party versus treating institution for evaluating quality of life after radical cystectomy. Eur Urol. 2004;46(2):195–9.
38. Litwin, M.S., et al., Differences in urologist and patient assessments of health related quality of life in men with prostate cancer: results of the CaPSURE database. J Urol, 1998. 159(6): p. 1988–92.
39. Sonn GA, et al. Differing perceptions of quality of life in patients with prostate Cancer and their doctors. J Urol. 2009;182:2296–302.
40. Svaboe Steinsvik EA, et al. Do perceptions of adverse events differ between patients and physicians? Findings from a randomized, controlled trial of radical treatment for prostate Cancer. J Urol. 2010;184:525–31.

13

Three novel methods to measure the postoperative displacement of lower urinary tract structures following radical prostatectomy in a sample of Korean patients

Hong Koo Ha[1,2,3], Henk B. Luiting[4,5], Petra L. Graham[6], Manish I. Patel[7,8], Jaspreet S. Sandhu[9], Oguz Akin[10] and Sean F. Mungovan[4,11,12*]

Abstract

Background: There is a change in the position of the remaining anatomical structures of the lower urinary tract system following radical prostatectomy. The aims of this investigation were to describe three novel methods used to measure the displacement of i) the vesico-urethral junction (VUJ), proximal membranous urethra (PMU) and anorectal junction (ARJ) and ii) the VUJ angle of displacement in men following radical prostatectomy and determine their intra- and interrater reliability.

Methods: Retrospective comparative measurement of twenty pre- and postoperative MRI scans was undertaken by one observer on two separate occasions and on one occasion by another observer. Three standardized midsagittal pelvimetry reference lines were used to describe three X, Y axis measurement systems. The displacement (mm) of the VUJ, PMU and ARJ, and the angle of displacement (degrees) of the VUJ was measured for each of the three methods. Interrater reliability of VUJ, PMU and ARJ displacement and the VUJ angle of displacement measurements was assessed using a two-way mixed-effects agreement intra-class correlation coefficient (ICC) with 95% confidence intervals (CI). Test-retest (intrarater) reliability was calculated using a two-way random effects consistency ICC with 95% CI for all displacement measures of the VUJ, PMU and ARJ for one observer between two days.

Results: The pubococcygeal line (PCL) axis measurement system demonstrated good to excellent intrarater and interrater reliability (ICC 95% interval lower bound > 0.75) for the VUJ and PMU displacement and the VUJ angle of displacement measurements. Other measurement systems were less reliable and more variable.

Conclusions: In this sample of 20 Korean patients with median prostate volume 27.5 mL and maximum volume 70 mL, the measurement methodology using the PCL consistently demonstrated good to excellent reliability and the lowest variability for the measurement of the displacement of the VUJ and PMU and the VUJ angle of displacement. The PCL methodology is recommended as the method of choice. Further studies should validate these results in patients with large prostate volumes.

Keywords: Displacement, Measurement, Reliability, Urethra, Urinary tract, Magnetic resonance imaging

* Correspondence: sean.mungovan@crinstitute.com.au
[4]The Clinical Research Institute, Sydney, Australia
[11]Westmead Private Physiotherapy Services, Westmead Private Hospital, Suite 6, 16-18 Mons Road, Westmead, NSW 2145, Australia
Full list of author information is available at the end of the article

Background

Radical prostatectomy (RP) is the primary surgical option for men with localised prostate cancer, providing definitive oncologic control. Following removal of the prostate gland, the position and function of the remaining anatomical structures of the lower urinary tract system are known to change. Typically, there is inferior displacement of the vesiculo-urethral junction (VUJ) and the intrapelvic displacement of the proximal membranous urethral stump (PMU), that allows for the formation of the urethrovesicular anastomosis [1, 2]. Despite modifications and improvements in the surgical technique, postoperative impairments of the lower urinary tract system, including urinary incontinence and erectile dysfunction occur in the majority of patients [3, 4].

Pre- and postoperative magnetic resonance imaging (MRI) can provide clinicians with high resolution and sharp depiction of the anatomical structures of the lower urinary tract system that are displaced following RP, including the VUJ, PMU and periprostatic structures such as the anorectal junction (ARJ) [5–8]. Preoperative MRI pelvimetry assessment has been used for surgical planning and to investigate the relationship between the position of the prostate and oncologic outcomes [9, 10]. Postoperative MRI pelvimetry assessment has reported lower urinary tract morphological changes within the pelvis in relation to continence outcomes [6, 7, 11, 12]. Similarly, using pre- and postoperative MRI images, changes in the size of anatomical structures including the membranous urethral length and variations in the thickness of the pelvic floor musculature following RP have also been reported [6, 7].

Quantifying the reliability of postoperative displacement (mm) of the VUJ, PMU and the ARJ and the direction of displacement (degrees) of the VUJ will allow the selection of the preferred measurement method for use in studies of the post-surgical displacement of anatomical structures and its relationship with urinary incontinence and erectile dysfunction. To our knowledge a reliability study of methods for measurement of anatomical displacement has not been reported.

In this investigation, we describe and assess the reliability of three new methods to measure the postoperative displacement of the VUJ, PMU and ARJ, and the postoperative angle of displacement of the VUJ.

Methods

The aim of this investigation was to examine the test-retest and inter-rater reliability of three novel MRI measurements of postsurgical displacement of lower urinary tract structures.

Patients

Following Pusan National University ethical approval (H-1707-009-057), we reviewed the pre-and three month postoperative MRI examinations of twenty randomly selected patients who underwent laparoscopic bladder neck sparing RP performed by a single surgeon (HKH). A simple random sample of patients was selected by using a computer to randomly shuffle identification numbers, then the first twenty numbers in the shuffled list were selected. Patient characteristics including age (years), preoperative prostate specific antigen (ng/mL), prostate volume (mL), membranous urethral length (MUL, mm) and Gleason grade grouping were recorded.

Magnetic resonance imaging

Pre- and postoperative sagittal, axial and coronal T2W MRI images were captured using a 1.5 T or 3 T MRI unit (Magnetrom Symphony; Siemens, Erlangen, Germany) with the patient positioned in the supine position.

We undertook the measurement of the pre- and postoperative MRI images for each patient using three standardised MRI measuring methods i) pubococcygeal line (PCL), ii) midsagittal horizontal line one (HOR-1) and iii) midsagittal horizontal line two (HOR- 2) (Fig. 1).

The measurement procedures were undertaken independently by two observers: on two separate occasions by one observer (HBL) and on a single occasion by another observer (SFM). Each of the three MRI measuring methods was used to conduct pelvimetry measurements of the postoperative displacement (mm) of the VUJ, PMU and the ARJ and the postoperative angle of displacement VUJ within the pelvic cavity.

Pelvimetry measurements

Reference Lines

Pre- and postoperative PCL [13], HOR-1 and HOR- 2 [14] provided separate X, Y axis systems for each respective MRI measuring method (Fig. 1)

Anatomical Landmarks

The VUJ, PMU and ARJ were identified on the pre- and postoperative T2W midsagittal MRI images (Fig. 2). T2W coronal and axial images were used to confirm the position of the VUJ, PMU and ARJ on the midsagittal images.

VUJ

The preoperative VUJ was located at the bladder neck and was defined as the midpoint between the ventral and dorsal aspect of the VUJ (Fig. 2a). The postoperative VUJ was located at the most distal section of the bladder neck at the urethrovesicular anastomosis (Fig. 2b).

PMU

The preoperative PMU was located at the junction between the membranous urethra and the apex of the prostate (Fig. 2a), and the postoperative PMU was

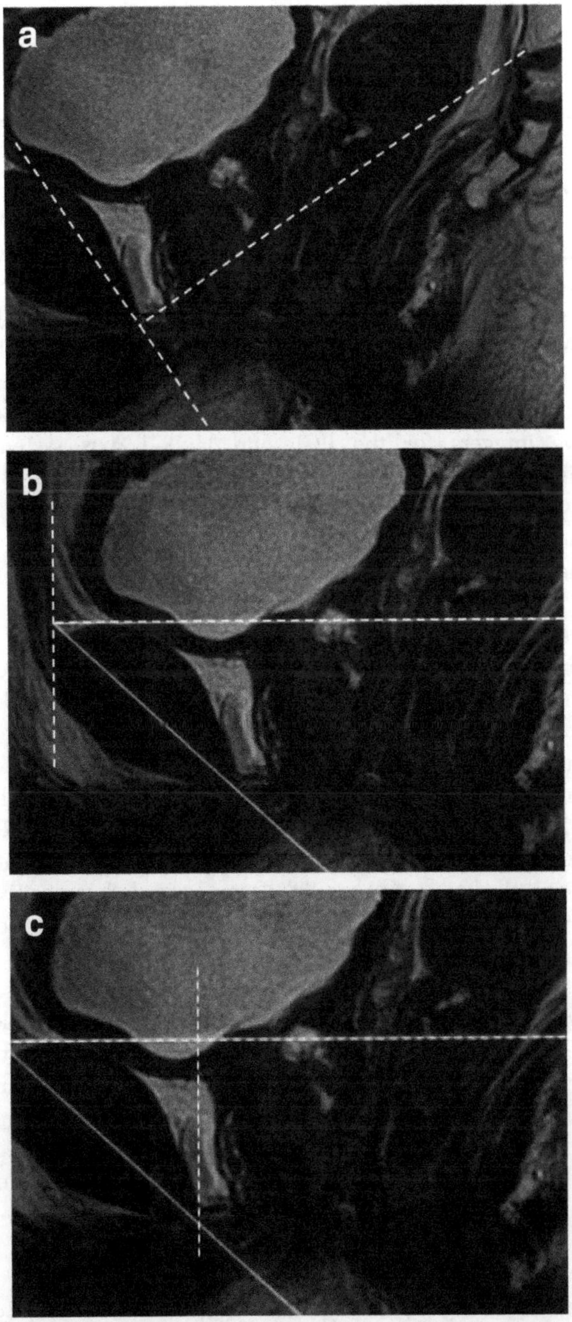

Fig. 1 The three common axis systems that were investigated. **a** The pubococcygeal line (PCL) axis system was comprised of the line formed between the inferior rim of the pubic symphysis and the sacrococcygeal joint (PCL line) (X) and the perpendicular line to the PCL at the inferior rim of the pubic symphysis (Y). **b** The HOR-1 axis system was comprised of the horizontal line of the symphysis angle (X) and the line perpendicular to the horizontal line at the symphysis angle (Y). **c** The HOR-2 axis system was comprised of the horizontal line of the symphysis angle (X) and the line perpendicular to the horizontal line at the inferior rim of the pubic symphysis (Y)

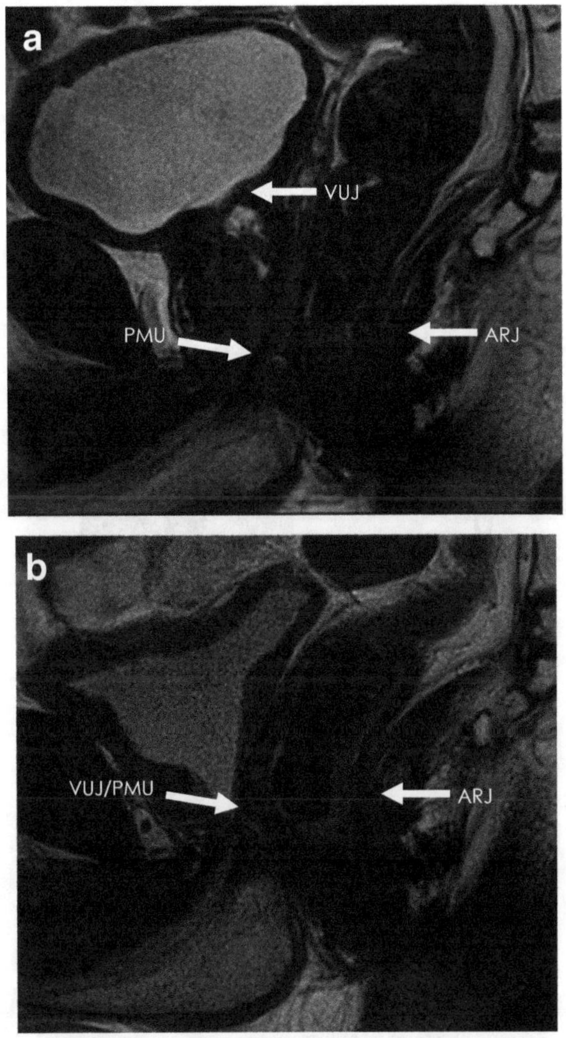

Fig. 2 The **a**) preoperative and **b**) postoperative T2W midsagittal MRI images showing the VUJ, PMU and ARJ anatomical landmarks

defined as the most proximal section of the membranous urethra at the VUJ (Fig. 2b).

ARJ

The ARJ was defined as the point of transition between the posterior wall of the rectum and the posterior wall of the anal canal. The ARJ was identified where there was an abrupt change in the orientation of the posterior wall of the rectum and the anal canal, where the puborectalis muscle could also be identified (Figs. 2a and b).

Pelvimetry X, Y axis system measurements

The pre- and postoperative horizontal and vertical positions of the VUJ, PMU and ARJ for the PCL (Fig. 3), HOR-1 (Fig. 4) and HOR-2 (Fig. 5) using the X, Y axis systems were determined.

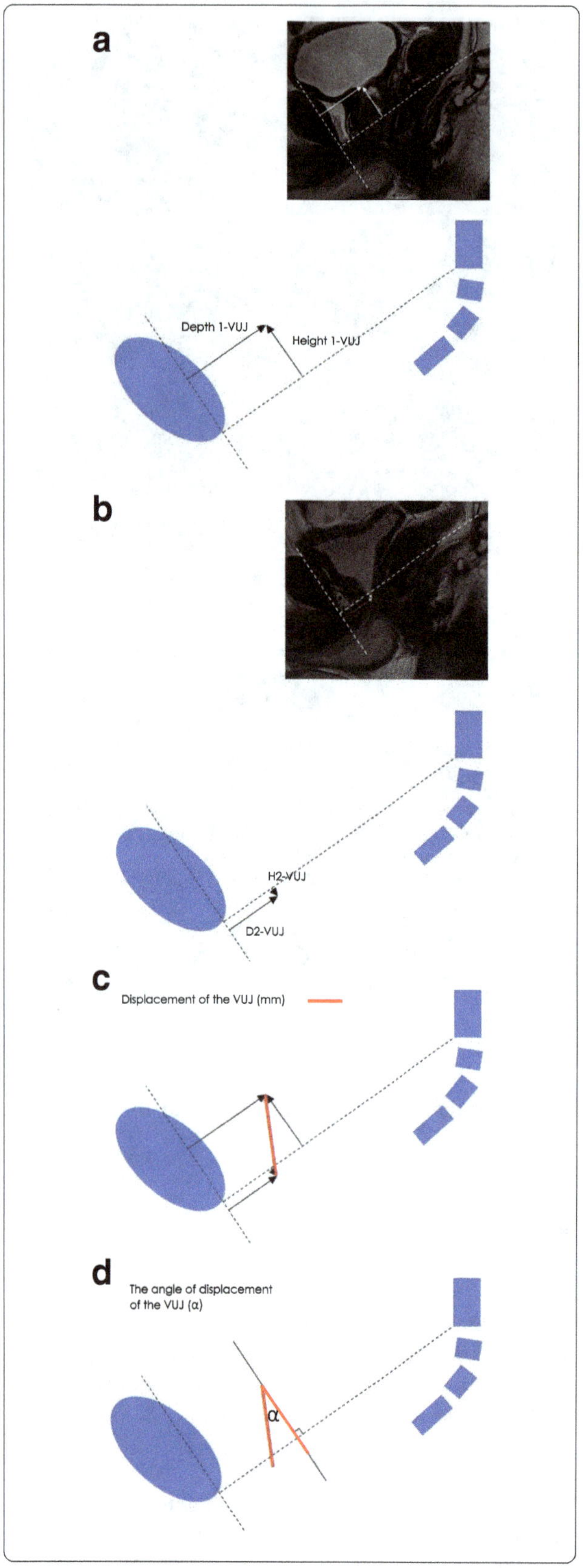

Fig. 3 PCL Axis System: The **a**) preoperative VUJ (Depth 1-VUJ and Height 1-VUJ), **b**) postoperative VUJ (Depth 2-VUJ and Height 2-VUJ) **c**) VUJ postoperative displacement **d**) postoperative angle of displacement

X Axis

The horizontal measurement along each X axis reference line, i.e. the depth within the pelvis from the pubic symphysis was measured (mm). The pre- and postoperative depth of the VUJ (Depth 1-VUJ and Depth 2-VUJ), PMU (Depth 1-PMU and Depth 2-PMU) and the ARJ (Depth 1-ARJ and Depth 2-ARJ) were measured. The X axis measurements of Depth 1 and Depth 2 were positive integers for the PCL and HOR-1 axis systems (Figs. 3, 4). Depth 1 and Depth 2 measurements for the HOR-2 X axis were negative integers when anterior to the perpendicular Y axis and positive when posterior to the perpendicular Y axis (Fig. 5).

Y Axis

The vertical measurements along each Y axis reference line, i.e. the height within the pelvis perpendicular to the X axis reference line, were measured (mm). The pre- and the postoperative height of the VUJ (Height 1-VUJ and Height 2-VUJ), PMU (Height 1-PMU and Height 2-PMU) and the ARJ (Height 1-ARJ and Height 2-ARJ) were measured. Height 1 and Height 2 measurements above all three reference lines were recorded as positive integers and measurements below the three reference lines were recorded as negative integers (Figs. 3, 4, 5).

Standard DICOM viewer software (Intelerad Medical Systems, Canada) was used for all VUJ, PMU and ARJ depth (X axis) and height (Y axis) measurements. Training was given to members of the investigating team (SFM and HL) by an experienced radiologist (OA) and three urologists (HKH, JSS and MIP). The observers (SFM and HL) were blinded to all identifiable patient data when undertaking all measurements.

Postoperative displacement calculation

The following equation was developed to measure the postoperative displacement (mm) of the VUJ, PMU and ARJ for the PCL, HOR-1 and HOR-2 axis systems:

$$\text{Displacement (mm)} = \sqrt{(\,Depth\ 1\text{–}Depth\ 2)^2 + (Height\ 1\text{–}Height\ 2)^2}$$

Depth 1 = Preoperative depth (mm) of the VUJ (Depth 1-VUJ), PMU (Depth 1-PMU) and ARJ (Depth 1-ARJ); Depth 2 = Postoperative depth (mm) of the VUJ (Depth 2-VUJ), PMU (Depth 2-MU) and ARJ (Depth 2-ARJ); Height 1 = Preoperative height (mm) of the VUJ (Height 1-VUJ), PMU (Height 1-PMU) and ARJ (Height 1-ARJ);

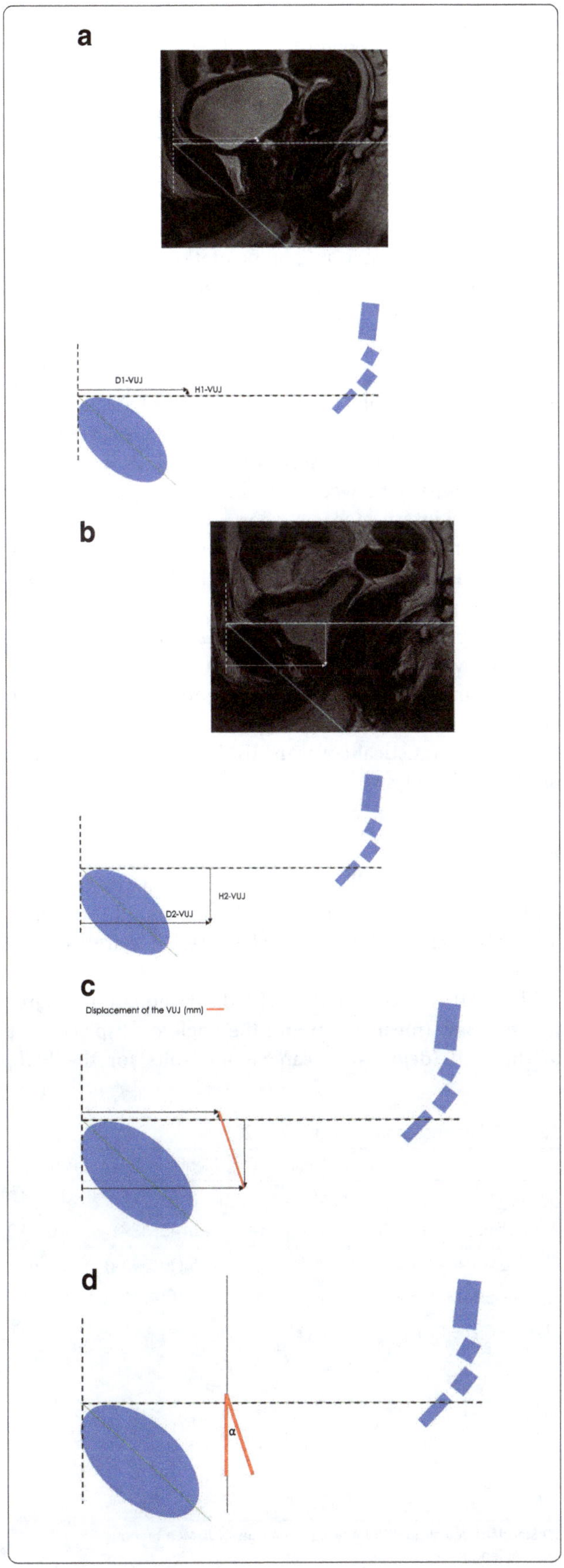

Fig. 4 HOR-1 Axis System: The **a**) preoperative VUJ (Depth 1-VUJ and Height 1-VUJ), **b**) postoperative VUJ (Depth 2-VUJ and Height 2-VUJ) **c**) VUJ postoperative displacement **d**) postoperative angle of displacement

Height 2 = Postoperative height (mm) of the VUJ (Height 2-VUJ), PMU (Height 2-PMU) and ARJ (Height 2-ARJ).

Postoperative angle of displacement calculation

The postoperative angle of displacement (α) of the VUJ was calculated as the angle that was formed between the intersection of two lines: i) the line connecting preoperative and postoperative position of the VUJ and ii) the perpendicular line from the preoperative position of the VUJ to either the PCL, HOR-1 or HOR-2 (Figs. 3, 4, 5). The postoperative angle of displacement (α) of the VUJ was calculated for each of the three reference lines using the following equation.

$$\text{VUJ Angle of displacement } (\alpha) = -\tan^{-1}\frac{(\text{Depth 1–VUJ}) - (\text{Depth 2–VUJ})}{(\text{Height 1–VUJ}) - (\text{Height 2–VUJ})}$$

Depth 1-VUJ = Preoperative depth of the VUJ (mm); Depth 2-VUJ = Postoperative depth of the VUJ (mm); Height 1-VUJ = Preoperative height of the VUJ (mm); Height 2-VUJ = Postoperative depth of the VUJ (mm).

The postoperative position of the VUJ is always inferior to the preoperative position i.e. the VUJ is deeper within the pelvis following RP surgery. The postoperative position of the VUJ can be either anterior or posterior relative to the preoperative position. When Depth 1-VUJ > Depth 2-VUJ, the angle of displacement of the VUJ following RP occurs in an anterior direction. When Depth 1-VUJ < Depth 2-VUJ, the angle of displacement following RP is in a posterior direction. When D1-VUJ > D2-VUJ the angle of displacement was recorded as a negative angle to describe the angle of displacement in an anterior direction. When Depth 1-VUJ < Depth 2-VUJ, the angle of displacement was recorded as a positive angle to describe the angle of displacement.

Statistical analysis

Means and standards deviations (SD) and/or medians with interquartile range (IQR) and range were used to describe continuous variables. Categorical variables were summarised using count with percentage (%) for each group. Kolmogorov-Smirnov tests [15] were used to check the normality of the displacement measures and the angle of displacement. Because of the multiple tests

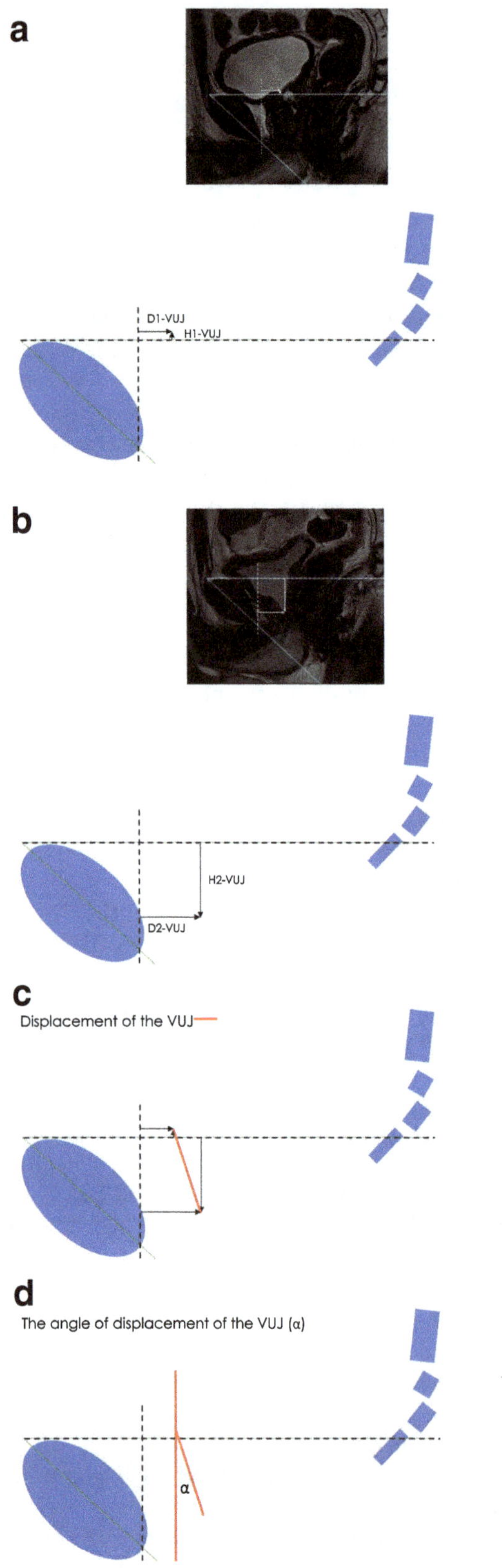

Fig. 5 HOR-2 Axis System: The **a**) preoperative VUJ (Depth 1-VUJ and Height 1-VUJ), **b**) postoperative VUJ (Depth 2-VUJ and Height 2-VUJ) **c**) VUJ postoperative displacement **d**) postoperative angle of displacement

a more stringent significance level of 0.01 was used for these tests. Interrater reliability of the VUJ, PMU and ARJ displacement measurements and the VUJ angle of displacement measurement was performed using a two-way mixed-effects agreement intra-class correlation coefficient (ICC) with 95% confidence intervals (CI). Test-retest (intrarater) reliability was calculated using two-way random-effects consistency ICC with 95% CI for all displacement measures of the VUJ, PMU and ARJ for one observer between two different days. Calculated ICC's were interpreted as: poor < 0.5, moderate 0.5 to 0.75, good 0.75 to 0.9 and excellent > 0.9 [16]. Using methods described by Walter et al. [17], with two raters (or two repeated measurements), a 5% significance level and 80% power to detect a hypothesised poor reliability (0.4, say) versus an alternative good reliability (0.8, say), a minimum sample size of 16 patients was needed. We decided to use a slightly larger sample size of 20 patients. The statistical software IBM SPSS version 24 was used for all analyses.

Results

Twenty patients, all of whom had laparoscopic RP underwent both preoperative and three-month postoperative MRI scans. The patient characteristics are listed in Table 1.

The VUJ, PMU and the ARJ displacement measurements (mm) (mean ± SD) and the angle of displacement of the VUJ (degrees) (mean ± SD) results for the PCL,

Table 1 Patient Characteristics (*n* = 20)

	Mean ± SD	Median (IQR)	Range
Age (years)	66.4 ± 5.5	66.5 (63.0, 71.5)	53.0–74.0
Preoperative PSA (ng.mL^{-1})	15.4 ± 23.4	7.0 (4.2, 13.4)	3.0–94.0
Prostate volume (mL)	30.7 ± 13.2	27.5 (20.6, 32.4)	16.5–69.3
Preoperative MUL (mm)	13.4 ± 3.5	12.8 (12.2, 15.4)	6.8–20.5
Gleason Grade Group	n (%)		
1	7 (35)		
2	4 (20)		
3	6 (30)		
4	1 (5)		
5	2 (10)		

SD Standard deviation, *IQR* Interquartile range, *MUL* Membranous urethral length

Table 2 The mean ± SD displacement (mm) of VUJ, PMU and ARJ and VUJ angle of displacement (degrees) measured using the pubococcygeal axis (PCL), HOR-1 and HOR-2 axis reference systems in 20 men following RP

	VUJ Displacement (mm)		PMU Displacement (mm)		ARJ Displacement (mm)		VUJ Angle of displacement (degrees)	
	Day 1	Day 2	Day 1	Day 2	Day 1	Day 2	Day 1	Day 2
PCL axis system								
Observer 1	34.1 ± 4.3	33.7 ± 4.7	4.1 ± 2.1	4.0 ± 1.6	3.5 ± 2.5	4.1 ± 2.6	−16.9 ± 11.6	−16.3 ± 11.4
Observer 2	33.9 ± 4.9		4.7 ± 2.0		4.4 ± 2.5		−16.8 ± 11.0	
HOR-1 axis system								
Observer 1	34.9 ± 4.4	34.4 ± 4.6	4.2 ± 2.3	4.6 ± 2.2	4.0 ± 2.0	3.7 ± 1.9	13.9 ± 10.7	12.7 ± 11.0
Observer 2	34.7 ± 5.0		5.3 ± 2.3		5.1 ± 2.6		11.8 ± 12.2	
HOR-2 axis system								
Observer 1	34.8 ± 4.3	34.6 ± 4.9	4.0 ± 2.0	3.7 ± 1.9	3.9 ± 2.2	4.6 ± 2.5	13.0 ± 11.1	13.6 ± 11.1
Observer 2	34.8 ± 5.1		4.2 ± 2.2		4.4 ± 2.44		13.6 ± 10.8	

VUJ Vesico-urethral junction, *PMU* Proximal membranous urethra, *ARJ* anorectal junction, *PCL axis system*: Pubococcygeal line axis system, *HOR-1 axis system*: Horizontal line 1 axis system, *HOR-2 axis system*: Horizontal line 2 axis system

HOR-1 and HOR-2 axis systems are presented in Table 2. None of these measures showed evidence of non-normality using the more stringent significance level because of multiple testing ($p > 0.02$).

The ICC (95% CI) results for the PCL, HOR-1 and HOR-2 axis systems are presented in Table 3. The PCL axis measurement system demonstrated good to excellent intrarater and interrater reliability for the VUJ and PMU displacement and the VUJ angle of displacement measurements. The intrarater and interrater reliability of the ARJ displacement measures was the most variable with intervals ranging from poor to excellent reliability across the three axis systems. Table 4 shows that the HOR-1 measurements are consistently more variable than the PCL and HOR-2 measurements except for the VUJ displacement. Small differences in variability were observed between PCL and HOR-2 measurements though the variability in PCL measurements was smallest of all of the measurement systems.

Discussion

This study has addressed the reliability of three new methods that can potentially be used to calculate the postoperative displacement of the VUJ, PMU and ARJ and the VUJ angle of displacement via the comparative measurement of pre- and postoperative MRI scans. Excellent reliability was demonstrated for the VUJ and PMU displacement measures and the VUJ angle of displacement for the PCL and HOR-2 measurement systems. The reliability of ARJ displacement measurements was highly variable regardless of the measurement system that was selected.

The displacement of the VUJ and PMU is an outcome of RP surgery. The newly formed urethrovesical anastomosis is created when traction is applied to the VUJ and PMU. The measurement of the VUJ and PMU anatomical change in position within the pelvis was possible by the incorporation of an X, Y axis system using standardized and previously reported pelvimetry reference lines

Table 3 Intra- and interrater reliability with 95% confidence interval (CI) for the measurement of displacement of the VUJ, PMU and ARJ (mm) and the VUJ angle of displacement (degrees)

	VUJ Displacement (mm)	PMU Displacement (mm)	ARJ Displacement (mm)	VUJ Angle of displacement (degrees)
Intrarater Reliability ICC (95%CI) Day 1 vs Day 2				
PCL axis system	0.97 (0.93, 0.99)	0.93 (0.84, 0.97)	0.78 (0.53, 0.91)	0.99 (0.98, 1.00)
HOR-1 axis system	0.96 (0.90, 0.99)	0.80 (0.58, 0.92)	0.71 (0.38, 0.88)	0.96 (0.89, 0.98)
HOR-2 axis system	0.96 (0.91, 0.99)	0.89 (0.74, 0.95)	0.78 (0.51, 0.91)	0.99 (0.97, 1.00)
Interrater Reliability ICC (95%CI) Observer 1 vs Observer 2				
PCL axis system	0.97 (0.93, 0.99)	0.89 (0.75, 0.96)	0.84 (0.63, 0.93)	0.99 (0.96, 0.99)
HOR-1 axis system	0.94 (0.85, 0.98)	0.64 (0.26, 0.83)	0.60 (0.22, 0.82)	0.95 (0.87, 0.98)
HOR-2 axis system	0.94 (0.86, 0.98)	0.85 (0.67, 0.94)	0.76 (0.48, 0.9)	0.98 (0.95, 0.99)

VUJ Urethrovesicular junction, *PMU* Proximal membranous urethra, *ARJ* anorectal junction, *ICC* Intra-class correlation coefficient, *CI* confidence interval, *PCL* axis system: Pubococcygeal line axis system, *HOR-1 axis system*: Horizontal line 1 axis system, *HOR-2 axis system*: Horizontal line 2 axis system

Table 4 Mean ± SD of the differences between and within raters for the measures of displacement of the VUJ, PMU and ARJ (mm) and the VUJ angle of displacement (degrees)

	VUJ Displacement mm	PMU Displacement (mm)	ARJ Displacement (mm)	VUJ Angle of displacement (degrees)
Mean difference within Observer 1 measurements. Day 1 vs Day 2				
PCL axis system	−0.3 ± 1.0	−0.1 ± 0.7	0.6 ± 1.6	0.6 ± 1.5
HOR-1 axis system	− 0.5 ± 1.1	0.4 ± 1.4	0.9 ± 1.7	−1.2 ± 3.1
HOR-2 axis system	−0.2 ± 1.3	−0.3 ± 0.9	0.6 ± 1.5	0.8 ± 1.3
Mean difference between Observer 1 and Observer 2 measurements				
PCL axis system	0.2 ± 1.1	0.5 ± 0.9	0.8 ± 1.4	0.0 ± 2.0
HOR-1 axis system	0.2 ± 1.6	1.1 ± 2.0	0.8 ± 2.3	−2.0 ± 3.7
HOR-2 axis system	0.0 ± 1.6	−0.2 ± 1.3	0.5 ± 1.6	0.8 ± 2.2

VUJ Vesiculo-urethral junction, *PMU* Proximal membranous urethra, *ARJ* anorectal junction, *PCL* axis system: Pubococcygeal line axis system, *HOR-1 axis system* Horizontal line 1 axis system, *HOR-2 axis system* Horizontal line 2 axis system

[13, 14]. To achieve reliable and reproducible comparative measurement of the lower urinary tract system [18] we used fixed anatomical structures that serve as stable reference points. The pelvic bony structures, including the pubic symphysis and the sacrococcygeal joint appear as clearly defined anatomical structures on T2W midsagittal MRI images.

The PCL, HOR-1 and HOR-2 MRI measuring systems all use the inferior edge of the pubic symphysis as a common stable bony point of reference [13, 14]. The PCL MRI measuring system has an advantage compared to the HOR-1 and HOR-2 MRI measuring systems by having the sacrococcygeal joint as the second stable bony point of reference. This may have been a contributing factor to the more consistent and reliable PCL measurements. The PCL has been previously used to measure the position of pelvic organs in men prior to and following RP and is related to urinary incontinence outcomes [12]. A potential limitation to the application of the PCL MRI measuring system occurs when the field of view for pre- and postoperative pelvic MRI images does not capture a clearly defined sacrococcygeal joint. Anatomical variations in the structure of the sacrococcygeal region, including fusion of the sacrococcygeal joint may potentially make accurate identification problematic [19]. The HOR-2 measurement system could be then used to provide an alternate approach when use of the PCL measurement system is not possible.

We acknowledge some limitations of this investigation. This study was a retrospective design involving a sample of twenty patients from a single facility in Korea and single surgeon series. While the sample size was small, a larger than required sample size was used. Increasing the sample size further was not possible due to time constraints and limited resources. The patient characteristics from this sample were similar to those observed in other studies [20–22] suggesting a reasonable range of anatomical variability was observed however it is possible that the results are not generalisable beyond the population studied. Larger studies that include, in particular, more patients with large prostate volumes, may provide valuable additional information regarding all measuring systems.

Conclusions

Comparative measurement of pre- and postoperative MRI scans can be used to assess the reliability of measurement of the displacement of the vesico-urethral junction and proximal membranous urethra, and the angle of displacement of the vesico-urethral junction in men following radical prostatectomy. In this study of 20 Korean patients with median prostate volume 27.5 mL and maximum volume 70 mL, the pubococcygeal line measurement system was preferred, providing the smallest differences in variability to quantify of the postoperative displacement of the anatomical structures that can affect urinary incontinence and erectile dysfunction following RP. Further studies should validate these results in patients with large prostate volumes.

Abbreviations

ARJ: Anorectal junction; BU: Penile bulb; CI: Confidence interval; Depth 1: Preoperative depth from either the PCL, HOR-1 or HOR-2 reference line; Depth 2: Postoperative depth from either the PCL, HOR-1 or HOR-2 reference line; Height 1 – ARJ: Preoperative height of the anorectal junction from either the PCL, HOR-1 or HOR-2 reference lines; Height 1 – PMU: Preoperative height of the proximal membranous urethra from either the PCL, HOR-1 or HOR-2 reference lines; Height 1 – VUJ: Preoperative height of the VUJ from either the PCL, HOR-1 or HOR-2 reference line; Height 1: Preoperative perpendicular distance from the PCL, HOR-1 or HOR-2 reference lines; Height 2 – ARJ: Postoperative height of the anorectal junction from either the PCL, HOR-1 or HOR-2 reference lines; Height 2 – PMU: Postoperative height of the proximal membranous urethra from either the PCL, HOR-1 or HOR-2 reference lines; Height 2 – VUJ: Postoperative height of the VUJ from either the PCL, HOR-1 or HOR-2 reference line; Height 2: Postoperative perpendicular height from either the PCL, HOR-1 or HOR-2 reference lines; HOR-1: Midsagittal horizontal line axis 1; HOR-2: Midsagittal horizontal line axis 2; ICC: Intraclass correlation coefficient; MRI: Magnetic resonance imaging; MUL: Membranous urethral length; PCL: Pubococcygeal line; PMU: Proximal membranous urethra; PV: Prostate volume; VUJ: Vesico-urethrol junction

Acknowledgements
Feedback on the manuscript was given by Prof Gregory C. Gass and support for completion of the research was given by C. Skowron and K. Sterns.

Authors' contributions
H-K.H.: Project development and manuscript writing; H.B.L.: Project development, data management, data analysis, manuscript writing; P.L.G.: Project development, statistical data analysis and manuscript writing, editing and revisions. M.I.P.: Project development and manuscript writing; J.S.S: Project development and manuscript writing; O.A.: Project development and manuscript writing; S.F.M.: Project development, data management, data analysis and manuscript writing, editing and revisions. All authors read and approved the final version of the manuscript.

Author details
[1]Department of Urology, Pusan National University Hospital, Busan, South Korea. [2]Pusan National University School of Medicine, Busan, South Korea. [3]Biomedical Research Institute, Pusan National University Hospital, Busan, South Korea. [4]The Clinical Research Institute, Sydney, Australia. [5]Faculty of Medical Sciences, University of Groningen, Groningen, The Netherlands. [6]Centre for Economic Impacts of Genomic Medicine (GenIMPACT), Macquarie University, Sydney, Australia. [7]Department of Urology, Westmead Hospital, Sydney, Australia. [8]Discipline of Surgery, Sydney Medical School, The University of Sydney, Sydney, Australia. [9]Urology Service, Department of Surgery, Memorial Sloan- Kettering Cancer Center, New York, USA. [10]Department of Radiology, Memorial Sloan- Kettering Cancer Center, New York, USA. [11]Westmead Private Physiotherapy Services, Westmead Private Hospital, Suite 6, 16-18 Mons Road, Westmead, NSW 2145, Australia. [12]Department of Health Professions, Faculty of Health, Arts and Design, Swinburne University of Technology, Melbourne, Australia.

References

1. Allen SD, Thompson A, Sohaib SA. The normal post-surgical anatomy of the male pelvis following radical prostatectomy as assessed by magnetic resonance imaging. Eur Radiol. 2008;18(6):1281–91.
2. Kadono Y, Machioka K, Nakashima K, Iijima M, Shigehara K, Nohara T, et al. Changes in penile length after radical prostatectomy: investigation of the underlying anatomical mechanism. BJU Int. 2017;120(2):293–9.
3. Carlsson S, Drevin L, Loeb S, Widmark A, Lissbrant IF, Robinson D, et al. Population-based study of long-term functional outcomes after prostate cancer treatment. BJU Int. 2016;117(6B):E36–45.
4. Mungovan SF, Huijbers BP, Hirschhorn AD, Patel MI. What makes men leak? An investigation of objective and self-report measures of urinary incontinence early after radical prostatectomy. Neurourol Urodyn. 2016; 35(2):225–9.
5. Coakley FV, Eberhardt S, Kattan MW, Wei DC, Scardino PT, Hricak H. Urinary continence after radical retropubic prostatectomy: relationship with membranous urethral length on preoperative endorectal magnetic resonance imaging. J Urol. 2002;168(3):1032–5.
6. Song W, Kim CK, Park BK, Jeon HG, Jeong BC, Seo SI, et al. Impact of preoperative and postoperative membranous urethral length measured by 3 tesla magnetic resonance imaging on urinary continence recovery after robotic-assisted radical prostatectomy. Can Urol Assoc J. 2017;11(3–4):E93–E9.
7. Sohn DW, Hong CK, Chung DJ, Kim SH, Kim SJ, Chung J, et al. Pelvic floor musculature and bladder neck changes before and after continence recovery after radical prostatectomy in pelvic MRI. J Magn Reson Imaging. 2014;39(6):1431–5.
8. Mungovan SF, Sandhu JS, Akin O, Smart NA, Graham PL, Patel MI. Preoperative membranous urethral length measurement and continence recovery following radical prostatectomy: a systematic review and meta-analysis. Eur Urol. 2017;71(3):368 78.
9. Matikainen MP, von Bodman CJ, Secin FP, Yunis LH, Vora K, Guillonneau B, et al. The depth of the prostatic apex is an independent predictor of positive apical margins at radical prostatectomy. BJU Int. 2010;106(5):622–6.
10. Hong SK, Lee ST, Kim SS, Min KE, Hwang IS, Kim M, et al. Effect of bony pelvic dimensions measured by preoperative magnetic resonance imaging on performing robot-assisted laparoscopic prostatectomy. BJU Int. 2009; 104(5):664–8.
11. Haga N, Ogawa S, Yabe M, Akaihata H, Hata J, Sato Y, et al. Factors contributing to early recovery of urinary continence analyzed by pre- and postoperative pelvic anatomical features at robot-assisted laparoscopic radical prostatectomy. J Endourol. 2015;29(6):683–90.
12. Soljanik I, Bauer RM, Becker AJ, Stief CG, Gozzi C, Solyanik O, et al. Is a wider angle of the membranous urethra associated with incontinence after radical prostatectomy? World J Urol. 2014;32(6):1375–83.
13. Madill S, Tang A, Pontbriand-Drolet S, Dumoulin C. Comparison of two methods for measuring the pubococcygeal line from sagittal-plane magnetic resonance imaging. Neurourol Urodyn. 2011;30(8):1613–9.
14. von Bodman C, Matikainen MP, Yunis LH, Laudone V, Scardino PT, Akin O, et al. Ethnic variation in pelvimetric measures and its impact on positive surgical margins at radical prostatectomy. Urology. 2010;76(5):1092–6.
15. Hollander M, Wolfe DA, Chicken E. Nonparametric statistical methods. Third edition/ed. Hoboken, New Jersey: John Wiley & Sons, Inc.; 2014. xiii, 819 pages p.
16. Portney L, Watkins M. Foundations of clinical research: applications to practice. New Jersey: Prentice Hall; 2000.
17. Walter SD, Eliasziw M, Donner A. Sample size and optimal designs for reliability studies. Stat Med. 1998;17(1):101–10.
18. Stafford RE, Ashton-Miller JA, Constantinou CE, Hodges PW. A new method to quantify male pelvic floor displacement from 2D transperineal ultrasound images. Urology. 2013;81(3):685–9.
19. Woon JT, Stringer MD. Clinical anatomy of the coccyx: a systematic review. Clin Anat. 2012;25(2):158–67.
20. Berges R, Oelke M. Age-stratified normal values for prostate volume, PSA, maximum urinary flow rate, IPSS, and other LUTS/BPH indicators in the German male community-dwelling population aged 50 years or older. World J Urol. 2011;29(2):171–8.
21. Park J, Lee DG, Suh B, Cho SY, Chang IH, Paick SH, et al. Establishment of reference ranges for prostate volume and annual prostate volume change rate in Korean adult men: analyses of a Nationwide screening population. J Korean Med Sci. 2015;30(8):1136–42.
22. Matsushita K, Kent MT, Vickers AJ, von Bodman C, Bernstein M, Touijer KA, et al. Preoperative predictive model of recovery of urinary continence after radical prostatectomy. BJU Int. 2015;116(4):577–83.

14

Oncological safety of intrafascial nerve-sparing radical prostatectomy compared with conventional process: A pooled review and meta-regression analysis based on available studies

Xiao Wang†, Yiqi Wu†, Jia Guo, Hui Chen, Xiaodong Weng and Xiuheng Liu*

Abstract

Background: Intrafascial prostatectomy was a modified technique from the conventional nerve-sparing surgery in order to improve patients' post-surgical continence and erectile function; however, ongoing controversy exists regarding the oncological safety of this technique. In this study we aimed to provide a critical and pooled analysis based on published literatures regarding the oncological outcomes after intrafascial nerve-sparing prostatectomy.

Methods: Database searches were performed for published articles till June 2018 on PubMed. Three reviewers screened fulfilled papers and extracted data independently. Main outcome was the positive surgical margins (PSMs) rates stratified by pathological stages. We performed both one-arm and comparative meta-analysis to evaluate the oncological safety of intrafascial technique. Moreover, we built meta-regression models to assess the confounding factors.

Results: We retrieved a total of 117 records after electronic search, of which 21 studies were finally included in this review. There were 15 controlled studies and 6 surgical series. Our one-arm meta-analysis demonstrated that the total PSM rates after intrafascial techniques ranging from 2.2 to 35%, with a pooled rate of 14.5% on average (480 of 3151 patients, 95% confidence interval[CI]: 11.2–17.5%). Meta-regression model showed that patients' age, pT2 cancer percentage and Selection Score of Oncological Safety (SSOS) were significantly associated with total PSM rate; moreover, each 1 point of SSOS could decrease the total PSM rate by 1.3% on average. Comparative meta-analysis demonstrated that there was no significant difference between intra- and inter-fascial group regarding PSM rates.

Conclusions: With stringent case selection and when performed by experienced surgeons, intrafascial prostatectomy could offer an acceptable or, at least, equivalent PSM rate compared with the conventional interfascial approach. Preoperative SSOS more than 7 points could be considered as an indication of intrafascial radical prostatectomy.

Keywords: Oncological safety, Radical prostatectomy, Intrafascial nerve-sparing, Systematic review, Positive surgical margins

* Correspondence: prof_liuxhmd@163.com
†Xiao Wang and Yiqi Wu contributed equally to this work.
Department of Urology, Renmin Hospital of Wuhan University, 238Jiefang Road, Wuhan 430060, People's Republic of China

Background

Radical prostatectomy is recommended as an effective treatment for clinically localized prostate cancer [1, 2], and used to cure patients with low/intermediate risk of disease [3]. Based on the updated anatomy understandings, the approaches to preserve peri-prostatic nerves have undergone many modifications from the conventional nerve-sparing surgery [4]. Intrafascial technique was a kind of refinements, characterized by developing a dissection plane medially/internally to the prostatic fascia, in order to maximally preserve peri-prostatic nerves and to enhance the post-surgical recovery of continence and potency. This technique is now applied worldwide in combination with different surgical approaches and procedures [5, 6].

Controversy about the intrafascial nerve-sparing technique has persisted since its introduction [7]. Most doubts were concentrated at its oncological safety, considering the necessity of removing all fascial coverings of the prostatic surface in resecting a tumor. It is generally recognized that the greater extent of structures spared, the higher is the risk of residual tumor; therefore, some surgeons would be concerned that intrafascial dissection would compromise its oncological safety and incur a risk of a higher rate of positive surgical margins (PSMs) [8].

There were obvious variations regarding the oncological results reported by different surgeons, which may be influenced by factors such as surgeon characteristics, surgical procedures, patient inclusion criteria, and outcome assessment methods. The purpose of this study was to critically summarize existing clinical trials and provide a detailed and comprehensive assessment of the oncological findings of intrafascial prostatectomy to guide urologists in selecting the appropriate technique.

Methods

Inclusion criteria

Inclusion criteria were set according to PICOS (patients, intervention, comparison, outcomes, and study design) principle as presented in Table 1. This review included trials designed as surgery series or controlled studies. Included studies had at least one arm that is performed using intrafascial techniques, including veil technique and other techniques approaching fascial planes close to the prostatic capsule and internal to the prostatic fascia, regardless of the types of surgery including retropubic radical prostatectomy (RRP), laparoscopic radical prostatectomy (LRP) and robot-assisted laparoscopic radical prostatectomy (RALRP). Study paralleling convetional interfascial technique was included in the comparative analysis as a control study. We excluded studies from the comparative assessment, including extra-fascial or wide-dissection or non-nerve-sparing prostatectomy, and for these studies we only extracted data from the intrafascial group.

Table 1 PICOS principle of inclusion criteria

Criteria	Description
Patients	Adult men diagnosed as prostate cancer undergoing radical prostatectomy
Intervention	Intrafascial nerve-sparing radical prostatectomy, including Veil, Leipzig, curtain dissection, or other techniques approaching fascial planes on the surface of the prostatic capsule or medial/internal to the prostatic fascia, regardless of surgery types
Comparison	Conventional interfascial nerve-sparing prostatectomy, regardless of surgery types
Outcomes	PSM rates stratified by pathological stages
Study design	Surgical series or prospective/retrospective controlled studies, including RCTs

PSM positive surgical margin, *RCTs* randomized controlled trials

Data sources and searches

Database searches were performed for published articles till June 2018 on PubMed. The following keywords were used across the "Title" and "Abstract" field including: ("intrafascial" OR "veil" OR "curtain dissection" OR "incremental nerve sparing" OR "high anterior release") AND "radical prostatectomy". Study characteristics were in accordance with our PICOS principle. There were no restrictions on the reporting characteristics of the publication status or language. In addition, there were no restrictions on the time of surgery or the date of publication. We manually checked the reference list of the included studies to further identify other relevant studies. Three reviewers (JG, HC, XW) independently screened the titles, abstracts and keywords of each search article. If the study met the inclusion criteria, we screened the full text for further evaluation. We excluded duplicate publications or superficially reported studies. Disagreements were resolved through open discussion.

Data extraction and synthesis

Data were independently extracted by three reviewers (JG, HC, XW) using standard formats, including study characteristics, patient characteristics, surgical information and outcomes. The authors of the original study were consulted for the missing data if needed. As surgical margins were confounded by patient selection, we evaluated and scored the patients' preoperative risk level according to the nomogram of Partin tables [9] along with D'Amico's study [10]. The scoring scale shown in Table 2 is stratified into 4 parts including clinical tumor stage, preoperative PSA level, Gleason score and invaded cores percentage. The scores of the 4 parts were summed up to the Selection Score of Oncologic Safety (SSOS). A high score indicated a more rigorous patient selection criteria and low risk of extraprostatic extension and margin involvement.

Table 2 Scoring scale of Selection Score of Oncologic Safety

Section	Clinical T stage						Preoperative PSA level (ng/ul)					
Item	T1c	T2a	T2b	T2c	T3	NS	0–2.5	2.6–4	4.1–6	6.1–10	> 10	NS
Score	5	4	3	2	1	0	5	4	3	2	1	0
Section	Biopsy Gleason score						Invaded cores percent (%)					
Item	2–4	5–6	3 + 4	4 + 3	8–10	NS	< 34	34–50		> 50		NS
Score	5	4	3	2	1	0	3	2		1		0

This scoring scale was according to the Partin table and D'Amico's study, stratified to 4 parts including clinical stage, preoperative PSA level, Gleason score and invaded cores percent. Scores of the 4 parts were summed to the Selection Score of Oncologic Safety (SSOS). High score means the more rigorous selection criteria for patients and low risk of extraprostatic extension and margin involvement. *PSA* prostate-specific antigen, *NS* not evaluated

With regard to a comparative analysis of the PSM rate, some studies had a selection bias between the intra- and inter-fascial groups. As surgeons often doubted the oncological safety of the intrafascial technique, they restricted the application of this technique to patients with early-stage tumors and lower risk of extraprostatic extension, but employed the interfascial procedure in high-risk disease. We considered this bias as a selection imbalance and, if surgeons made no exception in the selection of patients, we judged this as selection balance.

Bias assessment

The Cochrane Collaborative Bias Assessment Tool was used to assess the methodological quality of the included control studies. The following items were evaluated: (1) Adequate sequence generation? (2) Allocation concealment? (3) Binding? (4) Incomplete outcome data addressed? (5) Free of selective reporting? (6) Free of other bias? Each question was rated as "low risk", "high risk" or "unclear" and three reviewers (JG, HC and XW) independently assessed each trial. We used the funnel plot to evaluate publication bias. If there is a disagreement, judgment was made through public discussion.

Data analysis

All data extracted from the intrafascial arms were pooled using Open Meta-analyst software, stratified by surgical type. We performed one-arm meta-analysis using random effects models, and heterogeneity in the studies was assessed using Chi-square test and the I^2 index. Meta-regression analysis was performed with total PSM rate as a dependent variable, including patient age, preservation techniques, pT2 cancer percentage, and SSOS as covariate variables. An in-depth regression analysis was performed by including each part of the SSOS and excluding each part from the SSOS.

Comparative meta-analysis was conducted with the Cochrane Collaboration Review Manager. Heterogeneity among the studies was assessed using Chi-square test and the I^2 index statistic. When $p > 0.1$ and $I^2 < 50\%$, fixed-effect models were applied for the calculation of pooled effect index and only if $p < 0.1$ and $I^2 > 50\%$, the random-effect models were used. A comparative analysis of the PSM rates was performed by stratifying selection balance as a subgroup.

Results

This review was performed according to the Preferred Reporting Items of Systematic Reviews and Meta-analysis (PRISMA) statement. A total of 117 records were retrieved after electronic search strategy, which ultimately included 21 studies [6, 11–30]. Figure 1 present the PRISMA flowchart of literature searches and Table 3 provided detailed characteristics of the included studies. Among the 21 studies included, 15 were controlled studies and 6 were surgical series. Eight trials paralleling conventional interfascial technique as controlled groups were included for comparative meta-analysis. Additional file 1: Table S1 showed the risk of bias in individual studies.

One-arm meta-analysis

Figure 2 summarized the prevalence of total PSMs recorded in the intrafascial group of the published surgical series or controlled studies. The total PSM rate ranged from 2.2 to 35%, with a pooled rate of 14.2% (498/3351, 95% confidence interval [CI]: 11.0–17.3%). It was possible to calculate the heterogeneity among the included studies as I^2 was 86.38%. Three studies showed significantly higher PSM rates than the pooled rate, which included the studies of Curto 2006 [11], Choi 2012 [18], and Mortezavi 2012 [16], with a PSM rate of 30.8% (127/413, 95% CI: 26.3–35.2%), 34% (17/50, 95% CI: 20.9–47.1%), and 35% (28/80, 95% CI: 24.5–45.5%), respectively, whereas the VIP team reported a notably lower PSM rate of 1/46 [27]. No obvious differences could be detected among the 3 surgery types of LRP, RRP, and RALRP. PSM rates of intrafascial group stratified by pathological tumor stages could be found in Additional files 2 and 3, which showed that the pooled PSM rate was 9.7% (236/2423, 95% CI: 7.0–12.4%) in pT2 cancers (Additional file 2: Figure S1) and 44.0% (208/527, 95% CI: 34.9–53.2%) in pT3 cancer (Additional file 3: Figure S2). Overlapping higher rates could be seen in terms of the PSM rate in pT2 cancer that the studies of Curto (2006) [11] and Mortezavi (2012) [16],

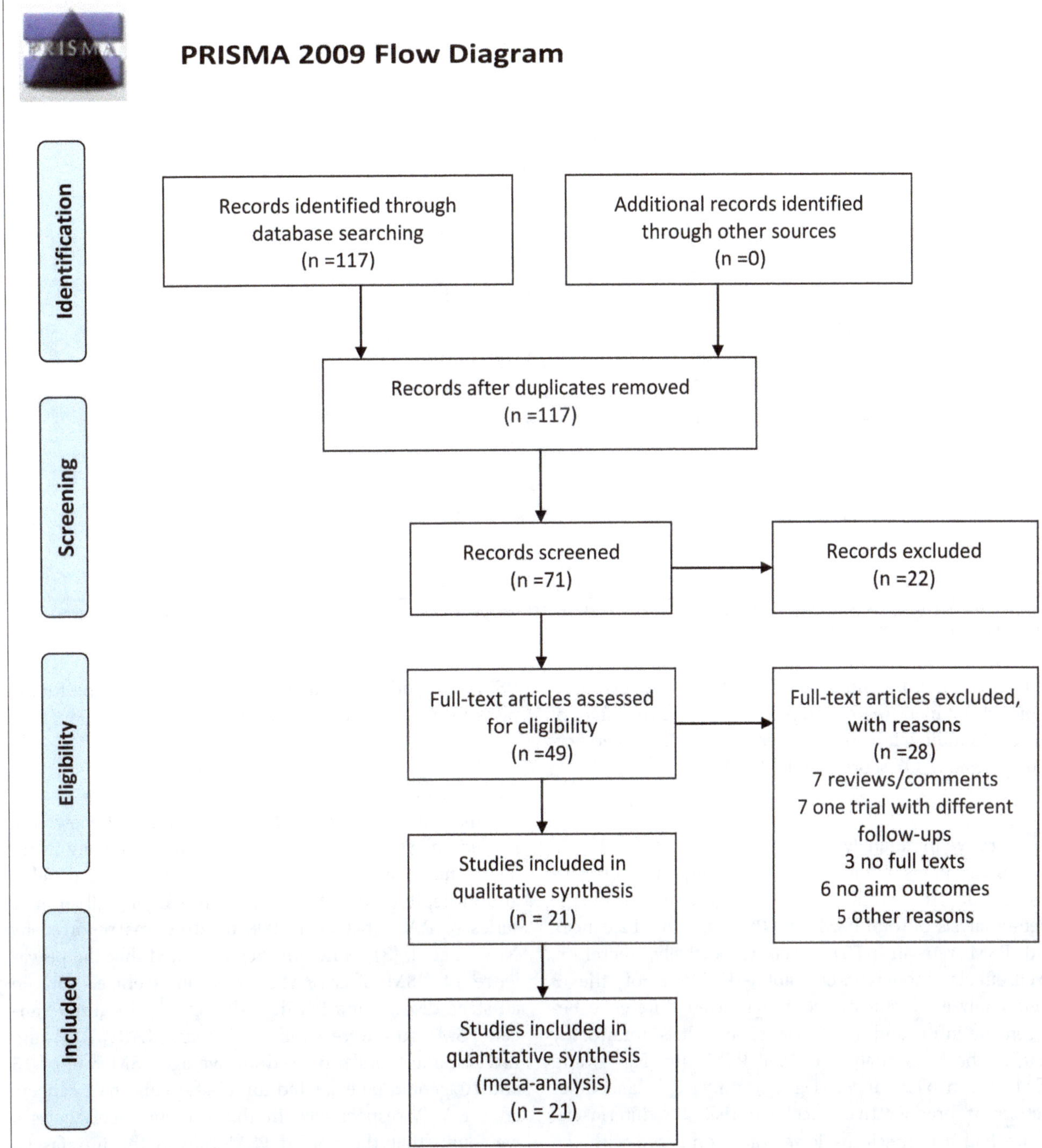

Fig. 1 PRISMA flowchart for identification and selection of studies for this systematic review

which also reported a significantly higher PSM rate than the pooled rate; however, this overlap was not observed with regard to the PSM rate in pT3 cancer.

Meta-regression analysis

Table 4 summarized the result of meta-regression evaluating the impact of confounding factors affecting PSM rates. Age, pT2 cancer percentage, and SSOS were significantly associated with the total PSM rate, and age was the only factor that affected the PSM rate in pT3 cancer. Regarding the total PSM rate, the regression model demonstrated that 1 more year to the mean age could increase the total PSM rate by an average of 1.2%, while each 1 point of SSOS could decrease it by an average of 1.3%. Moreover, preservation techniques including D-fascia preservation, puboprostatic ligament sparing, selective ligation of DVC,

Table 3 Characteristics of the included studies in meta-analysis

First author	Study design	Country	Surgery duration	Sample size for Intra-RP	Surgical type	Mean age in Intra-RP
Curto 2006	surgical series	France	2003.5–2005.3	425	LRP	62.0
Budaus 2009	surgical series	Germany	2005.4–2007.12	1150	RRP	63
Stolzenburg 2008	surgical series	Germany	2001.12–2007.11	150	LRP	60.2
Xylinas 2010	surgical series	France	2007.12–2008.6	50	RALRP	60.8
Asimakopoulos 2010	surgical series	Italy	2007.10–2009.3	30	RALRP	52
Khoder 2012	surgical series	Germany	2007.1–2009.12	231	RRP	63.3
Greco 2010	controlled	Germany	2005.1–2007.11	300	LRP vs RRP	61
Greco 2011	controlled	Germany	2005.1–2009.5	250	LRP	59
Asimakopoulos 2011	randomized controlled	Italy	2007.10–2008.10	128	LRP vs RALRP	60.4
Hoshi 2013	controlled	Japan	2009.1–2011.10	44	LRP	65.7
Stewart 2011	controlled	UK	2006.2–2009.12	102	LRP	61.5
Mortezavi 2012	controlled	Switzerland	2006.5–2008.8	80	RALRP	
VIP 2005	controlled	USA	2003.1–2003.12	35	RALRP	58.6
Neil 2009	controlled	UK	2000.3–2007.10	240	LRP	59
Potdevin 2009	controlled	New Jersey	2006.1–2007.12	70	RALRP	58.63
Stolzenburg 2010	randomized controlled	Germany	2004.6–2008.6	200	LRP	61
Choi 2012	controlled	Korea	2011.11–2012.4	50	LRP	66.5
Ihsan-Tasci 2015	controlled	Turkey	2009.8–2012.12	200	RALRP	60.8

Intra-RP intrafascial radical prostatectomy, *VIP* Vattikuti Institute Prostatectomy, *RRP* retropubic radical prostatectomy, *LRP* laparoscopic radical prostatectomy, *RALRP* robot-assisted laparoscopic radical prostatectomy

had no significant influence on PSM rate. Figure 3 depicted the meta-regression plot to describe the effect of the confounding factors of patient age, pT2 cancer percentage, and SSOS score on total PSM rate.

Comparative meta-analysis

As shown in Figs. 4 and 5, the I^2 standing for heterogeneity among the studies was 39, 47, and 0% in the meta-analysis of total PSM rate, PSM rate in pT2 cancer, and PSM rate in pT3 cancer, respectively, therefore, fixed-effects models were applied. None of the 3 meta-analyses demonstrated a significant difference between the intra- and interfascial groups. It is noteworthy that, in the meta-analysis of total PSM rate (Fig. 4) and PSM rate in pT2 cancer (Fig. 5a), under a balanced selection of preoperative oncologic risk, the interfascial group had a numerically lower rate compared with the intrafascial group, but interestingly, pooling the studies without a balanced baseline resulted in an observable significant difference in PSM rate in favor of the intrafascial group. This condition was not observed in the assessment of the PSM rate in pT3 (Fig. 5b), which showed consistency between the balanced and imbalanced studies, both indicating that the intrafascial group was associated with a higher PSM rate, although insignificant statistically. Table 5 provided characteristics of studies included in comparable meta-analysis reporting PSM and Additional file 4: Figure S3 showed the funnel plots for assessing the publication biases.

Discussion

In this study we conducted a systematic review and pooled analysis of oncological outcomes following intrafascial nerve-sparing prostatectomy. In 2012, a detailed and in-depth systematic review summarizing all surgical series of RALP between 2008 to 2011 was reported by Novara et al. [31], wherein they indicated that the prevalence of PSM after RALP was, on average, 15% in all-stage disease and 9% in pathologically localized cancer; PSM rates were similar following RARP, RRP, and LRP. The authors proposed an average PSM rate of 15 and 10% could be expected for all-stage and pT2 cancers after RALP, respectively. In this present meta-analysis, we found that the pooled PSM rate in the intrafascial group was, overall, 14.2% in all stages of prostate cancer and 9.7% in pT2 disease regardless of surgery types, which seemed to match the results of previous review. Comparative analysis revealed no significant difference in PSM rate between the intra- and inter-fascial groups, which was consistent with a previous meta-analysis [32]. From this point of view, oncological outcomes of intrafascial technique seemed acceptable, or at least not worse than with conventional approach. However, a hasty conclusion of the oncological safety of this

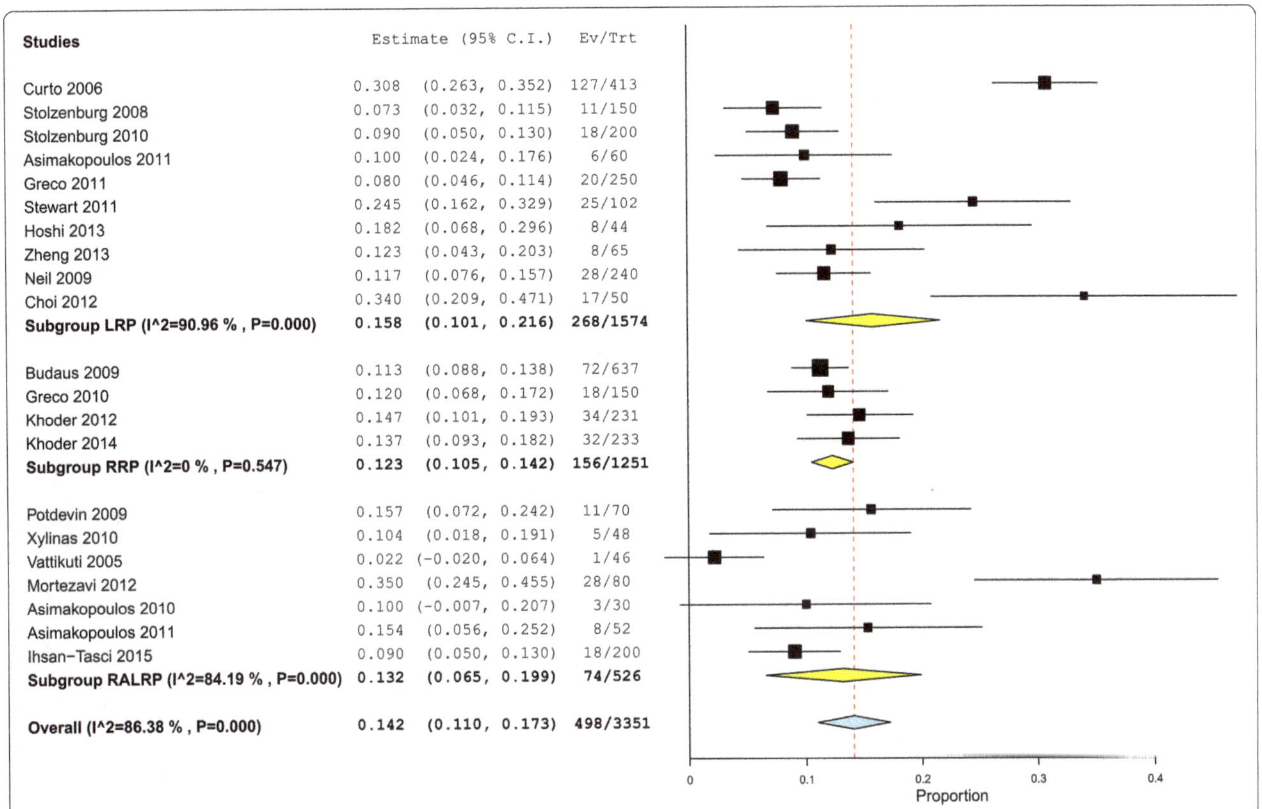

Fig. 2 Forest plot for one-arm meta-analysis of studies adopting the intrafascial technique in terms of total PSM rate in all-stage disease stratified by surgical types. PSM, positive surgical margin; LRP, laparoscopic radical prostatectomy; RRP, retropubic radical prostatectomy; RALRP, robot-assisted laparoscopic radical prostatectomy; VIP, Vattikuti Institute Prostatectomy

technique should be avoided, as there are additional issues worthy of critical appraisal.

Extracapsular extension of carcinoma could lead to higher PSM rate of radical prostatectomy compared with that associated with a localized tumor. The mean percentage of pT2 cancer in the intrafascial studies included in our present review was 84.5% (range: 58.6–98.1%), which is significantly higher than that in the 17 surgical series included in Novara's review [31] (t-test of independent samples: mean difference = – 7.91569, t = – 2.618, $p = .014$); this meant, surgeons selected more patients with localized disease to perform intrafascial approach, but only comparable total PSM rates were gained. Moreover, according to the guidelines of the European Association of Urology, radical prostatectomy could be extended for indications such as patients with intermediate-risk, localized prostate cancer with clinical stage T2b–T2c, Gleason score = 7, or PSA 10–20 ng/ml

Table 4 Meta-regression models evaluating the influence of the confounded factors to the PSM rate

Factor	Age		D-fascia preservation		Puboprostatic ligament sparing		Selective/no ligation of DVC		pT2 cancer percent		Selection Score of Oncologic Safety	
	β ± SE	*P*-value	β ± SE	P-value	β ± SE	P-value	β ± SE	P-value	β ± SE	P-value	β ± SE	P-value
Total PSM rate in all-stage	**0.013 ± 0.006**	**0.044**	–0.032 ± 0.037	0.385	–0.022 ± 0.039	0.561	0.021 ± 0.045	0.643	**–0.004 ± 0.002**	**0.012**	**–0.013 ± 0.005**	**0.012**
PSM rate in pT2 cancer	0.005 ± 0.005	0.303	0.011 ± 0.032	0.727	–0.050 ± 0.032	0.120	–0.044 ± 0.033	0.183	–	–	–	–
PSM rate in pT3 cancer	**0.041 ± 0.018**	**0.025**	–0.001 ± 0.097	0.990	0.111 ± 0.075	0.139	–0.111 ± 0.074	0.133	–	–	–	–

Each of the confounded factors including patients' age, preservation technique(D-fascia preservation, puboprostatic ligament sparing and selective/no ligation of DVC) was included respectively in the meta-regression models to assess the influence of the confounded factors to the PSM rate. If *p*-value was less than 0.05, the cofficient and *p*-value were showed as boldface in the table. *D-fascia* Denonvilliers fascia, *DVC* dorsal venous complex, *PSM* positive surgical margin, *β* coefficient, *SE* standard error

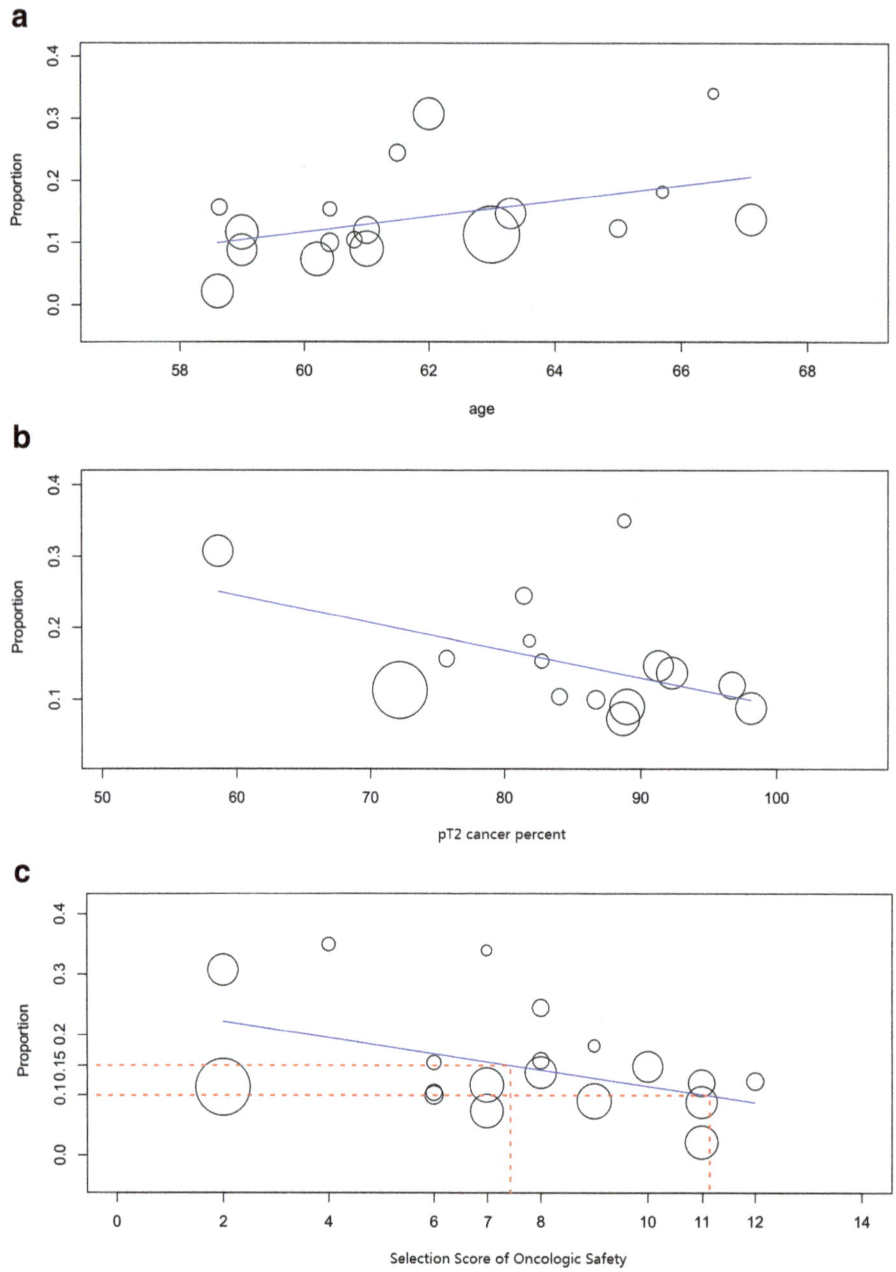

Fig. 3 Influence of (**a**) age, (**b**) pT2 cancer percentage, and (**c**) the Selection Score of Oncologic Safety on total PSM rate in all-stage cancer following intrafascial radical prostatectomy. PSM, positive surgical margin

[3]. However, our review found that most surgeons applied more rigorous selection criteria against generally recommended indications for radical prostatectomy. For example, the VIP team in 2005 reported a notably low PSM rate with a robot-assisted surgical system wherein only 1 case of positive margin was detected from among 46 patients who underwent intrafascial RALRP [27]. With regard to their selection criteria, only patients with clinical T1c stage cancer combined with a Gleason score ≤ 6 and preoperative PSA ≤10 were selected for the adoption of the intrafascial technique. Therefore, the currently acceptable low PSM rate following intrafascial prostatectomy could be attributed to more stringent patient selection and, subsequently, a higher proportion of localized disease; however, the oncological safety of this technique could not be confirmed. If intrafascial dissection is carried out among patients with a high risk of extracapsular invasion, the result may be unsatisfactory. For example, in 2006, Curto et al. reported a contemporary laparoscopic surgical series wherein a surgical team

Study or Subgroup	Intrafascial group Events	Intrafascial group Total	Interfascial group Events	Interfascial group Total	Weight	Odds Ratio M-H, Fixed, 95% CI	Year
2.1.1 Selection Balance							
Potdevin 2009	11	70	6	77	4.7%	2.21 [0.77, 6.32]	2009
Neil 2009	28	240	30	270	24.2%	1.06 [0.61, 1.83]	2009
Stolzenburg 2010	18	200	19	200	16.8%	0.94 [0.48, 1.85]	2010
Subtotal (95% CI)		**510**		**547**	**45.6%**	**1.13 [0.77, 1.67]**	
Total events	57		55				
Heterogeneity: Chi² = 1.89, df = 2 (P = 0.39); I² = 0%							
Test for overall effect: Z = 0.62 (P = 0.53)							
2.1.2 Selection imbalance							
VIP 2005	1	46	1	30	1.1%	0.64 [0.04, 10.71]	2005
Zheng 2013	8	65	21	130	11.9%	0.73 [0.30, 1.75]	2013
Khoder 2014	32	233	44	182	41.3%	0.50 [0.30, 0.83]	2014
Subtotal (95% CI)		**344**		**342**	**54.4%**	**0.55 [0.36, 0.85]**	
Total events	41		66				
Heterogeneity: Chi² = 0.55, df = 2 (P = 0.76); I² = 0%							
Test for overall effect: Z = 2.68 (P = 0.007)							
Total (95% CI)		**854**		**889**	**100.0%**	**0.82 [0.61, 1.09]**	
Total events	98		121				
Heterogeneity: Chi² = 8.19, df = 5 (P = 0.15); I² = 39%							
Test for overall effect: Z = 1.38 (P = 0.17)							
Test for subgroup differences: Chi² = 5.80, df = 1 (P = 0.02), I² = 82.7%							

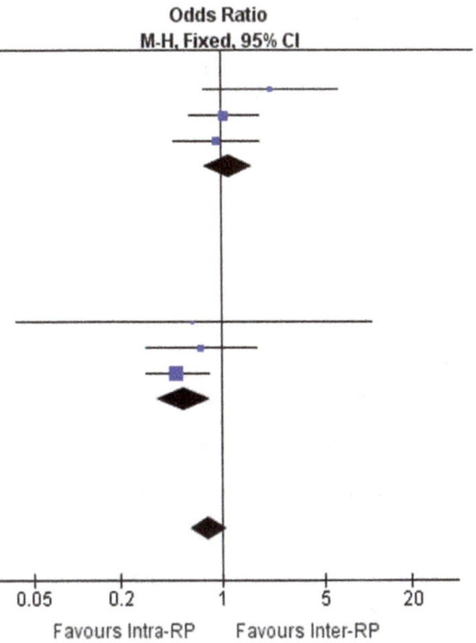

Fig. 4 Forest plots for comparative meta-analysis of studies comparing the intrafascial with the interfascial technique in terms of the total PSM rate in all-stage cancer stratified by whether selection balance was achieved. PSM, positive surgical margin; VIP, Vattikuti Institute Prostatectomy

experienced in over 2800 LRP performed intrafascial prostatectomies in patients with organ-confined prostate cancer (including 3 cases of cT3a disease) without other selection restrictions such as PSA level or Gleason score, for control of preoperative oncological risk. Subsequently, the percentage of pT2 cancer was only 58.6% and the overall PSM rate in all-stage tumors was as high as 30.7% (127/413) [11].

With regard to our regression model, the percentage of pT2 cancer was significantly associated with the total PSM rate, and high proportion of pT2 disease led to a low PSM rate. However, as preoperative pathological staging could not be obtained, the risk of extracapsular invasion was predicted on the basis of the patient's preoperative information. Clinical stage, PSA level, Gleason score, and positive biopsy cores could be used as independent predictors of this risk and, therefore, we scored each factor and summed to SSOS to quantitatively evaluate this risk preoperatively. We identified a significant correlation between the SSOS and pathological pT2 percentage (Pearson Correlation = 0.749, p = .001). Moreover, an obvious association could be identified from our meta-regression model by including SSOS as a confounding factor, indicating that, for intrafascial prostatectomy, stringent case selection was associated with low risk of PSM and quantitatively, each 1 point of SSOS could decrease the total PSM rate by 1.3% on average. Thus, based on our regression model, the preoperative SSOS should be more than 7 points to obtain a postoperative PSM rate of 15% on average and SSOS more than 11 points meant a postoperative PSM rate of 10%. Surgeons intending to adapt this technique should take cautions when setting criteria for patient selection and we, for the first time, proposed the SSOS as an indication of intrafascial prostatectomy.

SSOS had four components, by which we used to evaluate the patients' selection criteria for intrafascial prostatectomy of the included studies. We performed in-depth regression analysis setting total PSM rates as dependent variable by including each section and excluding each section from SSOS (see Additional file 5: Table S2). The result showed that section 1 (clinical T stage) was the most influential factor, as only section 1 could significantly affect PSM rates and when excluding section 1, the regression model became insignificant. Thus surgeons should make clinical T stage a priority when using SSOS as an indication.

A histological study by the VIP team indicated that 2/30 anterolateral zones of the prostate specimen after the Veil technique revealed capsular incision, compared with 0/40 for the standard technique [33]. In pathologically localized disease, the tumor does not invade beyond the limit of the prostatic capsule; thus, only intracapsular incision will lead to positive margins. Theoretically, intrafascial dissection should increase risk of capsular incision compared with the interfascial technique and, subsequently, with a localized tumor situated close to the capsule or having large volume, is likely to lead to PSM. This can be inferred from Curto's surgical series [11], wherein investigators found a higher PSM rate, especially for pT2c tumors, as compared with the previous largest series; however, this difference was not present for other pathological stages.

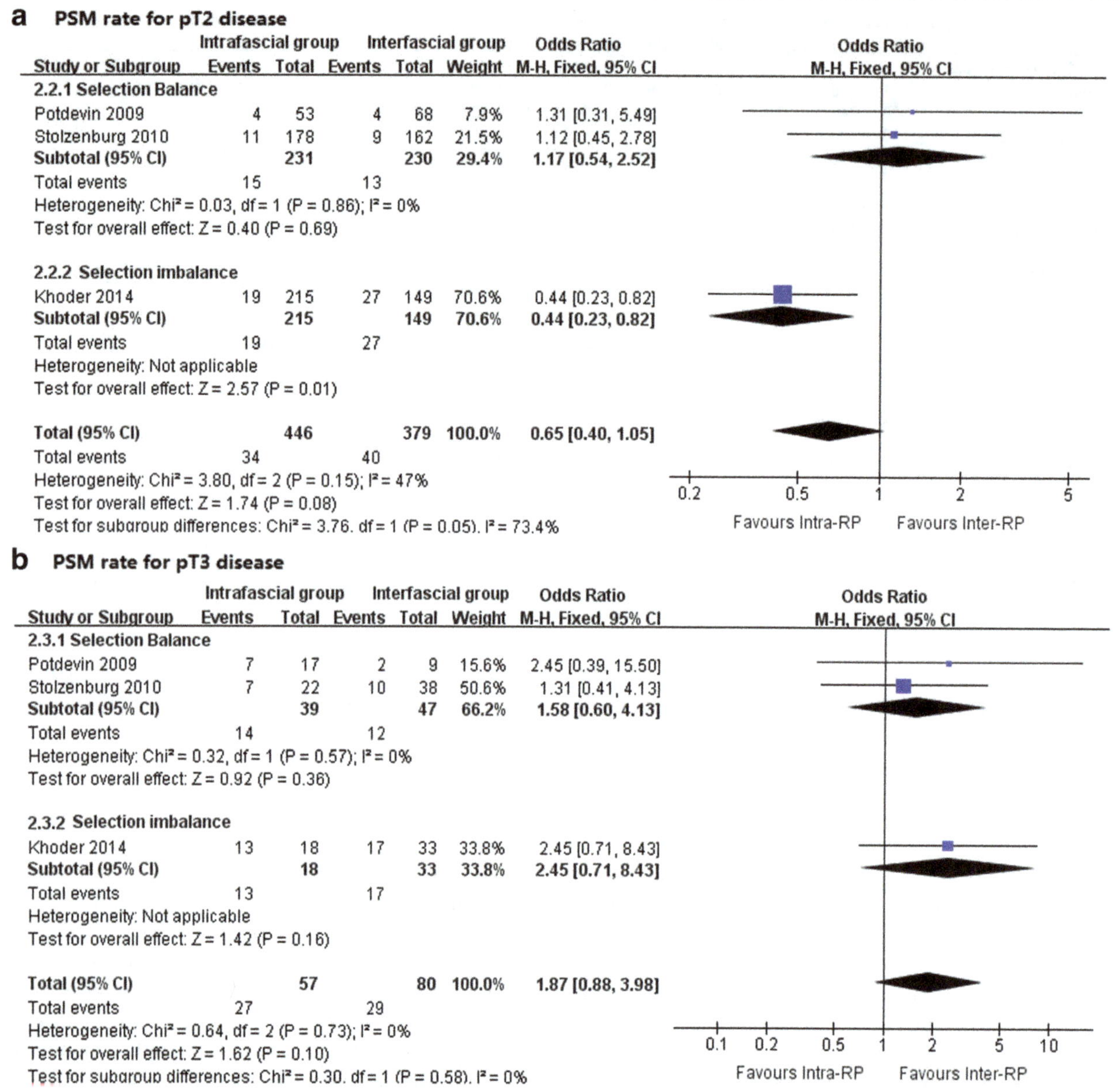

Fig. 5 Forest plots for comparative meta-analysis of studies comparing the intrafascial with interfascial technique in terms of (**a**) PSM rate for pT2 cancer and (**b**) PSM rate for pT3 cancer stratified by whether selection balance was achieved. PSM, positive surgical margin

For comparative analysis, we only included parallel-group studies including conventional interfascial nerve-sparing prostatectomy as the control. Several studies compared the outcomes of intrafascial prostatectomy with that of wide dissection or non-nerve-sparing prostatectomy, but as reported in some of these studies, wider preservation of the NVBs may be associated with a higher risk of PSM [34, 35]. Thus, for these studies, the oncological results could be confounded by the nerve-sparing technique, and, therefore, we did not include these studies in the comparative analysis. In our meta-analysis comparing intra- and interfascial groups, we stratified studies according to patient selection balance; however, the overall pooled result demonstrated there was no significant difference for PSM rate in all pathological stages of disease. Notably, in the study by Khoder et al. [12], patients were selected to undergo intrafascial prostatectomy only if biopsy Gleason scores were ≤ 6 and PSA ≤10 ng/mL with low tumor size; patients with relatively higher Gleason scores and PSA levels were allocated to the interfascial group, and this was considered as selection imbalance. These researchers ultimately reported that PSM rates for pT2 stage and all pathological stages were lower in the intrafascial group compared with the interfascial group; however, this advantage was not reported for pT3 cancer. From the subgroup results in our comparative analysis, a significantly lower PSM rate was

Table 5 Characteristics of studies included in comparable meta-analysis reporting PSM rate

First author	Selection balance	Criteria for Intra-RP	Criteria for Inter-RP	SSOS for Intra-RP	Percent of pT2 cancer, % (Intra-RP vs Inter-RP)	PSM rate, % (Intra-RP vs Inter-RP)		
						pT2	pT3	all-stage
VIP 2005	N	cT1c and PSA ≤ 10 and Gleason score ≤ 6	cT2a/b or PSA > 10 ≤ 20 or Gleason score = 7	11				2.2: 3.3
Zheng 2013	N	cT1/2a and PSA ≤ 10 and Gleason score ≤ 3 + 4 and positive cores≤3/12	cT2b/c or positive cores > 3/12 and PSA ≤ 10 and Gleason score ≤ 3 + 4	12				12.3: 16.2
Khoder 2014	N	cT1/2 and PSA ≤ 10 and Gleason score ≤ 6	cT1/2 and PSA ≤ 15 and Gleason score ≤ 7	8	92.3: 81.9	8.8: 18.1	72.2: 51.5	13.7: 24.2
Potdevin 2009	Y	cT1/2a and PSA ≤ 10 and Gleason score ≤ 7		8	75.7: 88.3	7.5: 5.9	41.2: 22.2	15.7: 7.8
Neil 2009	Y	cT1/2 and PSA ≤ 10 and absence of primary Gleason pattern 4/5		7				11.7: 11.1
Stolzenburg 2010	Y	cT1/2a and PSA < 10 and Gleason score ≤ 3 + 4		9	89: 81	6.2: 5.6	31.8: 26.3	9.0: 9.5

Intra-RP intrafascial radical prostatectomy, *Inter-RP* interfascial radical prostatectomy, *SSOS* Selection Score of Oncologic Safety, *VIP* Vattikuti Institute Prostatectomy, *Y* yes, *N* no.

identified in favor of the intrafascial technique in pT2 and all-stage disease for pooled studies with non-balanced selection criteria. All of these non-balanced studies applied additional more stringent patient selection criteria for the intrafascial technique, as compared with patient selection for the interfascial group. With regard to subgroup analysis of balanced studies, pooled results revealed a higher PSM rate, although statistically non-significant, with the intrafascial technique for pT2 and all-stage cancers. The variance between subgroups of balanced and non-balanced studies reconfirmed the crucial role of patient selection in controlling the PSM rate. In pT3 cancer, a higher PSM rate, although statistically non-significant, was detected for the interfascial group and may be attributable to insufficient sample size.

The PSM rate is known to be associated with surgeon-related characteristics, with surgical experience being the most important factor. Surgeons experienced in high-volume resections could decrease the PSM rate [36, 37]. A study evaluating the learning curve of radical prostatectomy indicated that increasing surgical experience was associated with substantial reductions in cancer recurrence: however, for LRP, the learning curve was slower than for RRP [38]. The relatively high PSM rate for LRP reported by Choi et al. in 2012 can be attributed to the learning curve [18]. In fact, the authors emphasized that, in the first 30 cases, the PSM rate was 51.7%, and then subsequently decreased to 9.5%. However, there are no published studies reporting an evaluation of PSM with the learning curve of the intrafascial technique.

Regarding on the dissection plane during procedure, surgeons supplied several technical variations, including VIP technique and Leipzig technique. We included all the intrafascial surgeries in this pooled study regardless of the variable techniques. Most authors described their dissection technique in the original manuscripts, but ignored pathological evaluation of the specimen regarding whether the utilized surgical technique was intra or interfacial nerve sparing. Thus we can only judge the classification depending on the authors' description. As the PSM rates were affected by the dissection plane, the quality of the original trials may confound our conclusion and this is a major limitation when we included these trials in our pooled analysis.

In the present review, no obvious evidence indicative of preserving technique, including D-fascia preservation, puboprostatic ligament sparing, or selective/no ligation of DVC, was detected in conjunction with increased PSM rate. In a retrospective controlled study reported by Hoshi et al. in 2013 [15], the authors reconfirmed that the DVC preserving technique would not increase the PSM rate, as compared with the conventional intrafascial technique. Further, we could not conclusively determine any significant differences among the 3 surgical types of RRP, LRP, and RALRP from our pooled results. Overlapping results could be identified from the studies of Asimakopoulos and Greco. Asimakopoulos et al. conducted a randomized comparison between LRP and RALRP and found no statistically significant differences for the PSM rate [21]. In the study of Greco et al. comparing RRP with LRP, results demonstrated that both surgical types had similar PSM rates [24]. In terms of our regression model, age was another relevant predictor of the PSM rate, demonstrating that older patients had higher PSM rates for pT3 and all-stage cancers.

Conclusions

In summary, intrafascial technique resulted in a total PSM rate of 14.2% for all-stage cancer and 9.7% in pT2 disease. With stringent case selection and conducted by experienced surgeons, intrafascial prostatectomy could offer an acceptable or, at least, equivalent PSM rate compared with the conventional interfascial approach. Current patient selection criteria are more stringent than those indicated for radical prostatectomy by guidelines, and we proposed SSOS as an indication of intrafascial prostatectomy. Preoperative SSOS should be more than 7 points to obtain an acceptable postoperative PSM rate of 15% on average.

Additional files

Additional file 1: Table S1. Risk of bias summary of included controlled studies. Review authors' judgments about each risk of bias item for included study. (DOCX 16 kb)

Additional file 2: Figure S1. Forest plots for one-arm meta-analysis of studies adopting the intrafascial technique in terms of PSM rate in pT2 disease stratified by surgical types. PSM, positive surgical margin; LRP, laparoscopic radical prostatectomy; RRP, retropubic radical prostatectomy; RALRP, robot-assisted laparoscopic radical prostatectomy. (TIF 2042 kb)

Additional file 3: Figure S2. Forest plots for one-arm meta-analysis of studies adopting the intrafascial technique in terms of PSM rate in pT3 disease stratified by surgical types. PSM, positive surgical margin; LRP, laparoscopic radical prostatectomy; RRP, retropubic radical prostatectomy; RALRP, robot-assisted laparoscopic radical prostatectomy. (TIF 1933 kb)

Additional file 4: Figure S3. Funnel plots for assessing publication biases of comparative meta-analysis of (a) total PSM rate, (b) PSM rate for pT2 disease and (c) PSM rate for pT3 disease. (TIF 5431 kb)

Additional file 5: Table S2. Meta-regression models evaluating each section of SSOS to the PSM rate. (DOCX 14 kb)

Abbreviations

D-fascia: Denonvilliers fascia; DVC: Dorsal venous complex; LRP: Laparoscopic radical prostatectomy; NS: Not evaluated; OR: Odds ratio; PICOS: Patients, intervention, comparison, outcomes, and study design; PRISMA: Preferred reporting items of systematic reviews and meta-analysis; PSA: Prostate-specific antigen; PSMs: Positive surgical margins; RALRP: Robot-assisted laparoscopic radical prostatectomy; RRP: Retropubic radical prostatectomy; SSOS: Selection score of oncologic safety; VIP: Vattikuti Institute Prostatectomy

Acknowledgements

Not applicable.

Authors' contributions

XW and XHL: Study conception and design, data collection and management; JG, HC and XDW: data collection and analysis, preparation of figures and tables; XW and YQW: Writing and revision of the manuscript. All authors read and approved the final manuscript

References

1. Walsh PC. Radical prostatectomy for localized prostate cancer provides durable cancer control with excellent quality of life: a structured debate. J Urol. 2000;163(6):1802–7.
2. Han M, Partin AW, Pound CR, Epstein JI, Walsh PC. Long-term biochemical disease-free and cancer-specific survival following anatomic radical retropubic prostatectomy. The 15-year Johns Hopkins experience. Urol Clin North Am. 2001;28(3):555–65.
3. Mottet N, Bellmunt J, Bolla M, Briers E, Cumberbatch MG, De Santis M, et al. EAU-ESTRO-SIOG guidelines on prostate Cancer. Part 1: screening, diagnosis, and local treatment with curative intent. Eur Urol. 2017;71(4):618–29.
4. Costello AJ, Brooks M, Cole OJ. Anatomical studies of the neurovascular bundle and cavernosal nerves. BJU Int. 2004;94(7):1071–6.
5. Stolzenburg JU, Rabenalt R, Tannapfel A, Liatsikos EN. Intrafascial nerve-sparing endoscopic extraperitoneal radical prostatectomy. Urology. 2006; 67(1):17–21.
6. Budaus L, Isbarn H, Schlomm T, Heinzer H, Haese A, Steuber T, et al. Current technique of open intrafascial nerve-sparing retropubic prostatectomy. Eur Urol. 2009;56(2):317–24.
7. Rassweiler J. Intrafascial nerve-sparing laproscopic radical prostatectomy: do we really preserve relevant nerve-fibres? Eur Urol. 2006;49(6):955–7.
8. Kaul S, Menon M. Robotic radical prostatectomy: evolution from conventional to VIP. World J Urol. 2006;24(2):152–60.
9. Partin AW, Mangold LA, Lamm DM, Walsh PC, Epstein JI, Pearson JD. Contemporary update of prostate cancer staging nomograms (Partin tables) for the new millennium. Urology. 2001;58(6):843–8.
10. D'Amico AV, Whittington R, Malkowicz SB, Wu YH, Chen M, Art M, et al. Combination of the preoperative PSA level, biopsy Gleason score, percentage of positive biopsies, and MRI T-stage to predict early PSA failure in men with clinically localized prostate cancer. Urology. 2000;55(4):572–7.
11. Curto F, Benijts J, Pansadoro A, Barmoshe S, Hoepffner JL, Mugnier C, et al. Nerve sparing laparoscopic radical prostatectomy: our technique. Eur Urol. 2006;49(2):344–52.
12. Khoder WY, Waidelich R, Buchner A, Becker AJ, Stief CG. Prospective comparison of one year follow-up outcomes for the open complete intrafascial retropubic versus interfascial nerve-sparing radical prostatectomy. Springerplus. 2014;3:335.
13. Zheng T, Zhang X, Ma X, Li HZ, Gao JP, Cai W, et al. A matched-pair comparison between bilateral intrafascial and interfascial nerve-sparing techniques in extraperitoneal laparoscopic radical prostatectomy. Asian J Androl. 2013;15(4):513–7.
14. Ko WJ, Hruby GW, Turk AT, Landman J, Badani KK. Pathological confirmation of nerve-sparing types performed during robot-assisted radical prostatectomy (RARP). BJU Int. 2013;111(3):451–8.
15. Hoshi A, Usui Y, Shimizu Y, Tomonaga T, Kawakami M, Nakajima N, et al. Dorsal vein complex preserving technique for intrafascial nerve-sparing laparoscopic radical prostatectomy. Int J Urol. 2013;20(5):493–500.
16. Mortezavi A, Hermanns T, Seifert HH, Wild PJ, Schmid DM, Sulser T, et al. Intrafascial dissection significantly increases positive surgical margin and biochemical recurrence rates after robotic-assisted radical prostatectomy. Urol Int. 2012;89(1):17–24.
17. Khoder WY, Schlenker B, Waidelich R, Buchner A, Kellhammer N, Stief CG, et al. Open complete intrafascial nerve-sparing retropubic radical prostatectomy: technique and initial experience. Urology. 2012;79(3): 717–21.
18. Choi YH, Lee JZ, Chung MK, Ha HK. Preliminary results for continence recovery after intrafascial extraperitoneal laparoscopic radical prostatectomy. Korean J Urol. 2012;53(12):836–42.
19. Stewart GD, El-Mokadem I, McLornan ME, Stolzenburg JU, McNeill SA. Functional and oncological outcomes of men under 60 years of age having endoscopic surgery for prostate cancer are optimal following intrafascial endoscopic extraperitoneal radical prostatectomy. Surgeon. 2011;9(2):65–71.
20. Greco F, Hoda MR, Wagner S, Reichelt O, Inferrera A, Magno C, et al. Bilateral vs unilateral laparoscopic intrafascial nerve-sparing radical prostatectomy: evaluation of surgical and functional outcomes in 457 patients. BJU Int. 2011;108(4):583–7.
21. Asimakopoulos AD, Pereira Fraga CT, Annino F, Pasqualetti P, Calado AA, Mugnier C. Randomized comparison between laparoscopic and robot-assisted nerve-sparing radical prostatectomy. J Sex Med. 2011;8(5):1503–12.
22. Xylinas E, Ploussard G, Salomon L, Paul A, Gillion N, Laet KD, et al. Intrafascial nerve-sparing radical prostatectomy with a laparoscopic robot-assisted extraperitoneal approach: early oncological and functional results. J Endourol. 2010;24(4):577–82.
23. Stolzenburg JU, Kallidonis P, Do M, Dietel A, Hafner T, Rabenalt R, et al. A comparison of outcomes for interfascial and intrafascial nerve-sparing radical prostatectomy. Urology. 2010;76(3):743–8.
24. Greco F, Wagner S, Hoda MR, Kawan F, Inferrera A, Lupo A, et al. Laparoscopic vs open retropubic intrafascial nerve-sparing radical prostatectomy: surgical and functional outcomes in 300 patients. BJU Int. 2010;106(4):543–7.
25. Neill MG, Louie-Johnsun M, Chabert C, Eden C. Does intrafascial dissection during nerve-sparing laparoscopic radical prostatectomy compromise cancer control? BJU Int. 2009;104(11):1730–3.

26. Stolzenburg JU, Rabenalt R, Do M, Schwalenberg T, Winkler M, Dietel A, et al. Intrafascial nerve-sparing endoscopic extraperitoneal radical prostatectomy. Eur Urol. 2008;53(5):931–40.
27. Menon M, Kaul S, Bhandari A, Shrivastava A, Tewari A, Hemal A. Potency following robotic radical prostatectomy: a questionnaire based analysis of outcomes after conventional nerve sparing and prostatic fascia sparing techniques. J Urol. 2005;174(6):2291–6 discussion 6.
28. Asimakopoulos AD, Annino F, D'Orazio A, Pereira CF, Mugnier C, Hoepffner JL, et al. Complete periprostatic anatomy preservation during robot-assisted laparoscopic radical prostatectomy (RALP): the new pubovesical complex-sparing technique. Eur Urol. 2010;58(3):407–17.
29. Potdevin L, Ercolani M, Jeong J, Kim IY. Functional and oncologic outcomes comparing interfascial and intrafascial nerve sparing in robot-assisted laparoscopic radical prostatectomies. J Endourol. 2009;23(9):1479–84.
30. Ihsan-Tasci A, Simsek A, Dogukan-Torer MB, Sokmen D, Sahin S, Bitkin A, et al. Oncologic results, functional outcomes, and complication rates of transperitoneal robotic assisted radical prostatectomy: single centre's experience. Actas Urol Esp. 2015;39(2):70–7.
31. Novara G, Ficarra V, Mocellin S, Ahlering TE, Carroll PR, Graefen M, et al. Systematic review and meta-analysis of studies reporting oncologic outcome after robot-assisted radical prostatectomy. Eur Urol. 2012;62(3): 382–404.
32. Weng H, Zeng XT, Li S, Meng XY, Shi MJ, He DL, et al. Intrafascial versus interfascial nerve sparing in radical prostatectomy for localized prostate cancer: a systematic review and meta-analysis. Sci Rep. 2017; 7(1):11454.
33. Savera AT, Kaul S, Badani K, Stark AT, Shah NL, Menon M. Robotic radical prostatectomy with the "veil of Aphrodite" technique: histologic evidence of enhanced nerve sparing. Eur Urol. 2006;49(6):1065–73; discussion 73-4.
34. Fromont G, Baumert H, Cathelineau X, Rozet F, Validire P, Vallancien G. Intraoperative frozen section analysis during nerve sparing laparoscopic radical prostatectomy: feasibility study. J Urol. 2003;170(5):1843–6.
35. Rassweiler J, Marrero R, Hammady A, Erdogru T, Teber D, Frede T. Transperitoneal laparoscopic radical prostatectomy: ascending technique. J Endourol. 2004;18(7):593–9 discussion 9-600.
36. Eastham JA, Kattan MW, Riedel E, Begg CB, Wheeler TM, Gerigk C, et al. Variations among individual surgeons in the rate of positive surgical margins in radical prostatectomy specimens. J Urol. 2003;170(6 Pt 1):2292–5.
37. Atug F, Castle EP, Srivastav SK, Burgess SV, Thomas R, Davis R. Positive surgical margins in robotic-assisted radical prostatectomy: impact of learning curve on oncologic outcomes. Eur Urol. 2006;49(5):866–71 discussion 71-2.
38. Vickers AJ, Savage CJ, Hruza M, Tuerk I, Koenig P, Martinez-Pineiro L, et al. The surgical learning curve for laparoscopic radical prostatectomy: a retrospective cohort study. Lancet Oncol. 2009;10(5):475–80.

15

Comparison of various continence definitions in a large group of patients undergoing radical prostatectomy

Sigrun Holze[1*], Meinhard Mende[2], Karl V. Healy[1], Norbert Koehler[3], Lutz Gansera[3], Michael C. Truss[4], Udo Rebmann[5], Stephan Degener[6] and Jens-Uwe Stolzenburg[1]

Abstract

Background: Due to the usage of various measurement methods and definitions, comparing continence rates after radical prostatectomy is a challenging task. This study compares continence rates based on different methods and aims to identify the definition for continence which agrees best with the patients' subjective assessment of continence. Additionally, continence was controlled for multiple influencing factors.

Methods: This prospective multicentre study was carried out in seven hospitals throughout Germany. Before and at 3, 6, and 12 months after surgery self-reporting questionnaires were completed and returned by 329 (84.4%) of 390 eligible patients. The questionnaires were independently evaluated and analysed by a third party. Association of continence with demographic, operative, and tumour factors in an ongoing comprehensive prostate cancer database was evaluated.

Results: The continence rate drops substantially for patients undergoing radical prostatectomy but increases again with time. Concrete numbers vary considerably depending on definition – 44% at 3 months and 68% at 12 months after surgery (0 pads) vs. 71 and 90% (0–1 pads). Significant confounding variables regarding continence rate are nerve-sparing procedure, categorized Gleason score, rehabilitative cure treatment, and pelvic floor training.
The definition of 0 pads for continence coincides greater than 0–1 pads with the patients' self-assessment of being continent.

Conclusion: A standardized definition for continence would be desirable, as it is one of the most important preconditions to guarantee sound comparison of continence rates. Since there are enough other factors that make comparison difficult, we suggest using the definition of "0 pads". It is easily measured objectively, leaves no room for interpretation, and agrees best with the patients' self-assessment.

Background

In Northern and Western Europe the carcinoma of the prostate is the third most frequent type of cancer and by far the most prevalent cancer among men. 128 and 140 out of 100,000 men are diagnosed with this disease, respectively [1]. As a curative treatment, radical prostatectomy (RP) is widely used.

Although RP assures a low morbidity rate [2], is very effective in reducing mortality [3], and the amount of postoperative complications have been reduced due to advances in surgical technique [4], treatment modalities generally cause two major side effects: urinary incontinence and erectile dysfunction [5–7]. Both have a considerable negative impact on the patients' postoperative quality of life [8, 9]. The former even more so than the latter [10]. Consequently, there is a large interest in evaluating incontinence's postoperative extent and its influencing factors (e.g., [11–14]).

However, no generally shared standard definition of continence exists. This strongly affects the reported number of patients considered continent. One meta-analysis has found continence rates ranging as far as 67

* Correspondence: sigrun.holze@medizin.uni-leipzig.de
[1]Department of Urology, University of Leipzig, Liebigstr. 20, 04103 Leipzig, Germany
Full list of author information is available at the end of the article

percentage points (from 5 to 72%) which has been attributed mainly to varying definitions [15]. This inconsistency in defining continence, exacerbated by the heterogeneity of used study designs and samples, data collection methods, measuring instruments, and lengths of follow-up, makes it extremely difficult to compare published results. This has been widely recognized among contemporary research literature (e.g., [16–18]). This paper's main objective is then to identify the best possible definition of continence and thus help prevent the distortion of reported outcomes. Secondary objectives are to investigate the development of the post-surgical continence rate and reveal additional factors that influence continence after RP.

Written informed consent was obtained from all patients prior to their participation. The study was approved by the Ethics Committee of the University of Leipzig, Faculty of Medicine (approval no. 219–2007) and has therefore been performed in accordance with ethical standards.

Methods

Study design

In this prospective longitudinal multicentre study patients with newly diagnosed localised prostate cancer undergoing radical prostatectomy were recruited between February 2008 and May 2009 from seven hospitals in Germany. Patients with other cancer types, pathological cancer stage of pT4, dementia, psychosis, or insufficient knowledge of the German language were excluded. Patients were initially asked to fill out a questionnaire in the hospital one day before surgery in hospital (baseline). Subsequent questionnaires were sent three, six, and twelve months after surgery via mail. These follow-up questionnaires are different from those necessary to fulfil the requirements of certified prostate cancer centres.

There have already been articles published based on the data of this study [19, 20] which have found no significant distinction in comparing the urinary continence rates of endoscopic extraperitoneal radical prostatectomy (EERPE) with open radical prostatectomy (ORP). Our analysis of the influence of continence definition on continence rates will add to these findings.

Continence data were evaluated as followed: (a) number of pads used per day (b) patients' subjective assessment of continence and (c) urinary symptom score according to the quality of life questionnaire EORTC QLQ-PR25.

Only patients reporting full continence prior to surgery were included in the analysis. Socio-demographic data, clinical data, prostate cancer characteristics (e.g. clinical stage, prostate-specific antigen, biopsy Gleason score, positive surgical margins), and surgical features (surgical approach, nerve-sparing) were recorded. Socio-demographic data were retrieved from the questionnaire and clinical data were compiled from the respective patient's record.

Patients

In total, 487 patients treated with RP were eligible to participate in the study. Ninety-seven patients refused study participation at baseline. Thus, the total number of valid preoperative questionnaires was 390 (baseline participation rate: 80.1%). Three hundred twenty-nine patients completed and returned a second, third, and fourth questionnaire at 3, 6, and 12 months after surgery (participation rate: 84.4%). Sixty-one patients did not fill out the questionnaires.

There were no statistically significant differences between respondents (study participants) and non-respondents (patients who were excluded from or refused participation) regarding age (65.3 vs. 64.8 years) and pelvic lymph node dissection (75% vs. 76%). The number of patients who underwent nerve-sparing surgery was significantly higher among respondents than non-respondents (64% vs. 55%, $p < 0.05$).

Instruments

For the assessment of urinary incontinence after radical prostatectomy, different criteria were used:

(a) Number of pads used in a 24-h period: Patients were categorized as either (completely) continent (requiring 0 pads), socially continent (0–1 pad per day), or incontinent (2 or more pads per day).
(b) Patient's self-assessment of continence: Patients answered the question: Do you suffer from urinary incontinence? (yes/no).
(c) Urinary and bowel symptoms: These are two scales from the validated EORTC QLQ-PR25 – a multidimensional questionnaire of the "European Organization for Research and Treatment of Cancer" to measure the prostate related quality of life [21]. The QLQ-PR25 was scored according to the EORTC scoring manual [22]. A high score on these 0–100 point scales indicates a high burden of symptoms.

Statistical methods

Continence was defined as 0 pads per day. Agreement between the different criteria for continence ("0 pads" vs. "0–1 pad") and the subjective assessment via questionnaire was measured by Cohen's Kappa. Kappa values between 0.61 and 0.8 indicate good agreement [23, 24].

The trial cohort was characterized by mean ± standard deviation for continuous and frequencies / percentages [Wilson 95% C.I.] for categorical data. Means of continuous data were compared by t-test (Welch) for independent samples, frequencies by chi-square or Fisher's exact tests, if appropriate.

With regard to continence in the follow-up, we juxtaposed the three categories 0, 1 and 2 and more pads at 3, 6 and 12 months. These frequencies were compared by McNemar test. We modelled continence at 3 months on the one hand by a simple logistic regression and on the other hand by a multiple model with all detected confounders (cf. Table 1).

The search for covariates multiple associated with continence at 3 months was done in several steps. We started with variables potentially associated with continence: therapy (ORP vs. EERPE), nerve-sparing technique, PSA, Gleason score (categorized max. 6 / 7 / 8 and more), age, TNM stage, pelvic lymph node dissection, pelvic floor training at 3 months, additional therapy, medical rehabilitation and school and university education (cf. Table 1). A LASSO procedure [25] was applied to select variables for fitting a multiple logistic model. While setting $\lambda 2 = 0$, the optimal $\lambda 1$ was found by maximising the cross-validated likelihood. We excluded further variables only weakly associated with continence to get a "sparse" and well interpretable standard logistic regression model for estimating and testing. The results of this model were depicted by means of a Forrest plot.

We performed data preparation and basis statistics by IBM SPSS Statistics, version 22. The LASSO procedure and the generation of the Forrest plot was done by R (R Core Team, Vienna, Austria) [26]. Alpha = 5% was globally determined as two-sided significance limit.

Table 1 Sociodemographic and clinical characteristics of the study population

Sociodemographic	Total $N = 329$	Mean / Proportion	95% CI
Age (Mean, SD)	329	65.3	[65, 65.7]
> 65 years	180	54.7%	[49.3, 60%]
Family Status: Married	283	86.0%	[81.9, 89.4%]
Partnership: Yes	314	95.7%	[92.6, 97.2%]
School Education: Higher Level	135	41.4%	[35.9, 46.4%]
University Education	124	38.2%	[32.6, 43%]
Health Insurance: Private	66	20.4%	[16.1, 24.7%]
Employment Status			
Employed	92	29.0%	[23.4, 33%]
Pensioner	225	71.0%	[63.2, 73.2%]
Clinical			
PSA ng/ml (Mean, SD)	329	8.4	[8.1, 8.8]
Surgery	152	46.2%	[40.9, 51.6%]
EERPE	177	53.8%	[48.4, 59.1%]
ORP			
Nerve-sparing			
none	119	36.2%	[31.2, 41.5%]
unilateral	57	17.3%	[13.6, 21.8%]
bilateral	153	46.5%	[41.2, 51.9%]
Pelvic Lymph Adenectomy	243	74.8%	[68.9, 78.3%]
Pathological Stage			
pT1a - pT1c	4	1.2%	[0.5, 3.1%]
pT2a - pT2c	235	71.4%	[66.3, 76%]
pT3a - pT3b	90	27.4%	[22.8, 32.4%]
Positive Surgical Margins			
R0	278	84.8%	[80.2, 88%]
R1	50	15.2%	[11.7, 19.5%]
Gleason Score			
Gleason ≤6	131	40.1%	[34.7, 45.2%]
Gleason 7	158	48.3%	[42.7, 53.4%]
Gleason 8–10	38	11.6%	[8.5, 15.5%]

Results

Socio-demographic and clinical factors

Table 1 characterises our study population.

The mean (SD, range) age of the patients was 65.3 (6.4, 45–81) years. One hundred forty-nine patients (45.3%) were ≤ 65 years and 180 patients (54.7%) were > 65 years (cf. Table 1). Two different surgery methods were used: EERPE and ORP. One hundred and fifty two patients (46.2%) were operated on using the former procedure, 177 (53.8%) using the latter. In total, 63.8% of patients received a nerve-sparing procedure. Of these, 72.9% received a bilateral nerve-sparing prostatectomy. Two hundred and eighty-three patients (86%) were married. One hundred thirty-five patients (41.4%) had an education of a higher level.

Continence rates at 3, 6, and 12 months

The analysis shows that the continence rate (0 pads) at 3 months after surgery increases significantly from 44% to 6 months (59%, $p < 0.001$) and 12 months (68%, $p < 0.001$, see Fig. 1, Additional file 2: Table S2). The continence rates were significantly higher ($P = 0.001$) after nerve-sparing surgery (3 months: 51%, 6 months: 68%, 12 months: 78%) compared to non-nerve-sparing surgery (31, 42, 52%) (not in Figure).

The social continence rate (being defined as 0–1 pad) at 3, 6, and 12 months was significantly higher (71, 85, 90%, $P < .05$) than the rates of complete continence (0 pads) and the continence rate according to the patients' self-assessment (44, 57, 64%, cf. Fig. 1).

The best definition of continence: comparison of different criteria

The high diversity of applied continence measures complicates the comparison of results. This is why this study

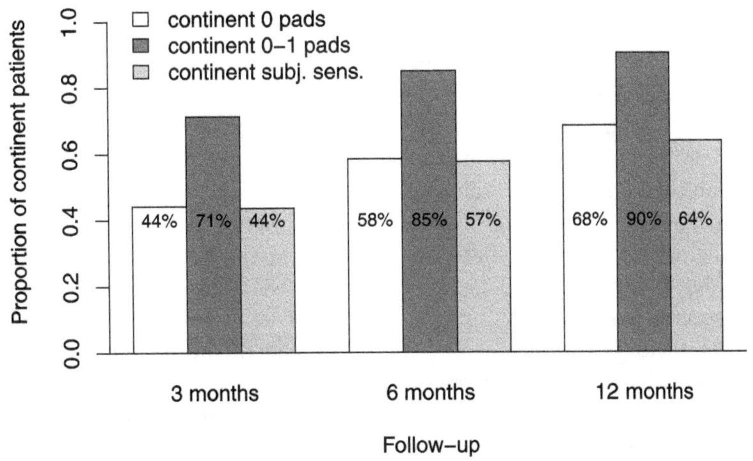

Fig. 1 Different assessments of continence

aims to identify criteria of continence which match best the patients' perception of continence. This was accomplished by collecting the number of pads as well as the patients' subjective assessment of continence.

It is controversially discussed if continence should be defined as the usage of "0 pads" or "0–1 pad". To clarify this issue, we calculated kappa coefficients measuring agreement between subjective sense of continence with assessment by the 0 and 0–1 criterion (cf. Table 2).

Kappa coefficients for 0 pads are higher than 0.61, indicating good agreement. At 3 and 6 months, even the lower 95% confidence bounds are over this threshold. On the other hand, kappa = 0.44 and 0.31 show only moderate to weak agreement of the 0–1 pad criterion with the subjective assessment of continence.

Table 2 (left panel) comparing the subjective assessment (in rows) with the evaluation by the respective criterion at 3 months (in columns) may illustrate this. The counts in the main diagonal are the numbers of patients for whom the subjective and objective assessments agree. That is, 140 and 122 patients feel continent and the 0–1 and 0 pads criterions respectively assess them continent, too. In the same manner, 91 and 162 patients feel incontinent in agreement with the evaluation by the 0–1 and 0 pads criterions. However, there are 94 patients feeling incontinent even though the 0–1-pads criterion determines them as continent. To summarize, there are 94 + 3 = 97 / 326 (30%) discrepant estimates by the 0–1 criterion in comparison to only 21 + 23 = 44 / 326 (13%) discrepant estimates by the zero pad criterion. The results at 6 and 12 months are similar.

Even though the 0 pads criterion is not perfect, it reflects the subjective sense of continence much better than the criterion of a safety pad (0–1 pads).

Factors associated with patients' post-surgical continence status

In our multivariate analyses, we observed a small disadvantage, albeit non-significant, of the ORP procedure compared to EERPE with respect to the binary endpoint

Table 2 Agreement between the different criteria and the subjective sense of continence at 3 (6 and 12) months

0/1-pads criterion					
Subjective sense of continence	continent 0–1 pads	incontinent 2+ pads	total	follow-up	kappa (95% c. i.)
Continent	140	3	143	3 mo.	0.44 (0.36, 0.52)
Incontinent	94	91	185	6 mo.	0.31 (0.22, 0.40)
total	234	94	328	12 mo.	0.31 (0.22, 0.40)
0-pads criterion					
Subjective sense of continence	continent 0 pads	incontinent 1+ pades	total	follow-up	kappa (95% c. i.)
Continent	122	21	143	3 mo.	0.73 (0.65, 0.80)
Incontinent	23	162	185	6 mo.	0.70 (0.62, 0.78)
Total	145	183	328	12 mo.	0.64 (0.56, 0.73)

Left panel: Agreement of subjective sense of continence (in rows) with actual use of pads at 3 months, above: 0/1-criterion, below: 0-pads criterion
Right panel: Estimated measure of agreement (kappa coefficient incl. 95% confidence interval) between subjective sense of continence and actual use of pads after 3, 6 and 12 months

continence at 3 months (odds ratio (OR) = 0.71, 95%C.I. 0.45–1.10). This alleged small disadvantage of ORP is only marginally changed by adjustment for confounders (OR = 0.63 [0.37–1.08], p = 0.092). TNM stage and PSA pre surgery, additional therapy, pelvic lymph node dissection, as well as social factors (marital status, in partnership or not, school and university education and employment state) are not predictive for continence. Thus, we got our final model with six variables after removing these confounders, but leaving age (cf. Fig. 2).

A second important question is which variables are bivariate and multiple associated with continence.

Of all covariates, the clear advantage of the nerve-sparing procedure is obvious. However, only the advantage of bilateral versus non-nerve-sparing technique is significant (OR 3.15 [1.55–5.98], p < 0.001). We could also observe a positive effect of the unilateral nerve-sparing procedure on the continence recovery rate (OR 1.86 [0.86–4.02] vs. non nerve-sparing, p = 0.113). However, there is no statistical evidence for this observation. Categorized Gleason score is significantly associated (p = 0.029), but none of the categories (Gleason =7: OR 1.68 [0.95–2.97], p = 0.073 against the reference category Gleason at most 6, Gleason ≥8: OR 0.55 [0.22–1.40], p = 0.208). Higher age is very weakly associated with risk of incontinence (OR 0.80 [0.53–1.21], p = 0.285). That is, odds for continence decrease by a factor of 0.8 per 10 years.

Finally, rehabilitative cure treatment (OR 0.47 [0.28–0.80], p = 0.005) and pelvic floor training (OR 0.16 [0.08–0.31], p < 0.001) are significantly negatively correlated with continence. Interpretation is difficult because statistics do not discriminate between risk factors for and responses on an outcome. We assumed that patients who are incontinent at 3 months are encouraged to participate in pelvic floor training. To check this assumption, we contrasted the continence rates at 6 and 12 months of patients who participated in pelvic floor exercises at three months vs. those who did not participate. Our data clearly shows the considerably steeper increase of continence rate at 6 and 12 months of patients who formerly exercised their pelvic floor (Additional file 1: Figure S1). This supports our hypothesis. The relationship of continence and rehabilitation could be similar. Only half of the patients continent at 3 months participated in rehabilitation (51%) but nearly ¾ (74%) of the incontinent patients. In other words, the portion of incontinence at three months is 65% in patients who participated in rehabilitation and only 40% in those who did not (OR 2.8). This difference in incontinence rates decreases up to six months (47% vs. 31%), giving an odds ratio of 1.9. This OR does not change essentially up to 12 months (37% vs. 22%, OR 2.1). This indicates that a fraction of patients, irrespective the method of surgery, has bad conditions for continence in spite of rehabilitation.

Urinary and bowel symptoms: EORTC QLQ-PR 25

There was a significant and clinically relevant worsening in urinary symptoms from a baseline score of 21.7 to 31.6 (− 9.9) points at 3 months (P < .001, Additional file 1: Table S1). Based on previous QoL research, a difference of at least 10 mean score points between different points in time is considered clinically relevant [27–29]. There was a gradual reduction of symptoms at 6 and 12 months after surgery.

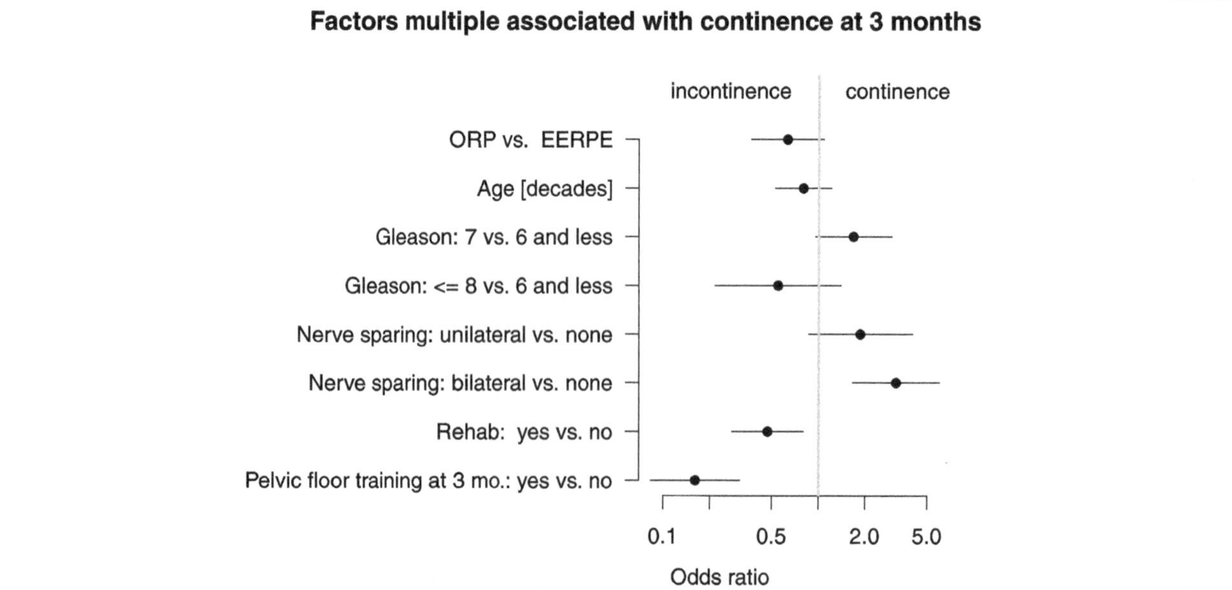

Fig. 2 Multivariate associations of several factors with continence at 3 months

In contrast, the burden of bowel symptoms was generally very low at all time-points. There was no statistically significant change over time.

Discussion

There are different reasons for the discrepancy between reported continence rates. Different clinical and sociodemographic characteristics of patients or the experience of the surgeon may be influencing factors [13, 30–32]. However, according to Sacco et al. [33] and Borregales et al. [16], it is the heterogeneity of methods and definitions that have the largest impact on the results. Trials using patient questionnaires for the evaluation of postoperative incontinence report lower continence rates than trials based on the physicians' assessment. For example, Lee et al. [34] have found continence rates varying from 14.7%, based on reports by patients, to 51.5%, based on reports by physicians at the same time. These numbers emphasize the problem of comparing continence rates if different measuring methods and/or definitions are used.

Some publications include patients using 1 pad per day in the group of complete continence. In this study, the strict definition of complete continence (0 pads) was used. Conflictingly, Krupski et al. [35] argue for a composite score to define continence. They find the 0 pads definition to be too superficial. An in-depth evaluation could surely reflect better the complex issue that is continence, but at the same time it would complicate the comparison of different study results. Krupski et al. acknowledge this themselves. Therefore, we strongly suggest the simple, yet conclusive definition of 0 pads per day. But keeping this objection in mind, the patients' self-assessment can be regarded as valuable supplemental information. Additionally, the standardized questionnaire EORTC QLQ-PR25 has been used as a part of this study to collect information on different aspects of urinary incontinence and its impact on the patients' quality of life for a deeper understanding. Nonetheless, other authors agree with adopting 0 pads per day as a standard. Borregales et al. [16] have systematically reviewed several articles on the subject and believe this definition to be optimal. Liss et al. [36] come to the conclusion that since there is a significant increase in quality of life with 0 pads in opposition to usage of 0 to 1 or a safety pad, this definition should be assumed universally. Incontinence and urinary symptoms are frequently associated with restrictions of social contacts and activities and have a high influence on the patients' quality of life. However, as our data also show, incontinence after RP is often a temporary problem. In the majority of patients, these symptoms decrease or disappear during the first postoperative year [37].

Patients who underwent nerve-sparing surgery were significantly less affected by urinary symptoms than patients who underwent non-nerve-sparing surgery. This effect can be observed for both unilateral and bilateral nerve-sparing techniques but is only of statistical significance for the latter. In regards to the effect of pelvic floor training, some articles state a positive outcome on the continence rate [38, 39]. A review conducted by Hunter et al. [40], on the other hand, elicits conflicting results. One of the seven articles considered in the review regarding this issue is in concordance with the aforementioned articles, "whereas the estimates from the others were consistent with no effect" [40] of pelvic floor training on continence rate. In our differentiated analyses, a positive correlation can be observed beyond the point of 3 months post-surgery. To assume that the negative correlation before that point in time is an artefact which results from increased training when incontinence stays consistent seems reasonable. Since the effect of rehabilitative cure treatment is most likely a mediator of pelvic floor training, similar assumptions can be made concerning its negative correlation with continence.

These results clearly show the superiority of the 0 pads usage definition. Firstly, defining continence as the usage of 0 pads has a higher objectivity and secondly, it shows good agreement with subjective assessments of continence.

Conclusion

Looking for a uniform continence criterion, the 0-pads criterion is advisable. It is clear and objective and does reflect the subjective sense of continence better than the criterion of 0–1 pads. We found the bilateral nerve-sparing procedure as only covariate clearly associated with continence.

Additional files

Additional file 1: Figure S1. Continence rates for patients who executed pelvic floor training or not at 3 months. **Table S1.** Symptom scales of the EORTC QLQ-PR25. (DOCX 70 kb)

Additional file 2: Table S2. Number of pads in the follow-up. (DOCX 15 kb)

Abbreviations

EERPE: Endoscopic extraperitoneal radical prostatectomy; EORTC QLQ: European Organization for Research and Treatment of Cancer Quality of Life Questionnaire; OR: Odds ratio; ORP: Open radical prostatectomy; RP: Radical prostatectomy

Acknowledgements

Not applicable

Authors' contributions

SH created the concept and design of the study together with JUW. Supported by LG and NK, they acquired the scientific data and implemented the clinical trial. Literature research was conducted by SH, KVH, MCT, UR, and SD. SH, KVH, and JUS also prepared the manuscript. Statistical data analysis was carried out by MM and SH. All authors reviewed and edited the manuscript.

Author details

[1]Department of Urology, University of Leipzig, Liebigstr. 20, 04103 Leipzig, Germany. [2]Coordination Centre for Clinical Trials, University of Leipzig, Härtelstr. 16-18, 04107 Leipzig, Germany. [3]Department of Medical Psychology and Medical Sociology, University of Leipzig, Philipp-Rosenthal-Str. 55, 04103 Leipzig, Germany. [4]Department of Urology, Klinikum Dortmund, Beurhausstr. 40, 44137 Dortmund, Germany. [5]Department of Urology, Diakonissenkrankenhaus Dessau, Gropiusallee 3, 06846 Dessau, Germany. [6]Department of Urology, Helios Klinikum Wuppertal, Heusnerstr. 40, 42283 Wuppertal, Germany.

References

1. Ferlay J, Steliarova-Foucher E, Lortet-Tieulent J, et al. Cancer incidence and mortality patterns in Europe: estimates for 40 countries in 2012. Eur J Cancer. 2013;49:1374–403.
2. Kirschner-Hermanns R, Jakse G. Quality of life following radical prostatectomy. Crit Rev Oncol Hematol. 2002;43:141–51.
3. Bill-Axelson A, Holmberg L, Ruutu M, et al. Radical prostatectomy versus watchful waiting in early prostate Cancer. N Engl J Med. 2005;352:1977–84.
4. Hoznek A, Menard Y, Salomon L, Abbou CC. Update on laparoscopic and robotic radical prostatectomy. Curr Opin Urol. 2005;15(3):173–80.
5. Litwin MS, Hays RD, Fink A, et al. Quality-of-life outcomes in men treated for localized prostate Cancer. JAMA. 1995;273(2):129–35.
6. Barry MJ, Gallagher PM, Skinner JS, Fowler FJ Jr. Adverse effects of robotic-assisted laparoscopic versus open Retropubic radical prostatectomy among a Nationwide random sample of Medicare-age men. J Clin Oncol. 2012; 30(5):513–8.
7. Haglind E, Carlsson S, Stranne J, et al. Urinary incontinence and erectile dysfunction after robotic versus open radical prostatectomy: a prospective, controlled, nonrandomised trial. Eur Urol. 2015;68:216–25.
8. Penson DF, McLerran D, Feng Z, et al. 5-year urinary and sexual outcomes after radical prostatectomy: results from the prostate Cancer outcomes study. J Urol. 2005;173:1701–5.
9. Miller DC, Sanda G, Dunn RL, et al. Long-term outcomes among localized prostate Cancer survivors: health-related quality-of-life changes after radical prostatectomy, external radiation and brachytherapy. J Clin Oncol. 2005; 23(12):2772–80.
10. Fowler FJ, Barry MJ, Lu-Yao G, et al. Effect of radical prostatectomy for prostate Cancer on patient quality of life: results from a Medicare survey. Urology. 1995;45(6):1007–15.
11. Ficarra V, Giacomo N, Rosen RC, et al. Systematic Review and Meta-analysis of Studies Reporting Urinary Continence Recovery After Robot-assisted Radical Prostatectomy. Eur Urol. 2012;62:405–17.
12. Geraerts I, Van Poppel H, Devoogdt N, et al. Influence of preoperative and postoperative pelvic floor muscle training (PFMT) compared with postoperative PFMT on urinary incontinence after radical prostatectomy: a randomized controlled trial. Eur Urol. 2013;64:766–72.
13. Kaye DR, Hyndman MF, Segal RL, et al. Urinary outcomes are significantly affected by nerve sparing quality during radical prostatectomy. Urology. 2013;82:1348–54.
14. Holm HV, Fossa SD, Hedlund H, et al. How should continence and incontinence after radical prostatectomy be evaluated? A prospective study of patient ratings and changes with time. J Urol. 2014;192:1155–61.
15. Boorjian SA, Eastham JA, Graefen M, et al. A Critical Analysis of the Long-Term Impact of Radical Prostatectomy on Cancer Control and Function Outcomes. Eur Urol. 2012;61:664–75.
16. Borregales LD, Berg WT. Tal O et la. 'Trifecta' after radical prostatectomy: is there a standard definition? BJU Int. 2013;112:60–7.
17. Patel VR, Coelho RF, Sanket C, et al. Continence, potency and oncological outcomes after robotic-assisted radical prostatectomy: early trifecta results of a high-volume surgeon. BJU Int. 2010;106:696–702.
18. Coelho RF, Bernardo R, Patel MB, et al. Retropubic, laparoscopic, and robot-assisted radical prostatectomy: a critical review of outcomes reported by high-volume centers. J Endourol. 2010;24(12):2003–15.
19. Köhler N, Gansera L, Stolzenburg JU, et al. Early continence in patients with localized prostate cancer: a comparison between open retropubic (RRPE) and endoscopic extraperitoneal radical prostatectomy (EERPE). Urol Oncol. 2012;30:798–803.
20. Köhler N, Gansera L, Holze S, et al. Cancer-related fatigue in patients before and after radical prostatectomy. Results of a prospective multi-Centre study. Support Care Cancer. 2014;22:2883–9.
21. Van Andel J, Bottomley A, Fossa SD, et al. An international field study of the EORTC QLQ-PR25: a questionnaire for assessing the health-related quality of life of patients with prostate cancer. Eur J Cancer. 2008;44(16):2418–24.
22. Fayers PM, Aaronson NK, Bjordal K, et al. The EORTC QLQ-C30 scoring manual. 3rd ed. Brussels, BE: European Organisation for Research and Treatment of Cancer; 2001.
23. Anthony JV, Joanne MG. Understanding Interobserver agreement: the kappa statistic. Fam Med J. 2005;37(5):360–3.
24. Landis TR, Koch GG. The measurement of observer agreement for Categorial data. Biometrics. 1977;33(1):159–74.
25. Goeman JJ. L1 penalized estimation in the cox proportional hazards model. Biom J. 2010;52:70–84.
26. R Development Core Team. R: A language and environment for statistical computing. Vienna, Austria: R Foundation for Statistical Computing. 2012. ISBN 3-900051-07-0. http://www.R-project.org. Accessed 6 Apr 2017.
27. King M. The interpretation of scores from the EORTC quality of life questionnaire QLQ-C30. Qual Life Res. 1995;5(6):555–67.
28. Osoba D, Rodrigues G, Myles J, et al. Interpreting the significance of changes in health-related quality-of-life scores. J Clin Oncol. 1998;16(1):139–44.
29. Rodrigues G, Bezjak A, Osob D, et al. The relationship of changes in EORTC QLQ-C30 scores to ratings on the subjective significance questionnaire in men with localized prostate cancer. Qual Life Res. 2004;13(7):1235–46.
30. Lee S, Yoon CJ, Park HJ, et al. The surgical procedure is the Most important factor affecting continence recovery after laparoscopic radical prostatectomy. World J Men's Health. 2013;31(2):163–9.
31. Magheli A, Busch J, Leva N, et al. Comparison of surgical technique (open vs. laparoscopic) on pathological and long term functional outcomes following radical prostatectomy. BMC Urol. 2014;14:18.
32. Mager R, Kurosch M, Hüsch T, et al. Verhinderung der Post-prostatektomieinkontinenz: Ätiologie und Risikofaktoren. Der Urologe. 2014; 53(3):327–32.
33. Sacco E, Prayer-Galetti T, Pinto F, et al. Urinary incontinence after radical prostatectomy: incidence by definition, risk factors and temporal trend in a large series with a long-term follow-up. BJU Int. 2006;97:1234–41.
34. Lee SR, Kim HW, Lee JW, et al. Discrepancies in perception of urinary incontinence between patient and physician after robotic radical prostatectomy. Yonsei Med J. 2010;51(6):883–7.
35. Krupski TL, Saigal CS, Litwin MS. Variation in continence and potency by definition. J Urol. 2003;170:1291–4.
36. Liss MA, Osann K, Canvasser N, et al. Continence definition after radical prostatectomy using urinary quality of life: evaluation of patient reported validated questionnaires. J Urol. 2010;183(4):1464–8.
37. Fritzsche K, Diederich D, Schultze-Seemann W. Psychooncology of prostate carcinoma - psychosocial distress and treatment approaches: a systematic review. Z Psychosom Med Psychother. 2008;54(4):329–53.
38. Mannassero F, Traversi C, Ales V, et al. Contribution of early intensive prolonged pelvic floor exercises on urinary continence recovery after bladder neck-sparing radical prostatectomy: results of a prospective controlled randomized trial. Neurourol Urodyn. 2007;26:985–9.
39. Tienforti D, Sacco E, Marangi F, et al. Efficacy of an assisted low-intensity programme of perioperative pelvic floor muscle training in improving the recovery of continence after radical prostatectomy: a randomized controlled trial. BJU Int. 2012;110:1004–10.
40. Hunter KF, Glazener CM, Moore KN. Conservative Management for Postprostatectomy Urinary Incontinence. Cochrane Database of Systematic Reviews. 2007.

16

Adherence and barriers to penile rehabilitation over 2 years following radical prostatectomy

Jeffrey Albaugh[1*], Brittany Adamic[2], Cecilia Chang[1], Nicholas Kirwen[1] and Joshua Aizen[2]

Abstract

Background: A variety of penile rehabilitation (PR) therapies are available to improve post-prostatectomy erectile dysfunction (ED) with mixed results. It is uncertain how adherent men are to PR therapies. The aim of this study is to determine adherence to and identify barriers to PR treatment.

Methods: A longitudinal cross-sectional approach was used in men who underwent radical prostatectomy over 2 years. Men were instructed to take a PDE5 inhibitor (PDE5i) three times per week, and if required, utilize a vacuum constriction device (VCD) daily. Outcomes were measured by multiple validated questionnaires. In addition, penile stretched length, side effects, compliance to PR regimen & barriers to participation were documented.

Results: Seventy-seven patients were enrolled, however only 49 completed evaluation at 3 or more timepoints and were included in analysis. This cohort was an average age of 58.1 years (±7.7), had robotic laparoscopic radical prostatectomy (91.7%), and had bilateral nerve sparing procedures (95.8%). Majority (62.5%) reported normal SHIM pre-operatively, however 79% used PDE5i. Erectile function as measured by IIEF and Erection Hardness Rating were negatively affected post-operatively, with gradual improvement in parameters throughout the 24 month follow up. Of the participants who had normal pre-op SHIM, only 23.1 and 28.6% regained baseline function at 1 and 2 years, respectively. Orgasm was significantly diminished immediately post-operatively, however, at the end of the study period only 37% of men reported diminished climax and no men reported absent orgasm. Adherence to penile rehabilitation therapies declined overtime. Men took oral PDE5i on average 2.3 times weekly at 12 and 24 months ($p < 0.001$). Men used the VCD 2.3–3.9 days a week, which declined overtime ($p = 0.014$).

Conclusions: Improvement in erectile and orgasm parameters was observed over time, but most men did not return to baseline function. Despite comprehensive instructions and a frequent follow up schedule, PDE5i and VCD adherence was poor. High attrition rates were noted with only 55.8% of men remaining at 12 months and 45% of men completing 24 months. The most common barriers to PR adherence were cost, inconvenience and perceived ineffectiveness.

Keywords: Penile rehabilitation, Radical prostatectomy, Erectile dysfunction, Adherence

* Correspondence: jalbaugh@northshore.org
[1]Northshore University HealthSystem, Evanston, IL, USA
Full list of author information is available at the end of the article

Background

Prostate cancer is the most commonly diagnosed non-skin cancer in men [1]. Men with clinically significant prostate cancer are required to decide between treatment options, each with side effects that may greatly affect quality of life [2]. Despite advances in nerve-sparing surgical techniques, the incidence of erectile dysfunction 2–15 years following radical prostatectomy has been reported to be as high as 78–87% in a large population-based study [3]. Erectile recovery following nerve-sparing radical prostatectomy can take two or more years [4].

The goal of penile rehabilitation (PR) after prostate cancer treatment is to maximally preserve preoperative erectile function through the use of medications and/or devices. PR success is determined by the ability to achieve and maintain erectile rigidity sufficient for satisfactory sexual relations without the use of any further ED treatments then used prior to surgery. Treatment options for PR include oral phosphodiesterase type 5 inhibitors (PDE5i), vacuum constriction devices (VCD), and intracavernosal injections (ICI). Men with comorbid medical conditions or those who utilized medications for erectile dysfunction prior to prostate cancer treatment are at greater risk for erectile dysfunction following radical prostatectomy [5].

Recommendations from the fourth International Consultation for Sexual Medicine suggest discussing erectile dysfunction and PR options with men prior to and after radical prostatectomy. The panel determined that inadequate data exist to recommend any specific PR regimen over another [6]. Thus, a critical need exists for further research in the realm of post-prostatectomy PR to determine the most effective strategies. This study aimed to assess rates of PR adherence and identify barriers to participation in PR. It also sought to assess the progression of erectile function and orgasm quality in men utilizing a post-prostatectomy PR regimen.

Methods

The study utilized a longitudinal cross-sectional approach in which men who underwent radical prostatectomy were followed for 2 years following surgery with assessment at 1, 3, 6, 12 and 24 month intervals after beginning penile rehabilitation. The Sexual Health Inventory for Men (SHIM) [7], a five-item subscale within the International Index of Erectile Function (IIEF) that assesses presence and severity of erectile dysfunction, was completed by all patients preoperatively [8]. Men underwent radical prostatectomy via a nerve-sparing approach when feasible from a technical and oncologic standpoint. Post-operatively, men initiated a PR regimen, consisting of PDE5i with or without VCD and/or ICI. Specifically, participants were instructed to take sildenafil with varied doses up to 100 mg or tadalafil up to 20 mg as needed at least three times per week. Participants could take doses of sildenafil or tadalafil, with dosing as needed as tolerated. Men were encouraged to take a dose a minimum of 3 times a week and did not take daily doses of tadalafil 5 mg. The men were encouraged to take varied doses three times a week as needed as tolerated rather than daily to determine if any doses were helping as compared to no medication. After taking sildenafil or tadalafil, patients were asked to complete an Erection Hardness Score (EHS), a scale ranging from 0 (no erection) to 4 (fully hard erection) [9]. If they were unable to achieve ≥3 on this scale with oral agents alone, they were instructed to add VCD to their regimen. Prescribed VCD routines consisted of 5–10 stretches per day, each held for 1–2 min within the device. If patients desired, they were also instructed to use intracavernosal injections as an adjunct erectogenic therapy.

Men were included in this study if they had undergone radical prostatectomy ≤12 weeks before initiating PR. Only men with preoperative SHIM of ≥16 were included, confirming at least moderate erectile function at baseline. Patients were required to have a sexual partner at the time of treatment. Finally, participants were excluded if they were unable to safely be treated with PDE5i and/or VCD. Informed consent was obtained from all participants for this institutional review board approved study.

Prior to the study, baseline preoperative clinical parameters were recorded from the medical record when available or from the patient, including co-morbidities, baseline erectile function and orgasm quality, and stretched penile length. During the course of the study, a variety of self-reported measures were completed by participants at the following time points: immediately post-surgery, 1 month, 3 months, 6 months, 12 months, and 24 months post-operatively. Some of the measures included the Erectile Dysfunction Inventory of Treatment Satisfaction (EDITS) [10], EHS, IIEF (15-item questionnaire measuring erectile function, orgasmic function, sexual desire, intercourse satisfaction, and overall sexual satisfaction) including the Sexual Health Inventory for Men (SHIM/IIEF-5), Self-Esteem and Relationship Questionnaire (14-item patient-reported assessment of sexual confidence and intimacy) [11], and stretched penile length. A list of the data collected/instruments/measures are described in the Appendix. The SHIM scores are collected with and without treatment. With treatment (treated SHIM) score means the men were responding to SHIM questions with the use of their erectile dysfunction treatment if needed (oral agents, vacuum device and/or injections) and without treatment (untreated SHIM) means they were not using anything to treat their erectile dysfunction (unless they were taking oral meds before surgery and then they would only be using what they used prior to surgery with the untreated score). In addition to these instruments, clinical data, PR side effects, compliance to PR regimen, and barriers to participation were documented at each follow up visit. Although it was not the main aim of the study, we also measured quality of life with the Quality of Life Index-Cancer Version (QLI- a validated measurement of overall quality of life, health and functioning, social and economic functioning, psychological/spiritual stability, and family role) [12] and the UCLA Prostate Cancer Index (measurement of health-related quality of life in men treated for prostate cancer) [13]. Categorical variables were analyzed using chi-squared test, whereas continuous variables were compared over time using ANOVA. All statistical analyses were conducted in SAS 9.4 (SAS Institute, Cary, NC).

Results

Seventy-seven men were enrolled in the study, however only 49 men were included in final analysis, as those who completed less than 3 evaluations were excluded. Table 1 describes the demographics of our cohort. The average age of our participants was 58.1 (SD = 7.74) and majority of men were Caucasian (89.8%). This cohort was well educated with 89.6% having a college level education or greater. Nearly all men underwent robotic nerve sparring radical prostatectomy (91.7%) with majority undergoing bilateral nerve sparring (95.8% bilateral and 4.2% unilateral). Seventy-nine percent of men reported treatment for erectile dysfunction (ED) pre-operatively with a PDE-5 inhibitor. The majority had a normal SHIM (62.5%) with a mean SHIM of 22.2 (SD = 2.59) and a mean erection hardness score of 3.41 out of 4 (SD = 0.37). Average stretched penile length was 13.7 cm (SD = 1.83) prior to prostatectomy.

Post-operative functional evaluations can be found in Tables 2 and 3. The treated SHIM at 3 months post-operatively was 12.13 (± 7.57) with only 21.7% of men reporting a normal erection. The SHIM and IIEF scores did improve over the 2 year follow up, with 40% of men reporting a normal treated SHIM at 2 years. Men without ED pre-operatively, as defined by a SHIM of 22–25, did not adequately return to baseline erectile function. Only 23.1 and 28.6% of these men reported a normal treated SHIM at 1 and 2 years respectively without ED treatment. Despite poor erectile function as measured by SHIM, mean treated erection hardness ratings returned to baseline at 2 years when using erectile dysfunction treatments. On average, loss of penile stretched length was 1.76 cm at the one-month post-operative visit. Average penile stretched length returned to within 0.5 cm of baseline after 6 months of penile rehabilitation and was maintained throughout the remainder of the follow up period. Overall, quality of life was not significantly impacted as measured by the Quality of Life Index, however, the health and functioning domain improved over the 2 year study period from 23.7 ± 4.10 to 26.1 ± 2.96 out of 30 ($p = 0.049$). The overall SEAR scores, measuring relationship satisfaction and sexual self-esteem were low following surgery but improved significantly over time as measures of erectile function improved.

Orgasm was also impacted by prostate cancer treatment. The orgasm function domain of the IIEF

Table 1 Initial Demographics

	Baseline ($N = 49$)	
	N	%
Age	58.12 ± 7.74	
< 50	8	16.33
50–59	20	40.82
60–69	17	34.69
≥ 70	4	8.16
Race		
Caucasian	44	89.80
African-American	5	10.20
Highest Education Level		
High School	5	10.42
Some College	6	12.50
Associate Degree	1	2.08
Bachelor's Degree	13	27.08
Master's Degree	15	31.25
Doctorate Degree	8	16.67
Type of Surgery		
Robotic	44	91.67
Open	4	8.33
Nerve Sparring		
Nerve Sparring	46	95.83
Non-nerve Sparring	0	0.00
Unilateral or Partial Nerve Sparring	2	4.17
ED Medications		
No	11	22.45
Yes	38	77.55
Any Treatment for ED		
No	10	20.83
Yes	38	79.17
Pre-Op SHIM	22.20 ± 2.59	
Abnormal	18	37.50
Normal (22–25)	30	62.50
Post-Op SHIM	4.78 ± 4.07	
Abnormal	49	100.00
Normal (22–25)	0	0.00

Table 2 Patient-Reported Outcomes of Erectile Function and Relationship Satisfaction over Time

	Pre-Op (*N* = 49)	Baseline (*N* = 49)	1 Month (*N* = 48)	3 Months (*N* = 46)	6 Months (*N* = 45)	1 Year (*N* = 43)	2 Years (*N* = 35)	*p*-value[b]
Treated SHIM Score[a]	22.20 ± 2.59	4.78 ± 4.07	9.88 ± 6.96	12.13 ± 7.57	14.80 ± 7.71	14.23 ± 8.80	16.66 ± 7.78	<.0001
Untreated SHIM Score			6.46 ± 5.04	7.70 ± 5.71	9.91 ± 6.32	12.55 ± 6.88	15.31 ± 6.92	<.0001
EDITS Score[e]			63.80 ± 18.83	62.04 ± 19.54	67.33 ± 22.35	71.75 ± 22.74	78.40 ± 20.93	0.0042
IIEF Score								
Erectile Function (EF)		5.80 ± 4.61	12.38 ± 8.35	15.20 ± 9.13	18.02 ± 9.52	17.51 ± 10.80	20.54 ± 9.48	<.0001
Orgasmic Function (OF)		4.10 ± 3.66	6.71 ± 2.68	6.93 ± 2.71	7.49 ± 2.42	6.63 ± 3.38	7.77 ± 2.45	<.0001
Climax/Orgasm								
Absent		8 18.60	2 4.26	0 0.00	3 6.67	1 2.33	0 0.00	0.0029
Diminished		20 46.51	21 44.68	17 36.96	15 33.33	11 25.58	13 37.14	
Normal		14 32.56	9 40.43	21 45.65	18 40.00	25 58.14	12 34.29	
Better		1 2.33	5 10.64	8 17.39	9 20.00	6 13.95	10 28.57	
Sexual Desire (SD)		6.43 ± 2.27	7.21 ± 1.57	7.02 ± 2.02	7.20 ± 1.74	6.65 ± 2.74	7.09 ± 1.99	0.3615
Intercourse Satisfaction (IS)		3.10 ± 3.20	5.77 ± 4.42	6.72 ± 4.51	8.16 ± 3.81	7.95 ± 4.65	8.57 ± 4.07	<.0001
Overall Satisfaction (OS)		4.90 ± 2.26	6.10 ± 2.41	6.09 ± 2.34	6.42 ± 2.49	6.16 ± 3.20	6.94 ± 2.61	0.0105
Treated EHR[c]	3.41 ± 0.37	1.15 ± 0.87	1.82 ± 1.02	2.56 ± 0.98	2.89 ± 0.85	3.21 ± 0.79	3.54 ± 0.42	<.0001
Untreated EHR			1.41 ± 0.87	1.68 ± 0.92	2.02 ± 1.06	2.55 ± 1.07	3.10 ± 0.70	<.0001
Penile Stretched Length	13.73 ± 1.83	11.97 ± 1.63	12.34 ± 1.48	12.98 ± 1.45	13.37 ± 1.38	13.42 ± 1.32	13.80 ± 1.24	<.0001
SEAR[d]		17.47 ± 8.75	20.60 ± 7.70	22.22 ± 8.49	24.91 ± 9.11	26.79 ± 8.62	32.34 ± 10.94	<.0001
Sexual Relationship Satisfaction		71.56 ± 19.77	70.05 ± 24.80	73.10 ± 24.11	80.69 ± 15.76	80.67 ± 15.30	84.82 ± 15.99	0.0021
Self-Esteem		78.06 ± 20.97	76.82 ± 20.14	78.80 ± 25.80	80.83 ± 17.80	81.10 ± 20.30	82.50 ± 20.83	0.8233
Overall Relationship Satisfaction		48.51 ± 18.79	53.50 ± 19.22	57.53 ± 21.51	64.80 ± 20.10	68.19 ± 18.60	74.49 ± 19.71	<.0001
Total		17.47 ± 8.75	20.60 ± 7.70	22.22 ± 8.49	24.91 ± 9.11	26.79 ± 8.62	32.34 ± 10.94	<.0001

[a]Data are presented as mean ± SD or N and %; [b]ANOVA for *p*-values over time from baseline to 2 years; [c]*EHR* Erection Hardness Rating; [d]*SEAR* Self Esteem and Relationship; [e]*EDITS* Erectile Dysfunction Inventory of Treatment Satisfaction

Table 3 SHIM Scores over Time

	1 Month ($N = 48$)		3 Months ($N = 46$)		6 Months ($N = 45$)		1 Year ($N = 43$)		2 Years ($N = 35$)		*p*-value
	N	%	N	%	N	%	N	%	N	%	
Treated SHIM Score[a]	9.88 ± 6.96		12.13 ± 7.57		14.80 ± 7.71		14.23 ± 8.80		16.66 ± 7.78		0.0010
Abnormal	42	87.50	36	78.26	31	68.89	30	69.77	21	60.00	0.0500
Normal (22–25)	6	12.50	10	21.74	14	31.11	13	30.23	14	40.00	
Untreated SHIM Score[a]	6.46 ± 5.04		7.70 ± 5.71		9.91 ± 6.32		12.55 ± 6.88		15.31 ± 6.92		<.0001
Abnormal	47	97.92	43	93.48	43	95.56	36	83.72	28	80.00	0.0176
Normal (22–25)	1	2.08	3	6.52	2	4.44	7	16.28	7	20.00	

SHIM scores similar to initial	1 Year ($N = 43$)		2 Years ($N = 35$)	
	N	%	N	%
Treated SHIM Score				
Dissimilar	36	83.72	30	85.71
Similar	7	16.28	5	14.29
Untreated SHIM Score				
Dissimilar	40	93.02	30	85.71
Similar	3	6.98	6	14.29

Normal Pre-Op SHIM scores ($N = 30$)	1 Year ($N = 26$)		2 Years ($N = 21$)	
	N	%	N	%
Treated SHIM Score				
Abnormal	18	69.23	14	66.67
Normal	8	30.77	7	33.33
Untreated SHIM Score				
Abnormal	20	76.92	15	71.43
Normal	6	23.08	6	28.57

[a]Data are presented as mean ± SD or N and %; Normal SHIM Score = (22–25)

Table 4 Treatment Adherence and Compliance over Time

	1 Month ($N = 48$)		3 Months ($N = 46$)		6 Months ($N = 45$)		1 Year ($N = 43$)		2 Years ($N = 35$)		p-value
	N	%	N	%	N	%	N	%	N	%	
Medications for ED											
No	0	0.00	0	0.00	0	0.00	1	2.33	4	11.43	0.0027
Yes	48	100.00	46	100.00	45	100.00	42	97.67	31	88.57	
How often? (per week)	3.02 ± 0.62		2.71 ± 0.86		2.75 ± 1.25		2.34 ± 1.32		2.30 ± 1.07		0.0104
Any Vacuum Device											
No	44	91.67	13	28.26	13	28.89	17	39.53	21	60.00	<.0001
Yes	4	8.33	33	71.74	32	71.11	26	60.47	14	40.00	
How often? (per week)	4.50 ± 1.73		3.86 ± 1.97		3.01 ± 1.81		2.28 ± 1.67		3.12 ± 1.73		0.0137
Any Other Treatments (Injections)											
No	46	100.00	46	100.00	41	91.11	36	83.72	30	88.24	0.0072
Yes	0	0.00	0	0.00	4	8.89	7	16.28	4	11.76	
How often? (per week)					1.06 ± 0.83		0.92 ± 0.97		0.56 ± 0.52		0.6892

(Questions 9–10 with maximum score of 10) was significantly diminished post-operatively (4.1 ± 3.66), however improved with a mean score of 7.77 ± 2.45 at 24 months. At the end of the study period, only 37% of men reported diminished climax, with no men reporting absent orgasm.

Satisfaction with treatment, as measured by the EDITS improved significantly over time from an average of 63.8 (SD = 18.8) at 1 month to 78.4 (SD = 20.9) at 24 months ($p = 0.004$). Adherence to the penile rehabilitation protocol declined with time after prostatectomy as seen in Table 4. Men were adherent to oral PDE5i, using them 3 times per week initially post-op, which declined to 2.3 times per week on average at 24 months. Men instructed to utilize a vacuum device daily reported use on average 4.5 days per week at 1 month post-operatively, declining to 3.12 days per week at 24 months. Only 2–5% of men utilized the VCD five or more times per week. The utilization of a VCD was highest between months 3–12 (60.5–71.7%).

Barriers to adherence to the penile rehabilitation protocol were assessed. Identified factors from most to least common were as follows: cost (17.8–32.6%), inconvenience (2.1–31.1%), treatment is not very helpful (2.0–23.3%), lack of insurance coverage (6.7–22.5%), treatment is cumbersome (2.1–19.6%), timing of treatment is difficult (2.1–18.6%), side effects (4.2–11.1%). Barriers of cost and insurance coverage were unique to oral PDE5i therapy and the treatment being cumbersome was identified in men using a vacuum device. Other patient reported barriers to treatment included partner factors, frustration with lack of sexual function recovery, time constraints, traveling with therapy, comorbid health problems, delayed recovery, surgical complications and/or family stressors. High attrition rates for the PR program were noted with only 55.8% of men remaining at 12 months and 45.5% of men completing 24 months.

At the conclusion of the study, 88.6% of men still required medical treatment of their erectile dysfunction ($p = 0.0027$). Forty percent were using a VCD and 11.7% of men required intracavernosal injections, using them about once every 2 weeks.

Discussion

Post-prostatectomy erectile dysfunction in a large population-based study revealed long term incidence of ED may be as high as 78–87% [3]. The role of oral PDE5i in penile rehabilitation has been called into question. The use of PR therapies has been found effective during utilization of the therapy, but it is uncertain if PR therapies can improve spontaneous erectile recovery [14]. Multiple variables may play a role in adherence to a PR therapy.

This observational cohort study followed a young population from a variety of prostate cancer surgeons from academic centers in the Chicago area for 2 years after radical prostatectomy. The majority of men underwent nerve sparing robotic assisted radical prostatectomy, which is consistent with current surgical trends [15, 16]. Continued improvement in erectile function was seen over the 24-month study period, as measured by SHIM, IIEF and erection hardness questionnaires. Erectile function is known to improve for 2 years post-operatively [17]. Pre-operatively, men were required to have a SHIM score of 16 to participate, and the average SHIM was 22.2 with 79% of men utilizing PDE5 inhibitors. Overall, the large majority of these men did not return to their baseline erectile function. Only 28.6% of men with normal erectile function pre-operatively (SHIM 22–25) returned to their baseline erectile function at 2 years. These results are similar to results from a recent study from Memorial Sloan Kettering, which determined erectile function returns in approximately 28% of post radical prostatectomy patients after 2 years [18]. The current study contributes further to the growing body of evidence that the majority of men do not recover their pre-operative erectile function and men undergoing nerve sparring radical prostatectomy should be counseled about this prior to treatment.

Penile stretched length was decreased by an average of 1.76 cm post-operatively and normalized after 6 months of penile rehabilitation which correlates with multiple studies [19, 20]. The men did regularly use PDE5i and the vacuum device if needed for penile rehabilitation and the improvement in penile length in the majority of patients could be due to this regimented rehabilitation program designed based on previous studies showing improvement [19, 21, 22]. Orgasm was described as absent or diminished in 65.1% of men post-operatively with return to normal or better in 62.9% of men at 24 months. These rates of anorgasmia and altered orgasmic sensation are consistent with available literature [23]. Men and their partners should be advised of these changes in orgasm prior to prostate cancer treatment.

Even amongst a highly educated population, adherence to therapy was less than expected. On average, men did not use the PDE5i at least 3 times a week, nor did they use the vacuum device daily. Barriers to adherence included cost of medications, side effects, remembering to utilize intermittent therapies, lack of perceived benefit, frustration with slow return of erectile function, inability to find time to use a cumbersome therapy, partner issues and life stressors. In general, the men in our program described many reasons why they were unable to consistently do penile rehabilitation as instructed. The more common reasons were consistent with previously reported barriers to therapy and adds further evidence about the challenges of doing penile rehabilitation and the reality of how much it can be done [24, 25]. Clinicians need to be realistic with men about what they can do with PR. It is important to identify barriers to treatment so they may be addressed in order to improve adherence. The most commonly identified barriers by men in our cohort were cost, perceived ineffectiveness of treatment and inconvenience.

Cost and insurance coverage were ongoing issues during the study period as the price of oral PDE5is continued to rise and Medicare no longer covered the vacuum device. Ultimately, men in the study were provided resources to obtain an affordable medical grade vacuum device and no participant in the study was without a vacuum device if they required one. Adherence to the penile rehabilitation protocol decreased with time for some men who reported improved erectile function, as expected. Conversely, some men identified frustration with lack of sexual function recovery as a barrier. Men who felt their progress was slow or inadequate were discouraged, reporting that rehabilitation treatments were a reminder of their erectile dysfunction, further deterring them from adhering to treatments. Inconvenience was a significant factor, with up to 31.1% of men stating that they were too busy for therapy. Additional inconveniences identified were related to travel and forgetfulness. One gentleman refused vacuum therapy due to his personal adversities. The challenges with adherence and the high attrition rate were also due to a number of reasons; need for adjuvant prostate cancer or other health issue treatments, partner factors, relationship issues, relocating away from the clinic, work environment and being too busy. At the conclusion of the study, nearly every participant continued to require therapy for ED. High attrition rates for the PR program were noted with only 44.5% completing the 24 month follow up.

Limitations of this study include the descriptive nature as well as selection bias. Only patients referred to our sexual health department were included. There was no control group in the study and this was not a randomized placebo trial, but rather a descriptive observational cohort study assessing sexual function before surgery, after surgery and with penile rehabilitation for 2 years. This is a major limitation of the study and randomized controlled studies are needed to assess the efficacy and safety of penile rehabilitation to be able to generalize findings to other populations. Following men for 2 years leads to attrition and the sample size was small and this was another limitation to the study.

Oral PDE5i medications are actually taken 2–3 time per week and VCD are often only used 2–4 time per week. Intracavernosal injections appeared to be used in an on-demand fashion, being utilized once every 1–2 weeks. This study describes how often patients are utilizing PR therapies. This information could be used in designing future studies and to help clinicians and patients be realistic about how often men are able to use oral PDE-5i, vacuum and injection therapy.

Conclusion

On average erectile dysfunction was severe immediately following nerve sparring radical prostatectomy and improved over the 2 years. Most men did not return to baseline erectile function. This study contributes further to the growing body of evidence that the majority of men do not recover their pre-operative erectile function after nerve sparring radical prostatectomy even with penile rehabilitation. Orgasm also was diminished after surgery and improved over time. Despite comprehensive instructions and a frequent follow up schedule, PDE5i and VCD adherence was less than anticipated. The men identified many factors that impacted adherence to the PR program and/or attrition. Ultimately, men and their partners need to clearly understand the sexual ramifications of prostate cancer surgery on erectile function and orgasm. This information may help them to make informed decisions about penile rehabilitation and erectile dysfunction treatment options after surgery.

Appendix

Instruments/Measures/Data Collection

Side Effects: Side effects were assessed through a checklist of side effects as identified in the prescribing information from the pharmaceutical company and the manufacturer of the vacuum device as well as a category of other where the participant can describe any other side effects from the medications or the vacuum device.

Participant's Perceived Barriers: The participant were asked the question: What (if anything) about the medication and/or vacuum device you are using would inhibit or stop you from using them for treating your erectile dysfunction? The participant were provided space to respond with any perceived barriers to the treatment.

Erection Hardness Grading Score (EHS): Erection strength as rated on a scale ranging from 0 to 4 with 0 (representing a 0% erection) being no erection at all and 4 (representing a fully hard 100% erection) being a completely hard erection.

The International Index of Erectile Function (IIEF) including the Sexual Health Inventory for Men (SHIM) and Overall Sexual Satisfaction: The International Index of Erectile Dysfunction consists of 15-item questionnaire measuring five domains including erectile function, orgasmic function, sexual desire, intercourse satisfaction and overall sexual satisfaction, which were determined by principal components analysis. The Sexual Health Inventory for Men (SHIM) is a five item subscale within the International Index of Erectile Function pertaining to erectile dysfunction and was developed to determine the severity and presence of erectile dysfunction.

The Self-Esteem and Relationship Questionnaire: The Self-Esteem and Relationship Questionnaire is a 14-item instrument developed as a patient-reported tool to assess sexual confidence and intimacy in the sexual relationship.[7]

Orgasm/climax: In addition to questions used from the IIEF in the orgasm domain, orgasm/climax quality was evaluated. In addition to questions used from the IIEF in the orgasm domain, patients were asked to compare the quality of their orgasm to orgasms experienced prior to treatment. Response in terms of the quality of orgasm could be classified as better than before treatment, similar to before treatment or worst then before treatment.

Other Documentation: Demographics and Health History: Demographics and health history were obtained from the participant and/or the medical record. The prostate treatment was recorded. The participant's health history in regards to factors that might affect erectile function was obtained from the participant or the medical record (i.e. cardiovascular disease, diabetes, neurological disorders, hyperlipidemia, medications that effect erectile function). The participant's preoperative IIEF was obtained from the medical record or patient to assess erectile function prior to surgery. The patient reported use of any and all erectile dysfunction treatments in terms of how much, how often and what was used. The patients were asked to respond to an open ended question about any barriers to treatment. The patient were asked about ability to climax after prostate cancer treatment, urinary leakage during climax and the quality of their climax. The patient's expectations and confidence about their erectile dysfunction treatment was assessed.

Penile stretched length: A ruler is pushed into the pubis directly above the penis and the stretched length was monitored for penile shrinkage during the clinical visit and that information as extracted from the patient visit.

Abbreviations

ED: Erectile dysfunction; EDITS: Erectile Dysfunction Inventory of Treatment Satisfaction; EHS: Erection Hardness Score; ICI: Intracavernosal injections; IIEF: International Index of Erectile Function; PDE5i: Phosphodiesterase Type 5 inhibitor; PR: Penile Rehabilitation; QLI: Quality of Life Index Cancer Versioin; SD: Standard deviation; SHIM: Sexual Health Inventory for Men; VCD: Vacuum Constriction Device

Acknowledgements

The authors wish to thank NorthShore University HealthSystem and the Foundation for support of this study. We would also like to thank all the participants from the study and Nathaniel Sufrin who was my original research coordinator helping with all IRB approval and reviews and entering data for the study.

Authors' contributions

JAI designed and implemented the study. He also collected all the data from each participant. He wrote the initial drafts of the manuscript and is the corresponding author. BA reviewed the design and data analysis and assisted with the writing of several drafts of the manuscript. CC was the statistician for the study who performed all statistical analysis, created the tables for the manuscript and reviewed/revised the manuscript. NK was the research coordinator for the study helping with coordinating data collection, obtaining institutional board approval and reviews, entered all data for the study and reviewed the manuscripts for publication. JAi helped with the writing of several drafts of the manuscript and helped review data/data analysis. All authors received and approved the final version of this manuscript.

Author details

[1]Northshore University HealthSystem, Evanston, IL, USA. [2]University of Chicago Medical Center, Chicago, USA.

References

1. Siegel RL, Miller KD, Jemal A. Cancer statistics, 2018. CA Cancer J Clin. 2018; 68(1):7–30.
2. Potosky AL, Davis WW, Hoffman RM, Stanford JL, Stephenson RA, Penson DF, et al. Five-year outcomes after prostatectomy or radiotherapy for prostate cancer: the prostate cancer outcomes study. J Natl Cancer Inst. 2004;96(18):1358–67.
3. Resnick MJ, Koyama T, Fan KH, Albertsen PC, Goodman M, Hamilton AS, et al. Long-term functional outcomes after treatment for localized prostate cancer. N Engl J Med. 2013;368(5):436–45.
4. Rabbani F, Schiff J, Piecuch M, Yunis LH, Eastham JA, Scardino PT, et al. Time course of recovery of erectile function after radical retropubic prostatectomy: does anyone recover after 2 years? J Sex Med. 2010;7(12): 3984–90.
5. McCullough AR. Prevention and management of erectile dysfunction following radical prostatectomy. Urol Clin North Am. 2001;28(3):613–27.
6. Salonia A, Adaikan G, Buvat J, Carrier S, El-Meliegy A, Hatzimouratidis K, et al. Sexual rehabilitation after treatment for prostate cancer-part 1: recommendations from the fourth international consultation for sexual medicine (ICSM 2015). J Sex Med. 2017;14(3):285–96.
7. Rosen RC, Cappelleri JC, Smith MD, Lipsky J, Pena BM. Development and evaluation of an abridged, 5-item version of the International Index of Erectile Function (IIEF-5) as a diagnostic tool for erectile dysfunction. Int J Impot Res. 1999;11(6):319–26.
8. Rosen RC, Riley A, Wagner G, Osterloh IH, Kirkpatrick J, Mishra A. The international index of erectile function (IIEF): a multidimensional scale for assessment of erectile dysfunction. Urology. 1997;49(6):822–30.
9. Mulhall JP, Goldstein I, Bushmakin AG, Cappelleri JC, Hvidsten K. Validation of the erection hardness score. The journal of sexual medicine. 2007;4(6): 1626–34.
10. Stanley E Althof, Eric W Corty, Stephen B Levine, Frederic Levine, Arthur L Burnett, Kevin McVary, Vera Stecher, Allen D Seftel, (1999) EDITS: development of questionnaires for evaluating satisfaction with treatments for erectile dysfunction. Urology 53 (4):793–799
11. Cappelleri JC, Althof SE, Siegel RL, Shpilsky A, Bell SS, Duttagupta S. Development and validation of the self-esteem and relationship (SEAR) questionnaire in erectile dysfunction. Int J Impot Res. 2004;16(1):30–8.
12. Ferrans CE, Powers MJ. Quality of life index: development and psychometric properties. Adv Nurs Sci. 1985;8(1):15–24.
13. Litwin MS, Hays RD, Fink A, Ganz PA, Leake B, Brook RH. The UCLA prostate Cancer index: development, reliability, and validity of a health-related quality of life measure. Med Care. 1998;36(7):1002–12.
14. Liu C, Lopez DS, Chen M, Wang R. Penile rehabilitation therapy following radical prostatectomy: a meta-analysis. J Sex Med. 2017;14(12):1496–503.
15. Lowrance WT, Eastham JA, Savage C, Mashino AC, Laudone VP, Dechet CB, al e. Contemporary open and robotic radical prostatectomy practice patterns among urologists in the United States. J Urol. 2012;187(6):2087–93.

16. Aggarwal A, Lewis D, Mason M, Purushotham A, Sullivan R, Meulen J. Effect of patient choice and hospital competition on service configuration and technology adoption within cancer surgery: a national, population-based study. Lancet Oncol. 2017;18:1445–53.
17. Sanda MG, Dunn RL, Michalski J, Sandler HM, Northouse L, Hembroff L, et al. Quality of life and satisfaction with outcome among prostate cancer survivors. N Engl J Med. 2008;358:1250–61.
18. Capogrosso P, Vertosick EA Benfante NE, Eastham JA Scardino PJ, Vickers AJ. Et. al. are we improving erectile function recovery after radical prostatectomy? Analysis of patients treated over the last decade. Eur Urol. 2018;75(2):221–8.
19. Kohler TS, Pedro R, Hendlin K, Utz W, Ugarte R, Reddy P, et al. A pilot study on the early use of the vacuum erection device after radical retropubic prostatectomy. BJU Int. 2007;100(4):858–62.
20. Kadono Y, Machioka K, Nakashima K, IiJima M, Shigehara K, Nohara T. Et. al. changes in penile length after radical prostatectomy: investigation of the underlying anatomical mechanism. BJU Int. 2017;120(2):293–9.
21. Brock G, Montorsi F, Costa P, Shah N, Martinez-Jabaloyas JM, Hammerer P, et al. Effect of Tadalafil once daily on penile length loss and morning erections in patients after bilateral nerve-sparing radical prostatectomy: results from a randomized controlled trial. Urology. 2015;85(5):1090–6.
22. Raina R, Agarwal A, Allamaneni SS, Lakin MM, Zippe CD. Sildenafil citrate and vacuum constriction device combination enhances sexual satisfaction in erectile dysfunction after radical prostatectomy. Urology. 2005;65(2):360–4.
23. Clavell-Hernández J, Martin C, Wang R. Orgasmic dysfunction following radical prostatectomy: review of current literature. Sex Med Rev. 2018;6(1): 124–34.
24. Lee DJ, Cheetham P, Badani KK. Penile rehabilitation protocol after robot-assisted radical prostatectomy: assessment of compliance with phosphodiesterase type 5 inhibitor therapy and effect on early potency. BJU Int. 2010;105(3):382–8.
25. Nelson CJ, Lacey S, Kenowitz J, Pessin H, Shuk E, Roth AJ, et al. Men's experience with penile rehabilitation following radical prostatectomy: a qualitative study with the goal of informing a therapeutic intervention. Psychooncology. 2015;24(12):1646–54.

17

Improvement in early urinary continence recovery after robotic-assisted radical prostatectomy based on postoperative pelvic anatomic features

Akihiro Nakane[1,2*], Hiroki Kubota[1,2], Yusuke Noda[1,2], Tomoki Takeda[1,2], Yasuhiko Hirose[1,2], Atsushi Okada[2], Kentaro Mizuno[3], Noriyasu Kawai[2], Keiichi Tozawa[2], Yutaro Hayashi[3] and Takahiro Yasui[2]

Abstract

Background: We investigated the impact of postoperative membranous urethral length and other anatomic characteristics of the pelvic floor shape as measured by magnetic resonance imaging on the improvement in continence following robotic-assisted radical prostatectomy.

Methods: We retrospectively reviewed data from 73 patients who underwent postoperative prostate magnetic resonance imaging following robotic-assisted radical prostatectomy between 2013 and 2018. Patient demographics; pre-, peri-, and post-operative parameters; and pelvic anatomic features on magnetic resonance imaging were reviewed. Patients who used no urinary incontinence pads or pads for protection were considered to have achieved complete continence.

Results: Urinary continence was restored in 27.4, 53.4, 68.5, and 84.9% of patients at 1, 3, 6, and 12 months after robotic-assisted radical prostatectomy, respectively. When patients were divided into early and late continence groups based on urinary continence at 3 months after robotic-assisted radical prostatectomy, no significantly different clinical characteristics or surgical outcomes were found. However, the mean membranous urethral length (18.5 mm for the early continence group vs. 16.9 mm for the late continence group), levator muscle width (7.1 vs. 6.5 mm, respectively), and bladder neck width on the trigone side (7.2 mm vs. 5.4 mm, respectively) were significantly different between groups (all $p < 0.05$). Multivariate logistic regression analysis showed that membranous urethral length (odds ratio, 1.227; 95% confidence interval, 1.011–1.489; $p = 0.038$) and bladder neck width (odds ratio, 1.585; 95% confidence interval, 1.050–2.393; $p = 0.028$) were associated with the period of early urinary continence.

Conclusions: Postoperative membranous urethral length and bladder neck width were significantly associated with early urinary continence recovery after robotic-assisted radical prostatectomy. It is highly recommended that surgeons focus on preserving the membranous urethral length and increasing the bladder neck width on the trigone side during surgery to achieve optimal continence outcomes after robotic-assisted radical prostatectomy.

Keywords: Robotic-assisted radical prostatectomy, Urinary incontinence, Pelvic anatomy, Magnetic resonance imaging

* Correspondence: aki-nakane@ams.odn.ne.jp
[1]Department of Urology, The Aichi Prefectural Federation of Agricultural Cooperatives for Health and Welfare Kainan Hospital, Yatomi, Japan
[2]Department of Nephro-urology, Nagoya City University Graduate School of Medical Sciences, 1 Kawasumi, Mizuho-cho, Mizuho-ku, Nagoya 467-8601, Japan
Full list of author information is available at the end of the article

Background

Robotic-assisted radical prostatectomy (RARP) has been widely used as the most advanced treatment for localized prostate cancer [1, 2]. Urinary incontinence after RARP arguably has the most significant impact on quality of life postoperatively [3], and 4–22% of patients reported not achieving urinary continence within 12 months after RARP [4–8]. Recent studies have reported that a patient's preoperative status and certain anatomic characteristics are predictors of urinary continence postoperatively, therefore, it is indicated that surgical techniques and urinary incontinence after RARP are significantly related [6, 9–12]. The membranous urethral length (MUL) is an important factor that directly correlates with the sphincter's functional mechanism. The urethral sphincter is composed of an external striated sphincter and an internal smooth muscle layer, both of which are important increasing urethral closure pressure [13]. Previous studies showed that MUL preservation is important because it relates to urinary continence after open or laparoscopic radical prostatectomy [9, 10]. Preoperative MUL has been shown to be an important predictor of urinary continence recovery [14]. Early recovery of urinary continence after RARP has been shown to depend on postoperative MUL [15]. However, MUL is almost completely determined by the anatomic characteristics of the patient's original pelvic floor shape [14].

Therefore, we investigated the impact of postoperative MUL on urinary continence recovery after RARP and the association between MUL and other anatomic characteristics of the pelvic floor shape, as measured with magnetic resonance imaging (MRI), with incontinence improvement after RARP.

Methods

Patient characteristics

Between May 2013 and March 2018, 301 patients who underwent RARP for prostate cancer were retrospectively reviewed. RARP was performed using the da Vinci Si surgical robot (Intuitive Surgical, Inc., Sunnyvale, CA, USA). In all cases, the Rocco stitch was used for posterior reconstruction of the Denonvillier's fascia [16, 17], and we did not routinely perform neurovascular bundle preservation, puboprostatic ligament preservation, and reconstruction of the distal apex. Postoperative pelvic MRI was performed on all patients who visited after RARP between May 2016 and November 2017, regardless of surgical procedure and pathological results, postoperative course. Postoperative pelvic MRI was routinely performed at 3 months postoperatively. Seventy-three patients who subsequently underwent postoperative pelvic MRI were identified. No patients had local recurrence or received salvage radiation therapy before undergoing postoperative pelvic MRI. None of these patients included neurovascular bundle preservation cases. All study protocols were approved by the Ethical Committee of the Aichi Prefectural Federation of Agricultural Cooperatives for Health and Welfare Kainan Hospital (approval no. 300214–01).

Clinical and pathological parameters

Patient demographics (age and body mass index [BMI]), preoperative parameters (preoperative prostate-specific antigen [PSA] level and Biopsy Gleason's score), perioperative parameters (operative time, console time, estimated blood loss, and prostate volume), and postoperative parameters (pathological T stage, positive surgical margin, catheter removal period, postoperative hospital stay, and postoperative continence status) were reviewed. A five-point scale was used to assess continence grade [10]. Patients with Level 1 who did not use urinary incontinence

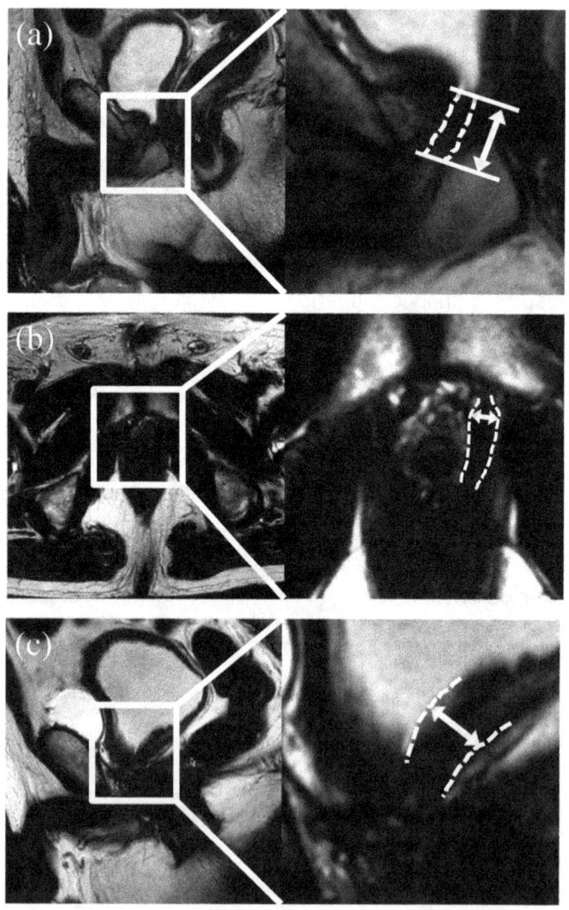

Fig. 1 Postoperative pelvic anatomic features on T2-weighted magnetic resonance imaging. **a** Membranous urethral length measured in the sagittal plane. The dashed lines show the membranous urethra. **b** Levator muscle width measured in the axial plane. The dashed lines show the levator muscle. **c** Bladder neck width on the trigone side measured in the sagittal plane. The dashed lines show the posterior bladder neck wall

pads or pads for protection were considered to have achieved complete continence.

MRI measurements

MRI was performed using a 1.5-T whole-body magnetic resonance scanner (Ingenia, Philips Healthcare, Best, the Netherlands). Images were obtained in 2 mm slices with T2-weighted sequences of the entire pelvis in the axial, sagittal, and coronal views. MUL was estimated in the midline sagittal plane (Fig. 1a). Levator muscle width (LMW) was estimated on axial images at the thickest portion of the urethral sphincter (Fig. 1b). Bladder neck width on the trigone side (BNW) was estimated on midline sagittal images (Fig. 1c).

Statistical analysis

Continuous variables were expressed as means (standard deviation, range) and compared using the independent t-test. Multivariate logistic regression analyses were performed to determine predictive factors associated with early recovery of urinary continence after RARP. All statistical analyses were performed using SPSS Statistics Ver. 22 (IBM, Armonk, NY, USA). Two-sided $p < 0.05$ were considered statistically significant.

Results

Baseline clinical and pathological characteristics of the 73 patients who underwent RARP and postoperative MRI and 301 patients in the whole series are summarized in Table 1. At 1 month after RARP, urinary

Table 1 Clinical characteristics and surgical outcomes

	Patients who underwent postoperative prostate MRI (*n* = 73)		Patients in the whole series (*n* = 301)	
Age (years; mean ± SD; range)	67.9 ± 5.4	(53–76)	68.7 ± 4.7	(53–76)
BMI (kg/m^2; mean ± SD; range)	24.1 ± 2.8	(18.9–30.7)	23.9 ± 2.8	(16.8–33.4)
Preoperative PSA level (ng/mL; mean ± SD; range)	9.9 ± 6.9	(4.0–43.4)	9.5 ± 6.6	(4.0–57.1)
Clinical T stage (n, %)				
cT1	23 (30.3)		148 (49.2)	
pT2	49 (67.1)		136 (45.2)	
pT3	1 (1.4)		17 (5.6)	
Biopsy Gleason's score (n, %)				
≦ 6	25 (34.2)		94 (31.2)	
= 7	30 (41.1)		137 (45.5)	
≧ 8	18 (24.7)		70 (23.3)	
Operative time (min; mean ± SD; range)	182.3 ± 48.8	(108–307)	187.3 ± 44.4	(103–313)
Console time (min; mean ± SD; range)	141.0 ± 41.7	(76–250)	145.6 ± 41.3	(74–289)
Estimated blood loss (mL; mean ± SD; range)	98.1 ± 76.6	(2–380)	93.3 ± 99.4	(1–650)
Prostate volume (mL; mean ± SD; range)	50.2 ± 24.2	(10–175)	44.1 ± 18.9	(10–175)
Pathological T stage (n, %)				
pT2	57 (78.1)		226 (75.1)	
pT3	16 (21.9)		75 (24.9)	
Positive surgical margins (n, %)				
All stages	11 (15.1)		62 (20.1)	
pT2	7 (12.3)		29 (12.8)	
pT3	4 (25.0)		33 (44.0)	
Catheter removal period (days; mean ± SD; range)	7.2 ± 0.8	(6–13)	7.5 ± 3	(4–45)
Postoperative hospital stay (days; mean ± SD; range)	10.7 ± 2.2	(8–20)	10.9 ± 4.9	(7–49)
% continence (%)				
≤ 1 month	27.4		31.7	
≤ 3 months	53.4		51.2	
≤ 6 months	68.5		70.3	
≤ 12 months	84.9		78.8	

Abbreviations: BMI Body mass index, *PSA* Prostate-specific antigen, *SD* Standard deviation

Table 2 Clinical characteristics and surgical outcomes for patients based on continence recovery at 3 months

	Early continece group	Late continece group
n	39	34
Age (years)	68.2 ± 6.2	67.6 ± 4.8
BMI (kg/m^2)	23.8 ± 3.0	23.1 ± 2.4
Console time (min)	179.0 ± 41.7	157.3 ± 37.8
Prostate volume (mL)	39.8 ± 12.6	43.7 ± 12.7
Catheter removal period (days)	7.0 ± 0.0	7.1 ± 0.3
Postoperative hospital stay (days)	11.3 ± 2.9	10.3 ± 1.4

Abbreviation: *BMI* Body mass index

continence was restored in 27.4% of 73 patients who underwent RARP and postoperative MRI. Urinary continence improved over time, with 53.4, 68.5, and 84.9% of patients achieving urinary continence at 3, 6, and 12 months, respectively. When patients were divided into two groups (early versus late recovery of continence) based on urinary continence at 3 months after RARP, no significantly different clinical characteristics or surgical outcomes were observed (Table 2). We evaluated the association between postoperative pelvic anatomic features on MRI and urinary continence at 3 months (Fig. 2). The mean MUL (18.5 mm for the early continence group vs. 16.9 mm for the late continence group), levator muscle width (LMW) (7.1 mm for the early continence group vs. 6.5 mm for the late continence group), and BNW (7.2 mm for the early continence group vs. 5.4 mm for the late continence group) were significantly different between groups (all $p < 0.05$).

Because 64 patients reached complete urinary continence after RARP during the observation period, multivariate logistic regression analysis was used to identify prognostic MRI measurements predicting early complete urinary continence at 3 months after RARP. Multivariate logistic regression analysis evaluated clinical characteristics and perioperative parameters together with MRI parameters, and the results are summarized in Table 3. On the multivariate analysis, MUL (odds ratio [OR], 1.227; 95% confidence interval [CI], 1.011–1.489; $p = 0.038$) and BNW (OR. 1.585; 95% CI 1.050–2.393; $p = 0.028$) were associated with the period of early complete urinary continence.

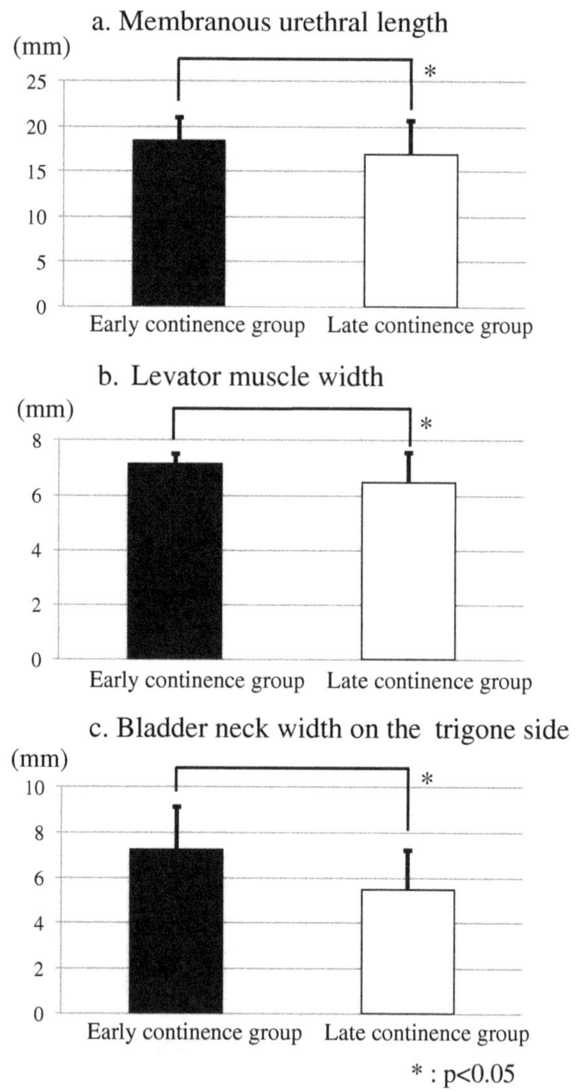

Fig. 2 Association between postoperative pelvic anatomic features and urinary continence after robot-assisted radical prostatectomy. Pelvic anatomic features were evaluated with magnetic resonance imaging and compared based on postoperative urinary continence. **a** Membranous urethral length. **b** Levator muscle width. **c** Bladder neck width on the trigone side

Discussion

A previous study reported that the most significant factor affecting quality of life after RARP was urinary incontinence [3]. In the present study, urinary incontinence was identified in 15.1% patients at 1 year after RARP, which was consistent with previous reports [4–8]. Recent studies have reported that several anatomic characteristics are preoperative predictors of postoperative urinary incontinence, and surgical techniques are

Table 3 Multivariate logistic regression analysis results for clinical characteristics, Perioperative parameters, and MRI measurements predicting the early urinary complete continence at 3 months after RARP

Clinical characteristics	Univariate analysis			Multivariate analysis		
	OR	95% CI	*p*-value	OR	95% CI	*p*-value
Age	0.924	0.841, 1.014	0.096	1.007	0.885, 1.146	0.912
BMI	1.110	0.932, 1.323	0.242	1.018	0.803, 1.290	0.884
Clinical T stage (cT1, cT2, cT3)	1.525	0.547, 4.248	0.420	2.354	0.469, 11.806	0.298
Biopsy Gleason's score (≦6, 7, 8≦)	0.813	0.456, 1.449	0.483	0.741	0.289, 1.904	0.534
Perioperative parameters						
Prostate volume	1.003	0.983, 1.023	0.783	0.996	0.965, 1.028	0.807
Catheter removal period	0.843	0.451, 1.576	0.593	1.001	0.510, 1.963	0.999
Postoperative hospital stay	0.955	0.767, 1.191	0.685	0.870	0.654, 1.156	0.335
Pathological T stage (pT2, pT3)	0.589	0.178, 1.950	0.386	0.783	0.147, 4.153	0.773
Pathological Gleason's score (≦6, 7, 8≦)	0.600	0.314, 1.144	0.121	0.495	0.179, 1.368	0.175
MRI measurements						
MUL	1.184	1.031, 1.359	0.017	1.227	1.011, 1.489	0.038*
BNW	1.617	1.181, 2.213	0.003	1.585	1.050, 2.393	0.028*
LMW	1.446	0.817, 2.561	0.205	1.087	0.486, 2.433	0.840

Abbreviations: *OR* Odds ratio, *CI* Confidence interval, *BMI* Body mass index, *BNW* Bladder neck width on the trigone side, *LMW* Levator muscle width, *MUL* Membranous urethral length

*On the multivariate analysis, MUL and BNW were associated with the period of early complete urinary continence

significantly associated with urinary incontinence after RARP [6, 9–12]. Recent advances in knowledge of the pelvic structure have led to increased understanding of the urinary continence mechanism [13]. In brief, the external striated sphincter is the main structure in maintaining a urethral closure pressure that is greater than bladder pressure. Several authors have evaluated the impact of pre- and postoperative MUL and found that continence recovery was slower in men with short MULs [10, 14, 18].

Postoperative MUL as measured on urethrovesicography has been reported to be the most important predictive factor for recovery of urinary continence in the early postoperative period after RARP, and it is greater with preservation of the neurovascular bundle, thus allowing early recovery of urinary continence [15]. However, the measurement of postoperative MUL and other anatomic characteristics of the pelvic floor shape on urethrovesicography seems to be inaccurate and limited; hence, we evaluated the postoperative MRI findings. The development of MRI has enabled more accurate measurement of anatomic characteristics of the pelvic floor shape. Furthermore, MRI allows a minimally invasive examination of anatomical structures at the points of radiation exposure and pain. MRI findings of MUL and LMW have been shown to be useful and independent predictors of postoperative continence recovery [9]. Pre- and postoperative MUL measured by MRI were significantly associated with urinary continence recovery after RARP, and pre- to postoperative MUL change was also associated with urinary continence recovery at 6 months after RARP [19]. Our results showed that postoperative MUL as evaluated on MRI was significantly associated with early urinary continence recovery, indicating that the residual MUL also influenced recovery of continence at 3 months after RARP.

Multiple intraoperative maneuvers have been proposed to improve urinary continence, including bladder neck preservation [20], and novel reconstruction of tissue around the vesicourethral anastomosis [21]. The posterior musculofascial plate plays a significant role as a dynamic support structure for the prostatomembranous urethra [22, 23]. Multilayer posterior reconstruction measured by postoperative MRI could potentially restore anatomic and functional defects more effectively and provide stronger posterior support to improve the recovery of urinary continence after RARP [24]. The posterior construction of bladder wall, including BNW thickness, also plays an important role as a dynamic support structure for early urinary continence recovery. Our results showed that postoperative BNW thickness on MRI was significantly associated with early urinary continence recovery. This study is the first to report that preserving MUL longer and making BNW thicker at surgery were important for early recovery continence after RARP.

Our study had several limitations. First, this study had a retrospective design and a relatively small sample size, and all surgeries were performed by the three different surgeons. However, the same RARP protocol was used during the study period. Second, urinary continence status was evaluated based on the number of pads that patients used, which is relatively subjective. Measurement of the 24-h pad weight is considered to be the most accurate test [25], but it is difficult to apply in practice. In this study, we evaluated whether patients used no pads or pads for protection; hence, the severity of urinary incontinence was measured by a self-reported number of pads used. Finally, other parameters affecting urinary incontinence might have been underestimated because we focused on the impacts of postoperative MUL, LMW, and BNW on urinary incontinence.

Conclusions

Postoperative MUL as measured on MRI was significantly associated with early urinary continence recovery after RARP. Postoperative MUL was longer and BNW was thicker in patients who experienced early continence recovery (by 3 months after RARP). MUL and BNW on postoperative MRI were also related to the period of complete continence. Thus, surgeons' efforts to preserve longer MUL and thicker BNW are recommended during surgery to achieve optimal continence outcomes after RARP.

Abbreviations

BMI: Body mass index; BNW: Bladder neck width on the trigone side; CI: Confidence interval; LMW: Levator muscle width; MRI: Magnetic resonance imaging; MUL: Membranous urethral length; OR: Odds ratio; PSA: Preoperative prostate-specific antigen; RARP: Robotic-assisted radical prostatectomy; SD: Standard deviation

Acknowledgements

None.

Authors' contributions

(AN, HK, YN, TT, YHi, AO, KM, NK, KT, YHa, TY.) Conception and design: AN and HK; enrollment of patients and acquisition of data: AN, HK, YN, TT, and YH1; drafting of the manuscript: AN, YH2 and TY; statistical analysis: AN and HK; analysis and interpretation of data: AO, KM, NK and KT; supervision: TY. We confirm that all authors read and approved the final manuscript.

Author details

[1]Department of Urology, The Aichi Prefectural Federation of Agricultural Cooperatives for Health and Welfare Kainan Hospital, Yatomi, Japan. [2]Department of Nephro-urology, Nagoya City University Graduate School of Medical Sciences, 1 Kawasumi, Mizuho-cho, Mizuho-ku, Nagoya 467-8601, Japan. [3]Department of Pediatric Urology, Nagoya City University Graduate School of Medical Sciences, Nagoya, Japan.

References

1. Ficarra V, Novara G, Rosen RC, Artibani W, Carroll PR, Costello A, et al. Systematic review and meta-analysis of studies reporting urinary continence recovery after robot-assisted radical prostatectomy. Eur Urol. 2012;62:405 17.
2. Porpiglia F, Bertolo R, Manfredi M, De Luca S, Checcucci E, Morra I, et al. Total anatomical reconstruction during robot-assisted radical prostatectomy: implications on early recovery of urinary continence. Eur Urol. 2016;69:485–95.
3. Katz G, Rodriguez R. Changes in continence and health-related quality of life after curative treatment and watchful waiting of prostate cancer. Urology. 2007;69:1157–60.
4. Patel VR, Sivaraman A, Coelho RF, Chauhan S, Palmer KJ, Orvieto MA, et al. Pentafecta: a new concept for reporting outcomes of robot- assisted laparoscopic radical prostatectomy. Eur Urol. 2011;59:702–7.
5. Lee DJ, Cheetham P, Badani KK. Predictors of early urinary continence after robotic prostatectomy. Can J Urol. 2010;17:5200–5.
6. Novara G, Ficarra V, D'Elia C, Secco S, Cioffi A, Cavalleri S, et al. Evaluating urinary continence and preoperative predictors of urinary continence after robot-assisted laparoscopic radical prostatectomy. J Urol. 2010;184:1028–33.
7. Ploussard G, de la Taille A, Moulin M, Vordos D, Hoznek A, Abbou CC, et al. Comparisons of the perioperative, functional, and oncological outcomes after robot-assisted vs. pure extraperitoneal laparoscopic radical prostatectomy. Eur Urol. 2014;65:610–9.
8. Martin AD, Nakamura LY, Nunez RN, Wolter CE, Humphreys MR, Castle EP. Incontinence after radical prostatectomy: a patient centered analysis and implications for preoperative counseling. J Urol. 2011;186:204–8.
9. Matsushita K, Kent MT, Vickers AJ, von Bodman C, Bernstein M, Touijer KA, et al. Preoperative predictive model of recovery of urinary continence after radical prostatectomy. BJU Int. 2015;116:577–83.
10. Paparel P, Akin O, Sandhu JS, Otero JR, Serio AM, Scardino PT, et al. Recovery of urinary continence after radical prostatectomy: association with urethral length and urethral fibrosis measured by preoperative and postoperative endorectal magnetic resonance imaging. Eur Urol. 2009;55: 629–37.
11. Hakimi AA, Faleck DM, Agalliu I, Rozenblit AM, Chernyak V, Ghavamian R. Preoperative and intraoperative measurements of urethral length as predictors of continence after robot-assisted radical prostatectomy. J Endourol. 2011;25:1025–30.
12. Hamada A, Razdan S, Etafy MH, Fagin R, Razdan S. Early return of continence in patients undergoing robot-assisted laparoscopic prostatectomy using modified maximal urethral length preservation technique. J Endourol. 2014;28:930–8.
13. Kojima Y, Takahashi N, Haga N, Nomiya M, Yanagida T, Ishibashi K, et al. Urinary incontinence after robot-assisted radical prostatectomy: pathophysiology and intraoperative techniques to improve surgical outcome. Int J Urol. 2013;20:1052–63.
14. von Bodman C, Matsushita K, Savage C, Matikainen MP, Eastham JA, Scardino PT, et al. Recovery of urinary function after radical prostatectomy: predictors of urinary function on preoperative prostate magnetic resonance imaging. J Urol. 2012;187:945–50.
15. Haga N, Ogawa S, Yabe M, Akaihata H, Hata J, Sato Y, et al. Factors contributing to early recovery of urinary continence analyzed by pre- and postoperative pelvic anatomical features at robot-assisted laparoscopic radical prostatectomy. J Endourol. 2015;29:683–90.
16. Rocco F, Carmignani L, Acquati P, Gadda F, Dell'Orto P, Rocco B, et al. Restoration of posterior aspect of rhabdosphincter shortens continence time after radical retropubic prostatectomy. J Urol. 2006;175:2201–6.
17. Rocco B, Gregori A, Stener S, Santoro L, Bozzola A, Galli S, et al. Posterior reconstruction of the rhabdosphincter allows a rapid recovery of continence after trans- peritoneal videolaparoscopic radical prostatectomy. Eur Urol. 2007;51:996–1003.
18. Song C, Doo CK, Hong JH, Choo MS, Kim CS, Ahn H. Relationship between the integrity of the pelvic floor muscles and early recovery of continence after radical prostatectomy. J Urol. 2007;178:208–11.
19. Song W, Kim CK, Park BK, Jeon HG, Jeong BC, Seo SI, et al. Impact of preoperative and postoperative membranous urethral length measured by 3 tesla magnetic resonance imaging on urinary continence recovery after robotic-assisted radical prostatectomy. Can Urol Assoc J. 2017;11:E93–9.
20. Braslis KG, Petsch M, Lim A, Civantos F, Soloway MS. Bladder neck preservation following radical prostatectomy: continence and margins. Eur Urol. 1995;28:202–8.
21. Menon M, Muhletaler F, Campos M, Peabody JO. Assessment of early continence after reconstruction of the periprostatic tissues in patients undergoing computer assisted (robotic) prostatectomy: results of a 2 group parallel randomized controlled trial. J Urol. 2008;180:1018 23.
22. Burnett AL, Mostwin JL. In situ anatomical study of the male urethral sphincteric complex: relevance to continence preservation following major pelvic surgery. J Urol. 1998;160:1301–6.

23. Rocco F, Rocco B. Anatomical reconstruction of the rhabdosphincter after radical prostatectomy. BJU Int. 2009;104:274–81.
24. Ogawa S, Hoshi S, Koguchi T, Hata J, Sato Y, Akaihata H, et al. Three-layer two-step posterior reconstruction using peritoneum during robot-assisted radical prostatectomy to improve recovery of urinary continence: a prospective comparative study. J Endourol. 2017;31:1251–8.
25. Bauer RM, Gozzi C, Hübner W, Nitti VW, Novara G, Peterson A, et al. Contemporary management of post-prostatectomy incontinence. Eur Urol. 2011;59:985–96.

18

Pelvic floor muscle training in radical prostatectomy: A randomized controlled trial of the impacts on pelvic floor muscle function and urinary incontinence

Joanne E. Milios[1,2*], Timothy R. Ackland[1] and Daniel J. Green[1]

Abstract

Background: Pelvic floor muscle training (PFM) training for post-prostatectomy incontinence (PPI) is an important rehabilitative approach, but the evidence base is still evolving. We developed a novel PFM training program focussed on activating fast and slow twitch muscle fibres. We hypothesized that this training, which commenced pre-operatively, would improve PFM function and reduce PPI, when compared to a control group.

Methods: This randomized trial allocated 97 men (63 ± 7y, BMI = 25.4, Gleason 7) undergoing radical prostatectomy (RP) to either a control group ($n = 47$) performing low-volume rehabilitation, or an intervention group ($n = 50$). Both interventions commenced 5 weeks prior to surgery and continued for 12 weeks post-RP. Participants were assessed pre-operatively and at 2, 6 and 12 weeks post-RP using 24 h pad weights, International Prostate Symptom Score (IPSS), Expanded Prostate Cancer Index Composite for Clinical Practice (EPIC-CP) and real time ultrasound (RTUS) measurements of PFM function.

Results: Following RP, participants in the control group demonstrated a slower return to continence and experienced significantly more leakage ($p < 0.05$), measured by 24 h pad weight, compared to the intervention group, suggesting an impact of the prehabilitation protocol. PFM function measures were enhanced following RP in the intervention group. Secondary measures (IPSS, EPIC-CP and RTUS PFM function tests) demonstrated improvement across all time points, with the intervention group displaying consistently lower "bothersome" scores.

Conclusions: A pelvic floor muscle exercise program commenced prior to prostate surgery enhanced post-surgical measures of pelvic floor muscle function, reduced PPI and improved QoL outcomes related to incontinence.

Keywords: Pelvic floor muscle, Prostatectomy, Men's health, Urinary incontinence, Quality of life

Background

Prostate cancer (PCa) is the most commonly diagnosed cancer in men [1]. Radical prostatectomy (RP) is highly effective, with 97% of patients surviving at least 5 years following surgery [2]. However, side effects can be severe and distressing [3, 4]. Stress urinary incontinence (SUI) is the most common presentation following RP and is provoked by activities such as sneezing, coughing, bending, lifting, positional change and exercise [5]. The current gold standard approach to the assessment of UI (urinary incontinence) involves collection of 24 h pad weight scores ('mild' < 100 g, 'moderate' 100–400 g, 'severe' > 400 g) [6]. Anxiety and post-traumatic stress are associated with the combination of PCa diagnosis, the need for surgery and resultant UI [7], with depression

* Correspondence: jomilios22@gmail.com
[1]School of Human Sciences (Exercise and Sport Science), The University of Western Australia, Crawley, Western Australia 6009, Australia
[2]Faculty of Science, School of Human Services (Sport Science, Exercise and Health), University of Western Australia, Parkway Rd, Crawley, Western Australia 6009, Australia

occurring four times more often in men with PCa than their healthy counterparts [8].

Randomized controlled trials have investigated the impact of pelvic floor muscle (PFM) training on post prostatectomy UI, providing conflicting evidence. Whilst some support the benefits of exercise [9] other studies (summarized in the recent Cochrane Review [10]) do not recommend PFM training as first line rehabilitation, suggesting that UI symptoms improve over time, irrespective of management. The disparity in these findings likely stems from variability in the type of assessment performed, instructions given to subjects, and mode of delivery of PFM training [11]. Protocols that include pre-operative PFM training that continues post-surgery, and that specifically target fast- and slow-twitch muscle training performed in the clinically relevant standing posture, have not been previously been undertaken. Our primary focus was to lessen the burden of post-prostatectomy UI, since early return to continence has been widely acknowledged as a major quality of life (QoL) outcome [3]. We hypothesized that a significant difference in UI would be observed 2, 6 and 12 weeks post-surgery, when RP patients were randomized to either a PFM training intervention, or a control ('usual care') group.

Methods

Participants were enlisted from a cohort referred sequentially by their Urologist for pre-prostatectomy PFM training to a single physiotherapy clinic, in line with standard procedure; no patient had surgery delayed as a result of enrolment in this study. We used a minimization approach to randomization, with each participant randomly allocated to one of two groups, 'usual care' or 'high intensity' upon presentation to a high-volume physiotherapy clinic following a diagnosis of PCa. If randomly allocated to usual care, for example, the very next patient was allocated to the high intensity intervention group and this sequence continued until the desired sample was achieved. No a priori consideration was given to other factors such as age, surgical approach, surgeon, aetiology, or BMI. Once consent was provided, enrolment in the study and interventions commenced without delay. Relevant notes were recorded in participant medical files, which were collated over the trial duration, with results subsequently analysed by a blinded, independent statistician.

Patients with pre-existing UI, prior prostate surgery, or a history of receiving radiation or androgen deprivation therapy, were excluded (see Table 1). Both open RP (Control 8, Intervention 5) and Robotic–Assisted Laparoscopic Prostatectomy (RALP) (Control 39, Intervention 45) surgical types, performed by highly experienced surgeons operating at two high volume institutions, were included. All participants were provided with usual care advice regarding bladder training (minimum time between voids 2 hourly where possible), caffeine (maximum 1 serve /day) and alcohol consumption (to be avoided until continent), and behavioural changes relevant to minimizing incontinence issues. In addition, pre-operative physical activity levels were recorded at the initial screening consultation. Type of exercise, frequency, duration and difficulty were recorded and activity levels were rated as 'low' (i.e. 40–50% maximum heart rate (MHR)), 'moderate' (50–70% MHR), or 'high' (70–85% MHR) [13] with the number of sessions per week noted. As part of both intervention arms of the study, all participants were encouraged to walk daily for 30 mins, 5 days per week.

Procedures

Pre-surgery PFM training

Five weeks prior to RP surgery, participants were randomized to the intervention or usual care group. Both groups received initial physiotherapy-directed PFM instruction over two sessions of 30 min and were then prescribed a daily PFM training program. This program differed in mode and intensity, depending on randomization. Subjects allocated to the usual care group were instructed and directed to perform three sets of PFM exercises per day, with 10 contractions per set, aiming to hold for a duration of 10 s, with an equal rest time, providing a total of 30 contractions per day. Daily exercise sets were performed once each, in supine, sitting, then standing, in accordance with previously reported interventions [14]. This intervention is in keeping with current clinical practice [15] and it was administered in preference to a 'no-exercise' intervention as we considered it unethical to withhold some level of

Table 1 Inclusion – Exclusion criteria

Inclusion criteria	Exclusion criteria
• Pre-operative radical prostatectomy • Open or robotic-assisted approaches • Age > 18 years • Diagnosed with prostate cancer and referred for pelvic floor muscle training • Fully continent	• Acute illness • Prior urinary incontinence • Current smokers • Diabetes: type 1 or 2 • Alcohol consumption > 21 units/week • Impaired mental status • Prior prostate surgery • Undergoing or had prior radiation therapies • Undergoing or had prior androgen deprivation therapy

training. Nonetheless, it did not specifically target fast and slow-twitch muscle function and the intensity, number and duration of contractions were modest relative to the intervention group.

Exercise protocols in the intervention group targeted both slow and fast-twitch muscle fibres and participants were required to perform six sets of PFM exercises per day, with each set comprising 10 fast (1 s duration) and 10 slow (10 s duration) contractions with an equal rest time, providing a total of 120 contractions per day. All sets were performed in a standing posture for this group. Participants were blinded to group allocation; in that they were not exercised as a group and were not aware of the existence of the alternative exercise intervention.

During the initial instruction sessions, participants were given written and verbal instructions on correct PFM exercise technique [16] to ensure a full contraction and relaxation cycle was implemented with the cue to *"stop the flow of urine and shorten the penis while continuing to breathe"* [16]. Cues to relax abdominal muscles and avoid breath holding were also communicated, and confirmation of correct technique provided with real time ultrasound (RTUS) used as a biofeedback tool. Participants completed a PFM training diary to record the number, type and position of exercises undertaken on a daily basis. Adherence to the training program in both groups was assessed via individual diary entries during fortnightly physiotherapy appointments.

Post-surgery PFM training

Post–operative PFM training recommenced following removal of the catheter. Members of the control group performed three sets per day of the same exercises performed pre-surgery, while members of the intervention group continued their exercise regime with six sets per day of fast and slow-twitch training. Both groups exercised in the postures described above and these protocols were maintained throughout the 12-week assessment period.

Outcome measures

Bladder diaries for recording 24 h pad weight (the primary outcome variable) were assessed post-surgery at 2, 6 and 12 weeks as the primary outcome. No participant was incontinent prior to surgery, however, all wore pads after surgery and applied their first pad of the day with an empty bladder. Used pads were placed in a single plastic bag and sealed, then stored in a refrigerator to avoid evaporation. Net weight was calculated by deducting dry pad weight, using a single calibrated digital scale. Any positive net weight, recorded to the nearest 1 g, was deemed indicative of incontinence, with 'zero' net weight assessed as no leakage and full continence.

Physical activity, fluid intake and pad weights were recorded in the 24-h bladder diary for each participant. Re-test measures were recorded on the same day of the week to account for variable activity levels, thus avoiding any potential discrepancy between sedentary and more physically active days of the week. Six surgeons, working from two high volume hospitals and all with minimum of 7 years' experience in performing RP, referred patients into the study. Similar numbers per group were achieved for each surgeon. Nerve sparing was a primary goal of all surgeons who participated in this study as it is usual care practice in this population. Resected nerve matter was stained and weighed by a blinded, independent pathologist within 24 h of surgery, and reported in the Results section. A similar number of unilateral, bilateral and no nerve sparing was achieved in both groups (see Table 2).

Secondary measures of QoL using the International Prostate Symptom Score (IPSS) [17] and Expanded Prostate Cancer Index Composite for Clinical Practice (EPIC-CP) [18] questionnaires were recorded at baseline (approximately 5 weeks prior to surgery) and again at each post-surgery time point. Participants completed the questionnaires in a quiet private room at the completion of a scheduled appointment within the physiotherapy clinic.

Additional secondary measures of RTUS guided tests of PFM function, including the Rapid Response Test (RRT) and Sustained Endurance Test (SET) [19, 20] were performed by a single operator for each measurement using a commercially available point-of-care ultrasound machine (3.5 MHz sector probe, Mindray DP-30 Ultrasound, 6 U-42000440, China) at each post-surgery time point. Details of the methods used in each of these tests, along with their validity and reliability, are available in recent publications [19, 20].

Statistics

Outcome data were entered into SPSS (v22.0, SPSS, Chicago, IL) for analysis. A series of two-factor, repeated measures ANOVA (Group x Time) were performed and significance was accepted for all analyses at $p < 0.05$. Where necessary, post-hoc t-tests for independent samples were performed to determine the time points at which group scores differed.

The sample size of 101 participants was based on power calculations derived from previous studies utilizing 24-h pad weight as an objective measure of UI. Of 45 RCT studies investigated in the most recent Cochrane review [10], very few recorded 24-h pad weight as an objective measure, resulting in a recommendation for its use in future studies to enhance efficacy. Our study design, which randomized men to intensive pelvic floor muscle (PFM) training versus a usual care intervention, where each group received their intervention both pre- and post-surgery, is novel. For

Table 2 Participant characteristics

Characteristics	Control group ($n = 47$)	Intervention group ($n = 50$)
Age (y)	63.5 ± 6.8	62.2 ± 6.8
BMI	25.4 ± 2.7	25.3 ± 2.7
Pre-surgery training (weeks)	5.1 ± 3.2	5.2 ± 2.8
Gleason score	7	7
Prostate size (g)	49.5 ± 15.5	50.8 ± 18.6
Operation type	8 Open 39 Robotic-assisted	5 Open 45 Robotic-assisted
Nerve sparing procedure	5 Unilateral 39 Bilateral 4 Nil	12 Unilateral 36 Bilateral 2 Nil
Catheter in situ (days)	8.6 ± 3.0	8.1 ± 2.7
Pre-operative Activity Levels[a]		
Low (40–50% MHR)	25	27
Medium (50–70% MHR)	20	20
High (70–85% MHR)	2	3

[a]*MHR* Maximum heart rate

power estimation we selected the paper of Centemero et al. [12] as the closest exemplar. This trial randomized 118 men to a pre-surgery PFM intervention, versus no intervention pre-surgery. Both groups received the same post-surgical PFM training intervention [12]. Pad weight and continence were primary outcome measures, as in the current study. Centemero et al. indicated that 44.1% of subjects in the prehab group were continent at 1 month post–surgery, whereas this number was 20.3% in the no intervention group (ES = 23.8) [12]. This difference was statistically significant ($P = 0.018$). Given a priori assumptions of $\alpha = 0.05$, a two-tailed test and a sample size of 50 per group (100 total), our study possessed > 70% power to detect a similar effect size observed by Centemero et al. [12].

Results

Of the 101 participants recruited, 97 (63 ± 7 y, BMI = 25.4, Gleason 7) completed the study, with three participants from the usual care group ($n = 47$) and one participant from the intervention group ($n = 50$) unable to finish due to medical complications, including the need for radiation therapy ($n = 2$) and corrective surgery ($n = 2$). Participants were recruited over a 12-month period from April 2016 until April 2017 with follow up over a subsequent 12 months, until April 2018 when sufficient participant numbers were achieved. There were no appreciable differences in baseline characteristics between the groups, with only a few in each group having open RP rather than robotic-assisted surgery (see Table 2). No participant in either group was incontinent prior to surgery. Prostate size, Gleason score and days of catheterization were also similar between groups, as was rate and type of cavernosal nerve sparing.

Figure 1a represents the number of dry participants (continence = no pads or 0 g net pad weight), with all participants being continent at the baseline, pre-surgery assessment. At 2, 6 and 12 weeks post-surgery, the percentage of dry participants was greater across all time points in the intervention, compared to control (usual care) group, with the former group demonstrating a faster return to continence. At 2 weeks post-surgery 14% of the intervention group subjects, compared to 4% of the control group, were dry. At 6 weeks, this percentage increased to 32 and 11% respectively, then 74 and 43% by 12 weeks post-surgery.

Figure 1b displays the measured 24 h pad weights for the control and intervention groups pre-surgery and at 2, 6 and 12 weeks post-RP. The ANOVA results showed a significant main effect for Group ($F = 7.251$; $p = 0.008$), Time ($F = 82.318$; $p < 0.001$) and the Group x Time interaction ($F = 4.204$; $p = 0.016$). Post-hoc t-tests demonstrated that group differences occurred at each of the post-surgery time point ($p < 0.05$), however the significant interaction also indicates that rates of improvement differed between groups, favoring enhanced recovery in the intervention group. As we were interested to know whether operation type (RALP vs OPR) influenced the outcome for incontinence, we re-ran the analysis for pad weight using an Analysis of Covariance (ANCOVA) to compare the intervention groups whilst controlling for the effects of operation type. The ANCOVA outputs showed main effects for Time, Group and Group x Time (interaction) remained significant ($p < 0.05$).

In Fig. 2a, IPSS scores that measure urinary symptoms and QoL perceptions indicated similar levels at baseline, but significant ($p < 0.05$) between-group differences at 6 weeks post-surgery, with the intervention group scores

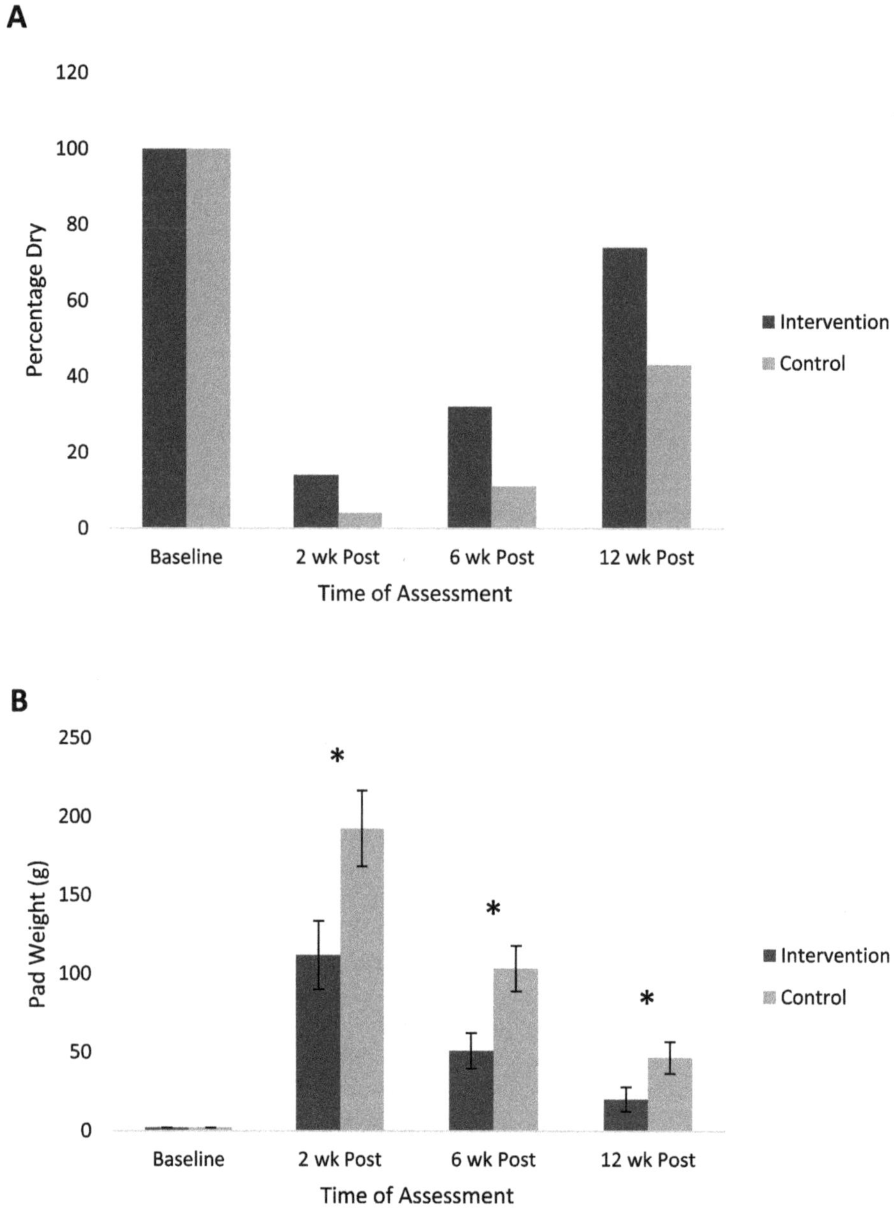

Fig. 1 The number of "dry" patients (panel **a**) and changes in 24-h pad weight (panel **b**) for patients following radical prostatectomy within the intervention and control groups at baseline, then at 2, 6 and 12 weeks post-surgery. All participants were fully continent at the pre-operative assessment (baseline). * indicates a significant difference ($p < 0.05$) between groups at the relevant time points

being superior to those for the control group. The ANOVA results showed a significant main effect for Time ($F = 25.45$; $p < 0.001$), but not for Group ($F = 3.17$; $p = 0.078$) or the Group x Time interaction ($F = 1.261$, $p = 0.288$).

Figure 2b describes EPIC-CP urinary incontinence scores (maximum score = 12) for impact on QoL. Pre-surgery EPIC-CP scores were similar, but the intervention group scored significantly better ($p < 0.05$) at 2 weeks post-surgery. There were no other group differences at 6 and 12 weeks post-surgery, although the intervention group retained some advantage. The ANOVA results show a significant main effect for Group ($F = 5.344$; $p = 0.023$) and Time ($F = 13.844$; $p < 0.001$), but not the Group x Time interaction ($F = 0.486$, $p = 0.487$).

Results for physiological assessments of pelvic floor muscle function are shown in Fig. 3a and b. Pre-surgery RTUS assessments were not performed so as to avoid any possible training effect for members of the control group participants. However, at all time points post-RP, (Fig. 3a) the intervention group recorded faster ($p < 0.05$)

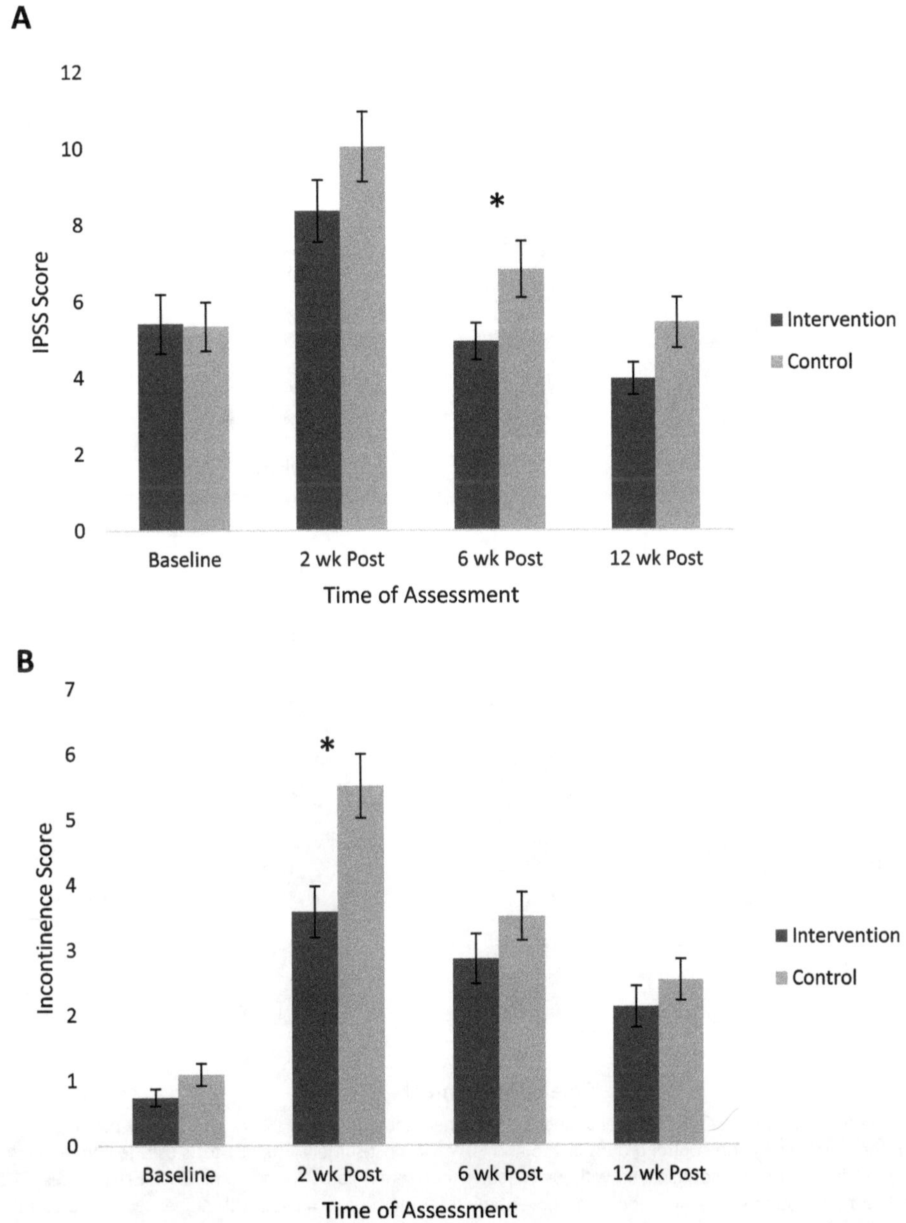

Fig. 2 Changes in the International Prostate Symptom Score (panel **a**) and the EPIC-CP (panel **b**) for patients following radical prostatectomy within the intervention and control groups at baseline, then at 2, 6 and 12 weeks post-surgery. The IPSS (maximum score = 12) is as a measure of self-reported urinary symptoms and quality of life, with lower scores indicating better outcomes. The EPIC-CP is a health related quality of life measure for men following treatment for prostate cancer, wherein the urinary continence domain (maximum score = 12) assesses self-reported bother of urinary incontinence symptoms, with lower scores indicating better outcomes. * indicates a significant difference ($p < 0.05$) between groups at the relevant time points

repeated muscle contraction (RRT scores), compared to the control group. The ANOVA results showed significant main effects for Group ($F = 16.132$; $p < 0.001$) and Time ($F = 69.790$; $p < 0.001$), but not the Group x Time interaction ($F = 2.12$; $p = 0.123$). Figure 3b provides results for the sustained pelvic floor muscle endurance test (SET). At all post-surgery time points, the intervention group recorded longer sustained ($p < 0.05$) contraction scores, compared the control group. The ANOVA results show significant main effects for Group ($F = 12.605$; $p = 0.001$) and Time ($F = 137.671$; $p < 0.001$), but not the Group x Time interaction ($F = 0.679$; $p = 0.508$).

Discussion

The incidence of UI prior to RP surgery is very low, affecting only 1–2% of the male population to age 75 y

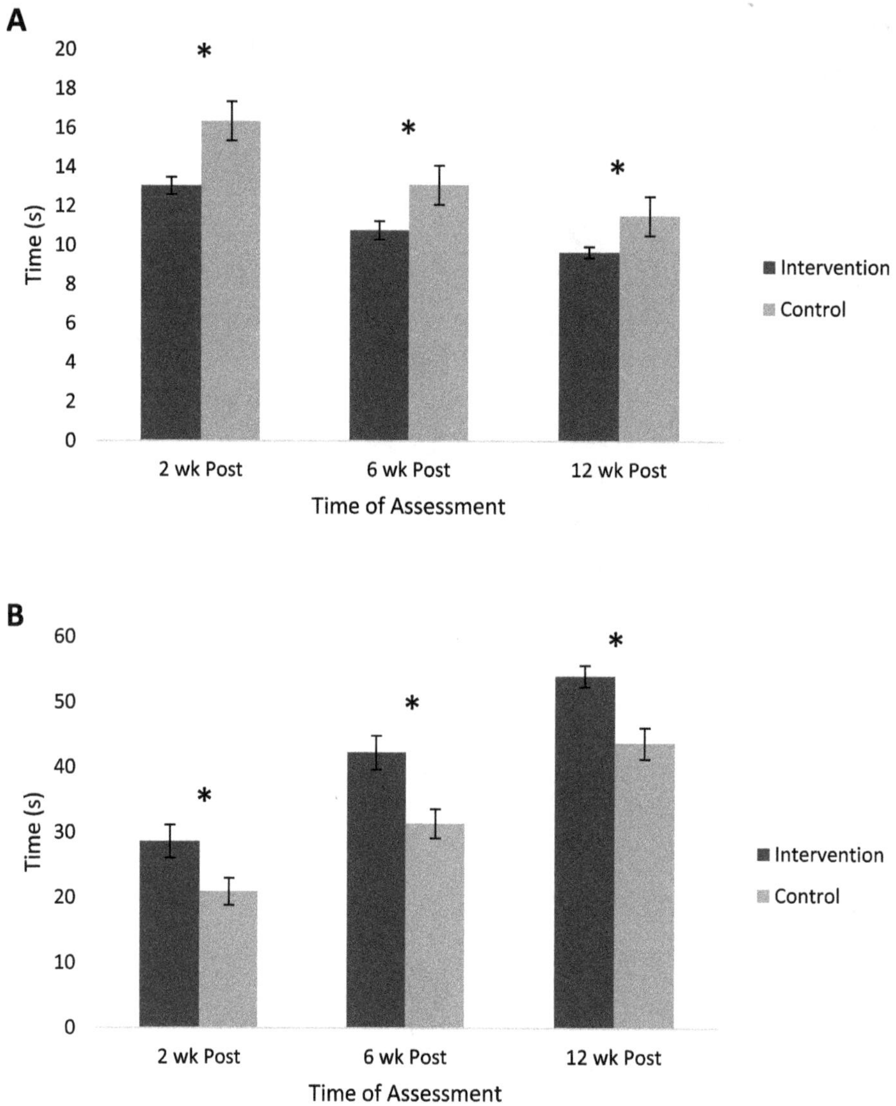

Fig. 3 Changes in the Rapid Response Test (RRT – panel **a**) and the Sustained Endurance Test (SET – panel **b**) for patients following radical prostatectomy within the intervention and control groups at 2, 6 and 12 weeks post-surgery. The RRT tests uses real time ultrasound (RTUS) to measure the speed of pelvic floor muscle contractions, with lower scores representing a better outcome. The SET also uses RTUS to measure the endurance of pelvic floor musculature to sustain a contraction over time (maximum score = 60 s), with higher scores representing a better outcome. * indicates a significant difference ($p < 0.05$) between groups at the relevant time points

[21]. Following RP surgery, however, this changes to 69–98% men affected with urinary leakage for some duration [22]. Fear and anxiety of the potential for UI is generally high before surgery, but levels of distress decline as symptoms improve. However, if continence is slow to recover, the long-term negative impact on QoL can remain substantial [23] and with an average 16–51% of men remaining incontinent at 12 months post-surgery, the long term impact on the patient and his partner can be significant [24].

The pre-operative period provides an opportunity to intervene and minimize the impact of UI. With the recommendation of a 6-week period between prostate biopsy and subsequent RP surgery to avoid complications, patients can be referred for pre-operative PFM training. A recent meta-analysis was only able to find five heterogenous papers which had addressed the question of prehabilitation benefit for UI in RP patients and concluded that insufficient data were available to warrant conclusive interpretation [25]. Our results indicate clear outcomes of less leakage, reduced time to return to continence and improved QoL in patients who received more intensive PFM training, utilizing standing postures, compared to the comparator control group protocol. This finding is in keeping with some previous studies which indicate that PFM training of longer duration prior to surgery, or of higher frequency and/or intensity, is more likely to be beneficial [26]. Recent developments in male pelvic floor assessment, utilizing RTUS, ensure that correct muscle activation is executed, with greater focus on anterior PFM, rather than the previously recommended anal sphincter approach. Mastery of PFM control was a novel aspect and focus of our intervention methodology [27, 28], alongside the quantification of pelvic floor muscle adaptation utilizing functional testing with RTUS-informed visual confirmation. Repeated one-on-one physiotherapy training sessions pre-surgery afforded the opportunity to correct any errors in PFM training technique, to progress each patient to sustain 10 s maximal contractions and to allay any participant concerns.

Providing all participants in our study with some level of pre-operative PFM training had the potential to reduce the impact of the group differences we observed and may have been a limitation. However, given the suggestion that PFM training should be recommended as a first line option for the treatment of UI [11], we considered it inappropriate to withhold PFM training altogether in the "control" group. Our intervention group received exercise specifically designed to focus on both fast and slow-twitch fibre training, completed in the upright posture, since this is the posture most often related to the clinical presentation of UI. UI is associated with increases in intra-abdominal pressure during cough, sneeze and sit to stand actions, so it is intuitive for training to be specific to rapid responses to pressure change.

Using RTUS tests that directly visualized and quantified function of the pelvic floor muscles during standardized tests, we were able to demonstrate lower RRT scores across all time points for the intervention versus control group, reflecting faster development of urethral closing pressure. This finding provides physiological and functional data supporting the more clinically orientated outcomes presented above which relate to decreased leakage post-surgery and a quicker return to continence for men who undertook the intervention training protocol. Similarly, training the slow-twitch PFM fibres in the standing posture, as quantified by the SET, resulted in higher scores for the intervention group across post-surgery time points. This was also reflected in reduced leakage and time to continence for the intervention group. No previous PFM exercise research has combined functional imaging-based tests of pelvic floor muscle function with clinical data related to UI to cross-validate findings. Our study is also novel in that we adopted a training protocol targeting both fast and slow-twitch muscle function for men following RP surgery.

Maintaining urethral closure pressure in the standing posture is more demanding than in supine postures, and this is seen clinically with few men leaking in the horizontal position. Upon catheter removal, however, most men will experience significant leakage in transitions from supine to sit, sit to stand, and when bending, lifting and walking. By initiating training in standing postures, the intervention group was able to experience reduced UI in all domains assessed. Matching PFM training to clinical presentations was considered an important issue for our study to address, as opposed to previous studies recommending PFM exercises be performed in sitting or lying postures. Whilst these recommendations may serve patients' needs when PFMs are weak, the opportunity to train patients pre-surgery may greatly reduce this problem. Furthermore, in physiological studies designed for strength training it is recognized that maximal force generation is achieved by performing three to four sets of 8–12 repetitions per day, which also results in greater hypertrophy of type 2a muscle fibres on biopsy testing [29]. In the context of PFM training in men who experience the complete removal of the prostate, exercise training to achieve some functional change may require more intensive approaches than that previously considered to be 'usual care'.

Fatigue is one of the major issues of PFM dysfunction and patients routinely complain of worsening incontinence with increased activity, and as the day progresses. To address this issue, participants in the intervention group were prescribed 120 individual maximum PFM contractions per day, compared to only 30 for the control group. Our aim to improve PFM endurance and strength as quickly as possible for the intervention group was achieved by increasing the frequency, number of sets, position and exercise type, versus the usual standard care. Training to increase muscle endurance requires the performance of high numbers of repetitions with decreased recovery time between sets. For example, Kraemer and Ratamess [30] reported greater increases in cross sectional area and strength when participants exercised twice, compared to only once per day. In PFM training studies published to date, wide variability exists in the prescription of exercises for endurance gains, with recommendations to hold PFM contractions ranging from sub-maximal to maximal efforts. In the present study, we chose to prescribe maximal contractions in an effort to increase exercise intensity. Participants recorded their daily PFM exercise regime in a diary which indicated 92% adherence with the PFM training program.

Urinary function and its impact on QoL measures were assessed using the EPIC-CP and IPSS domains, with significant differences found at 2 weeks and 6 weeks, respectively. Men in the intervention group reported less urinary leakage, less irritation, less pad use and less impact on overall QoL. Patients often report a sense of shame, loss of control, fear of bladder accidents and a need for hypervigilance with pad application, fluid consumption and social activity, all of which can affect aspects of daily life. Given the higher levels of depression and anxiety associated with UI post-RP, any measures to reduce these potential outcomes should be encouraged.

There have been many previous studies of PFM training in post prostatectomy patients, delivered both before and after surgery [9, 10, 12]. Many distinct interventions have been assessed and participants have differed in terms of clinical condition and status. Whilst some studies reported positive results and concluded an important role for PFM training, others, including a prominent and large clinical trial and a Cochrane review which included it, suggested that an active intervention did not substantially accelerate the degree of spontaneous recovery. Our findings demonstrated a benefit of the prehabilitation intervention performed at a higher intensity, but we also observed evidence for spontaneous post-op recovery in the control group. There was an increase in the speed of recovery in the more active rehabilitation intervention targeting physiological PFM function of fast and slow-twitch muscle fibres.

There were some limitations in our study, with the first related to sample size. Our power test was based on the paper of Centemero et al. [12] which a priori indicated that a sample size of 50 per group would provide >70% power to detect a similar effect size for the pad weight and continence outcomes observed in that study. In fact, we observed a larger effect size, with 74% of participants in the intervention group continent at 12 weeks post-surgery, versus 43% in the usual care group (ES = 31), indicating that our study was 87% powered for the groups sizes we achieved (n = 50 and 47). Our intervention was more intense that used by Centemero et al. [12] and our index follow-up was longer. We also calculated pad weight in absolute grams and observed a difference between the groups of 20 ± 54 g versus 47 ± 70 g at 12 weeks, indicating that we had 90% power to detect this difference with our sample size [12]. Although the numbers we recruited were adequate for statistical power, we may nonetheless have shown even greater benefit with a larger cohort. In addition, our intervention was for a period of 12 weeks post-operatively, after which, any men who were still incontinent were offered the high intensity PFM protocol. A longer period of intervention may have resulted in further differences between the two groups, with even clearer guidelines for protocol development.

Nerve sparing in our study, was assessed by volume of cavernosal nerve resected with the usual care group having marginally less nerve resected than the intervention group. The relationship between nerve sparing and continence is still emerging, however if this was a critical factor, it may have influenced our results. However, we can conclude in our study, that nerve sparing did not appear to negatively impact the effect of PFM training on continence. Investigations relating to erectile function may display a more significant relationship and this represents another opportunity for research in similar populations.

Conclusion

In conclusion, an intensive PFM training intervention, applied prior to surgery, improved post-surgical pelvic floor muscle function and decreased UI, compared to a control group. Group differences were also apparent for perceived UI and QoL post-surgery. Continence and PFM functional recovery was observed post-surgery for both groups, with some evidence for more rapid recovery by 12 weeks as a consequence of the more intense intervention. Our findings provide support for further investigation, in larger trials, of the impact of relatively intensive prehabilitative approaches to enhancing PFM function in men with prostate cancer.

Abbreviations

BMI: Body Mass Index; EPIC-CP: Expanded Prostate Cancer Index Composite for Clinical Practice; IPSS: International Prostate Symptom Score; PCa: Prostate Cancer; PFM: Pelvic floor muscle; QoL: Quality of life; RALP: Robotic Assisted Laparoscopic Prostatectomy; RP: Radical Prostatectomy; RRT: Rapid Response Test; RTUS: Real Time Ultrasound; SET: Sustained Endurance Test; SUI: Stress Urinary Incontinence; UI: Urinary Incontinence

Acknowledgements

Not applicable.

Authors' contributions

All authors read and approved the final manuscript. JEM was involved in the project and protocol development, data collection and had a minor role in data analysis. DJG was involved in the protocol and project development, data management and data analysis. TRA was involved in the data management and data analysis and oversaw the project development.

References

1. www.globocan.iarc.fr. Prostate cancer: estimated incidence: mortality and prevelance worldwide in 2012. 2018. https://www.iarc.fr/en/media-centre/pr/2018/pdfs/pr263_E.pdf. Accessed 8 Aug 2018.
2. Walsh PC, Partin AW, Epstein JI. Cancer control and quality of life following anatomical radical prostatectomy: results at 10years. J Urol. 1994;152(5, part 2):1831–6.
3. Shikanov S. Urinary and sexuality QOL 1 year following RARP. J Urol. 2008; 180(2):760–66.
4. Shikanov SA. A prospective report of changes in prostate cancer related quality of life after robotic prostatectomy. J Psych Oncol. 2011;29:1157–67.
5. www.ics.org. https://www.ics.org/terminology/580. 2018. Accessed 8 Aug 2019.
6. Nitti VW, Mourtzinos A, Brucker BM, SUFU Pad Test Study Group. Correlation of patient perception of pad use with objective degree of incontinence measured by pad test in men with post-prostatectomy incontinence: the SUFU Pad Test Study. J Urol. 2014;192:386–842.
7. Mehnert A, Lehmann C, Graffen M, Huland H, Kock U. Depression, anxiety, post-traumatic stress disorder and health related quality of life and its association with social support in ambulatory prostate cancer patients. European J Cancer Care. 2010;19(6):736–45.
8. Weber BA, Roberts BL, Mills TL. Physical and emotional predictors of depression after radical prostatectomy. Amer J Mens Health. 2008;2(2):165–71.

9. Prota C, Gomes CM, Ribeiro LH, et al. Early postoperative pelvic-floor biofeedback improves erectile function in men undergoing radical prostatectomy: a prospective, randomized, controlled trial. Int J Impot Res. 2012;24(5):174–8.
10. Anderson CA, Omar MI, Campbell SE, Hunter KF, Cody JD, Glazener CM. Conservative management for post-prostatectomy urinary incontinence. Cochrane Database Syst Rev. 2015; Available from: http://onlinelibrary.wiley.com/doi/10.1002/14651858.CD001843.pub5/full 2015. Accessed 8 Aug 2018.
11. Hall L, Alujuraifani R, Hodges PW. Design of programs to train pelvic floor muscles in men with urinary dysfunction: systematic review. Neuro Urod. 2018;37(7):2053–7.
12. Centemero A, Rigatti L, Giraudi D, Lazzeri M, Lughhezzeni G, Zugna D, Montorsi F, Rigatti P, Guazzoni G. Preoperative pelvic floor muscle exercise for early incontinence after radical prostatectomy: a randomised controlled study. Eur Urol. 2010;57:1039–43.
13. www.mayoclinic.org. Exercise intensity: How to measure it. 2019. https://www.mayoclinic.org/healthy-lifestyle/fitness/in-depth/exercise-intensity/art-20046887. Accessed 20 July 2019.
14. Glazener C, Boachie C, Buckley B, et al. Conservative treatment for urinary incontinence in Men After Prostate Surgery (MAPS): two parallel randomised controlled trials. Health Technol Assess. 2011;15(24):1–290 iii-iv.
15. Continence Foundation of Australia. Continence and prostate: a guide for men undergoing prostate surgery. In: Australian Government, Prostate Cancer Foundation of Australia, Australian Physiotherapy Association, Urological Society of Australia and New Zealand, ed. Pamphlet. Victoria: Commence Press; 2019.
16. Stafford RE, Ashton-Millar JA, Constantinou C, Couglin C, Lutton NJ, Hodges P. Pattern of activation of pelvic floor muscles in men differs with verbal instructions. Neuro Urod. 2015. https://doi.org/10.1002/nau.22745 Wylie online.
17. Barry MJ, Fowler FJ Jr, O'Leary MP, et al. The American Urological Association symptom index for benign prostatic hyperplasia. The Measurement Committee of the American Urological Association. J Urol. 1992;148(5):1564.
18. Chang P, Syzmanski K, Dunn R, et al. Expanded prostate cancer index composite for clinical practice: development and validation of a practical health related quality of life instrument for use in the routine clinical care of patients with prostate cancer. J Urol. 2011;156:865–72.
19. Milios JE, Atkinson CL, Naylor LN, et al. Pelvic floor muscle assessment in men's health: Comparing traditional and novel approaches in radical prostatectomy patients. ANZ Cont J. 2018; (In press).
20. Milios JE, Atkinson CL, Naylor LH, et al. Application of novel pelvic floor muscle function tests in men following radical prostatectomy: relationship to urinary incontinence. ANZ Cont J. 2018; (In press).
21. Pinnock CB, Stapleton AMF, Marshall VR. Erectile dysfunction in the community: a prevalence study. Med J Aust. 1999;171(7):353–7.
22. Ficarra V, Novara G, Artibani W, et al. Retropubic, laparoscopic, and robot-assisted radical prostatectomy: a systematic review and cumulative analysis of comparative studies. Euro Urol. 2009;55(5):1037–63.
23. Al-Ali BM, Ponholzer A, Augustin H, Madersbacher S, Pummer K. The long term effect of radical prostatectomy on erectile function, urinary continence and lower urinary tract symptoms: a comparison to age-matched healthy controls. BioMed Res Int. 2017. https://doi.org/10.1155/2017/9615080.
24. Reeves F, Preece P, Kapoor J, et al. Preservation of the nuerovascular bundles is assosciated with improved time to continence after radical prostatectomy but not long term continence rates: results of a systematic review and meta-analysis. Euro Urol. 2015;68(4):692–704.
25. Wang W, Huang QM, Liu FP, Mao QQ. Effectiveness of preoperative pelvic floor muscle training for urinary incontinence after radical prostatectomy: a meta-analysis. BMC Urol. 2014;14:99.
26. Patel MI, Yao J, Hirschorn AD, Mungovan SF. Preoperative pelvic floor physiotherapy improves continence after radical retropubic prostatectomy. Int J Urol. 2013;20:986–92.
27. Stafford R, Ashton-Miller JA, Constantaniou CE, Hodges PW. Novel insight into the dynamics of male pelvic floor contractions through transperineal ultrasound imaging. J Urol. 2012;188(4):1224–30.
28. Stafford RE, Ashton-Miller JA, Constantinou C, Coughlin G, Lutton NJ, Hodges PW. Pattern of activation of pelvic floor muscles in men differs with verbal instructions. Neurourol Urodyn. 2016;35(4):457–63.
29. Campos GE, Luecke TJ, Wendeln HK. Muscular adaptations in response to three different resistance-training regimens: specificity of repetition maximum training zones. Eur J Appl Physiol. 2002;88(1–2):50–60.
30. Kraemer WJ, Ratamess NA. Fundamentals of resistance training: progression and exercise presecription. Med Sci Sport Exerc. 2004;36(4):674–88.

19

Retzius-sparing robot-assisted laparoscopic radical prostatectomy: Functional and early oncologic results in aggressive and locally advanced prostate cancer

Joanne Nyaboe Nyarangi-Dix[1†], Magdalena Görtz[1*†], Georgi Gradinarov[2], Luisa Hofer[1], Viktoria Schütz[1], Claudia Gasch[1], Jan Philipp Radtke[1] and Markus Hohenfellner[1]

Abstract

Background: Retzius-sparing robot-assisted laparoscopic radical prostatectomy (rsRARP) allows entire prostatectomy procedure via the pouch of Douglas. In low- and intermediate-risk prostate cancer (PCa) there is level 1 evidence that the Retzius-sparing approach impacts early continence recovery. Since specific data on aggressive and locally advanced cancer is lacking and avoiding rsRARP is presently suggested, we investigated urinary and sexual recovery, perioperative complications and early oncologic outcomes after rsRARP in this particular cohort.

Methods: Prospectively collected data of 50 consecutive men (median age 66 years) with high-risk PCa who underwent rsRARP in a single institution was analysed retrospectively. The follow-up for all patients was 12 months after surgery.

Results: 3 vs. 12 months after surgery, 82% vs. 98% of men used no pad or one safety pad and 50% vs. 72% used no pad. 89% of patients did not observe a decline of continence if postoperative radiotherapy was carried out. Considering the 17 preoperatively potent patients who underwent bi- or unilateral nerve-sparing surgery, 41% reported their first sexual intercourse within 1 year after rsRARP.
84% of patients had ≥pT3a disease and 42% positive surgical margins. A lymphadenectomy was done in 94% of patients with a median lymph node removal of 15 and lymph node metastasis in 13%.
34% underwent adjuvant radiotherapy and 22% adjuvant androgen deprivation therapy (ADT). 1-year recurrence-free survival was 96%, including 25% of patients on adjuvant or salvage ADT.

Conclusions: RsRARP in high-risk PCa is feasible and results in excellent continence rates, even after postoperative radiotherapy. The potency rates are promising but need further clarification in larger cohorts. Reliable oncologic outcomes require longterm follow-up and are awaited.

Keywords: High risk prostate cancer, Retzius-sparing robot-assisted radical prostatectomy, Urinary continence, Erectile function

* Correspondence: magdalena.goertz@med.uni-heidelberg.de
†Joanne Nyaboe Nyarangi-Dix and Magdalena Görtz contributed equally to this work.
[1]Department of Urology, University Hospital Heidelberg, Im Neuenheimer Feld 110, 69120 Heidelberg, Germany
Full list of author information is available at the end of the article

Background

After Binder and Kramer [1] reported the first robot-assisted laparoscopic radical prostatectomy (RARP) in 2001, RARP proceeded to become a widespread and accepted surgical approach for prostatectomy [2]. Meanwhile, the "holy grail" in routine RARP consists of a complete tumor resection and optimal functional results [3]. With oncological outcomes after RARP in localized prostate cancer (PCa) being steadfast, focus is currently shifting towards improvement of perioperative morbidity and functional results.

Reports suggest that surgical techniques involving membranous urethral length preservation [4], posterior musculofascial reconstruction [5] and/or bladder neck preservation [6] may further improve continence. In 2010, Bocciardi et al. reported an innovative posterior Retzius-sparing RARP (rsRARP) approach avoiding bladder detachment [7] thereby presumably minimizing surgical trauma and preserving normal pelvic anatomy maximally. The continence rate reported within the first year of surgery was 96% [8]. In another prospective study, 71% of men after rsRARP were continent 1 week after catheter removal vs. 48% after conventional RARP [9]. These promising results were reported in studies that entirely focused on low- or intermediate-risk PCa collectives. Unknown for this novel technique is whether these functional outcomes can be replicated alongside good oncological outcomes in the challenging setting of high-risk and locally advanced PCa [10].

Men with PCa and a prostate-specific antigen (PSA) > 20 ng/ml, Gleason score 8–10 or clinical-stage ≥T3 are recognized by the major international guidelines to be advanced PCa and constitute the high-risk PCa group [11]. This advanced high-risk-group warrants RP with a clear need for radical/wider dissection, which may compromise functional outcomes [12]. Concerns in these high-risk tumors also regard positive surgical margins (PSMs), inadequate disease control and increased side effects [13]. Recently, accompanied by advances in surgical technology, RP alone or as an initial step within a multimodal concept has gained acceptance in locally advanced PCa [14]. Men with locally advanced PCa treated with RP plus radiotherapy have a lower risk of prostate cancer-specific death compared to men treated with radiotherapy plus androgen deprivation therapy (ADT) alone [15]. EAU guidelines now recognize the role of RP in men with locally advanced PCa, if required in combination with additional treatments such as radiotherapy or ADT [11].

Since rsRARP promotes early continence recovery without an impact on biochemical failure in low- and intermediate-risk PCa, we investigated rsRARP in high-risk PCa. We report the functional, early and midterm oncologic results of our first 50 RARP-patients with high-risk PCa treated by the Retzius-sparing approach.

Methods

Patient cohort

This study was a retrospective review of prospectively collected data at the Department of Urology at Heidelberg University Hospital. The study was approved by the ethical committee of the University of Heidelberg (S-403/2012). Our analytic cohort included 50 consecutive patients with aggressive and/or locally advanced PCa undergoing routine rsRARP between July 2016 and September 2017. Men were classified as high-risk when PSA level > 20 ng/ml, Gleason score 8–10 and/or a pathological stage ≥T3 was met, according to recent EAU guidelines [11].

Surgical technique

All prostatectomies were performed by 3 experienced surgeons routinely performing over 100 RARPs per year. Our rsRARP technique was largely similar to that first described by Galfano et al. [7]. Modifications used in our technique are as described below:

A standard, four-arm da Vinci Si surgical robot was used. Surgeons began with a 0° surgical lens and mostly switched to a 30°-upwards lens beginning at the preparation of the bladder neck henceforth. As a slight technical modification, in contrast to Galfano et al. [7, 8], there was no use of two or four cardinal stitches into the bladder for the identification of the bladder neck orifice during the urethrovesical anastomosis.

Evaluated clinical and oncological parameters

For each patient, we collected the following clinical and pathologic information: age, preoperative total PSA level, prostate volume, preoperative International Prostate Symptom Score (IPSS), International Index of Erectile Function-5 (IIEF-5) score, biopsy Gleason score, clinical cancer stage (cTNM), prostatectomy Gleason score, pathological cancer stage (pTNM) and PSM rate. Furthermore, the following perioperative variables were evaluated: perioperative transfusion rate, bilateral or unilateral nerve-sparing, intraoperative status of the vesicourethral anastomosis, intraoperative and early postoperative complications, length of hospital stay and time to catheter removal.

Postoperative complications were recorded using the Clavien-Dindo classification [16].

Follow-up

All patients completed a questionnaire the day before surgery, including the IPSS and the IIEF-5 questionnaire. During the first year after surgery an institutional questionnaire was sent by mail to inquire postoperative complications, the PSA level and the continence and potency recovery. Additionally, patients were interviewed by telephone to complete outstanding information. Minimum follow-up was 12 months.

Patients were considered continent when they used ≤1 safety pad/day. The date on which the patient stopped using more than 1 safety pad was considered the recovery time of continence. Time to recovery of erectile function in preoperatively potent men (IIEF-5 score > 17) was considered the date of the first sexual intercourse after surgery. All men with PSA ≥0.2 ng/ml at analysis were considered biochemically recurrent [11].

Statistical analysis

Median and interquartile ranges (IQRs) were used to report nonparametric continuous variables. Continence recovery was demonstrated using a Kaplan-Meier plot (IBM SPSS Statistics 24).

Results

Perioperative results

Demographic data are summarized in Additional file 1. The median age was 66 years and the median hospitalization was 4 days. The urethrovesical anastomosis was intraoperatively watertight in 92% of patients. A cystogram was performed in all cases on postoperative day 10 to 14. In case of extravasation, a new cystogram was planned. The Foley catheter was removed at a median of 12 days (IQR: 10–14 days).

Complications were classified according to the Clavien-Dindo system. Clavien-Dindo grade I, II and III complications took place in 2, 2 and 6% of cases, respectively. None of the cases required conversion to open surgery. Intraoperative or postoperative blood transfusions were not needed. There was 1 case of rectal perforation which was detected and sutured intraoperatively. Peripheral pulmonary embolism occured in 1 patient. Owed to anastomotic-insufficiency, 1 man was catheterised for 2 months. There were 3 cases of symptomatic lymphoceles, 2 of them requiring percutaneous drainage (Clavien-Dindo grade IIIa) and one requiring laparoscopic lymphocele-marsupialization (Clavien-Dindo grade IIIb).

Oncologic results

Postoperatively, pathological evaluation revealed 32% with a Gleason score of ≥8 and 84% with extraprostatic extension (pT3-disease). The overall PSM rate was 42% (21 of 50 patients). Eleven patients were identified to have an anterior index tumor in imaging. 8 of 11 (73%) patients with anterior tumors had pT3-disease and 5 of 11 (45%) had PSM. A lymphadenectomy was done in 94% of patients with a median lymph node removal of 15 (IQR 10–21). Lymph node metastasis was documented in 6 of 47 patients (13%).

Postoperative PSA persistence (defined as a PSA level ≥ 0.2 ng/ml at 3 months after surgery) was documented in 5 of 48 (10%) patients. 34% of patients underwent adjuvant radiotherapy and 22% of patients adjuvant ADT.

During 1-year follow-up 2 (4%) patients experienced biochemical recurrence. 2 (4%) patients received salvage treatments: radiotherapy alone or radiotherapy plus ADT. 1-year biochemical disease-free survival with a PSA ≤0.2 ng/ml was 96%. Among them, 12 (25%) patients were on ADT.

Continence results

The urinary continence rate was 38% at 1 week after catheter removal. Three months after surgery, 82% were continent. Figure 1 shows the recovery curve for continence.

Twelve months postoperatively, 98% were continent: while 73% used no pad, 27% used one safety pad per day. One man (2%) used two pads per day. 17 of 19 (89%) who had received adjuvant or salvage radiotherapy observed no decline of continence after radiotherapy. To date, no anastomotic stricture has been detected.

Erectile function results

Detailed information about sexual function recovery is shown in Additional file 2. 29 (58%) patients were preoperatively potent with an IIEF-5 score > 17. In those patients, bilateral and unilateral nerve-sparing was performed in 12 (41%) and 5 (17%) men, respectively. 7 of the 17 (41%) who underwent bilateral or unilateral nerve-sparing surgery reported to have regular and consistent sexual intercourse within the first year of surgery. 2 of the 7 (29%) postoperatively potent patients used phosphodiesterase type 5 inhibitors on-demand. Median time to recovery of erectile function was 8 months (IQR: 6–11 months). For the 7 postoperatively potent patients, the median IIEF frequency score (Q3) to maintain the erection during sexual intercourse was 4 (IQR: 3–4) and the median IIEF satisfaction score (Q5) was 4 (IQR: 4–5).

Discussion

Since the Bocciardi group described their technique of a Retzius-sparing approach of RARP in 2010, excellent functional and oncological outcomes have been reported [7, 8]. A recent review found that rsRARP is associated with earlier continence recovery compared to conventional RARP without significant impact on oncological outcomes [17]. Beyond the initiator group, subsequent studies focused on low- and intermediate-risk PCa, leaving a gap in reporting for the high-risk and locally advanced disease cohort [9]. Consequently, due to the lack of data on the outcomes in higher-risk PCa, it has been advised to limit the Retzius-sparing approach to low- or favorable intermediate-risk disease [18]. Since adapting Retzius-sparing prostatectomy in our centre, all men

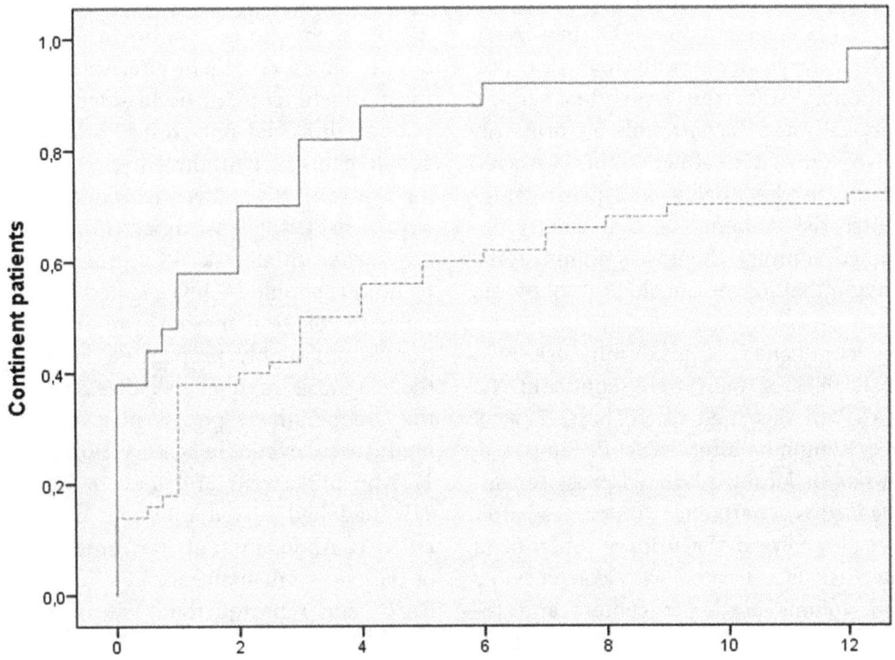

Fig. 1 Kaplan-Meier curve of continence recovery. Blue continuous line = no pad or one safety pad; green dashed line = no pad. Time to continence is expressed in months

viable for RARP were operated in this manner, regardless of preoperative oncological characteristics. We hereby present the first report that focuses on the perioperative, functional and oncologic results after rsRARP in a small purely aggressive PCa-collective.

Our perioperative results show that Retzius-sparing prostatectomy is not only feasible but safe in aggressive and locally advanced PCa. According to the Clavien-Dindo classification, only Grade III complications or less were detected. Grade III complications occurred in 3 (6%) patients and were due to extended lymphadenectomy yielding up to 40 lymph nodes per patient. Lymphadenectomy is mandatory in this cohort, since it improves the accuracy of cancer staging [19] and may be oncologically beneficial [20]. The lymphocele rate in our study was in accordance with another series reporting occurance in 10% of patients undergoing extended pelvic lymph node dissection [21].

As would be expected in an aggressive and locally advanced collective with PSA level > 20 ng/ml, Gleason score > 7 and/or pathological stage ≥T3, PSMs were higher than in a normal/mixed cohort. In the present analysis, 84% of patients harbored extraprostatic ≥pT3a disease. The present PSM rate (42%) is within range of other reports including a review on high-risk PCa treated with conventional RARP that reported a 16–58% PSM rate [22]. Harty and colleagues performed conventional RARP in a cohort more similar to the present study (high risk and locally advanced PCa). In their cohort with 78% ≥ pT3a disease, 50% had PSMs [23]. An explanation for a reduced PSM rate in rsRARP may be the possibility to dissect antegradely allowing improved visualization of the prostate base and posterior margin of the prostate, which are common sites of PSMs in conventional RARP [24].

Despite knowledge of higher likelihood of PSMs and biochemical recurrence in locally advanced PCa, studies have shown overall survival rates of > 75% at 10 years after RP [22]. Adjuvant therapies following prostatectomy play an important role in surviving locally advanced and high-risk PCa. Reduced biochemical recurrence, distant metastases and longer survival rates of high-risk patients have been repeatedly proved after adjuvant radiotherapy [25]. The role of hormonal manipulation therapy in the high-risk collective is embedded in all national and international guidelines [11]. In our cohort, 34 and 22% of patients underwent adjuvant radiotherapy and adjuvant ADT, respectively. Adjuvant radiotherapy was initiated in men at a high risk of progression according to the histopathological results, e.g. extracapsular extension and positive margins in final pathology specimen results. Adjuvant ADT was initiated in men with lymph node metastasis or with very high-risk localized disease. Twelve months after surgery, 4% of men had received salvage radiotherapy and 2% salvage ADT.

1-year progression-free survival in our cohort was 96%; this included 12 (25%) patients on ADT. In a previously published study on patients with high-risk PCa treated by conventional RARP, the 1-year biochemical recurrence-free survival was 81%, with only 6% primarily scheduled to receive adjuvant treatment [26]. However, current data support the view that overall progression-free survival of high-risk patients is significantly increased when planned adjuvant therapy is administered [25]. It is clear though, that longer oncological follow-up must be awaited.

Defining urinary continence as maximum use of a safety pad per day, 98% of men were continent 12 months after rsRARP in this high-risk cohort. 72% of men were pad free 12 months after rsRARP. Studies of patients with high risk or locally advanced prostate cancer show heterogeneous continence outcomes after RARP. Abdollah et al. analyzed the urinary function of 769 men with high-risk PCa treated with conventional RARP at two high-volume academic centers and revealed urinary continence recovery in 85% of men at 12 months after surgery (defined as the use of no pad or one safety pad per day) [12]. Gandaglia et al. found a 1-year urinary continence recovery rate of 64% after conventional RARP in locally advanced cancer (defined as the use of no pad) [27].

Regarding early continence recovery, 38% of men in our study were continent 1 week after catheter removal and 82% of men 3 months after surgery. With rsRARP in low- and intermediate-risk PCa, early continence was reported in 71% of men 1 week after catheter removal and in 95% of men 3 months after surgery [9]. One explanation for this discrepancy is that our cohort included locally advanced disease with 84% harboring extraprostatic extension in contrast to the previous predominantly pT2-cohort study [9, 28]. The oncological necessity of a more radical and wider dissection plane may explain generally reduced continence rates in high-risk collectives [12]. At the same time, prolonged postoperative catheterisation in the present cohort may have played a vital role. Furthermore, the proneness of high-risk cancer patients to delayed recovery of urinary continence after prostatectomy may also be due to the broader lymphadenectomy template necessary in high-risk PCa; increasing possible damage to nerve fibers innervating the pelvic floor [29]. Nevertheless, Retzius-sparing prostatectomy appears to substantially improve continence rates, rendering a great proportion (84%) of this high-risk cohort, ready for further multimodal therapies like adjuvant radiotherapy.

Men receiving postoperative radiotherapy are known to have a higher overall incontinence rate [30]. Interestingly, only 2 of 19 (11%) patients who received radiotherapy after rsRARP observed a decline in continence after radiotherapy. Previous studies revealed that only 22% of men who are continent at the start of radiotherapy remained continent afterwards [31]. During rsRARP most attachments of the bladder remain untouched and pubourethral and pubovesical attachments remain intact avoiding bladder/urethral hypermobility [32]. This may have a protective effect for continence after radiotherapy. Considering this impact for the adjuvant radiotherapy prone high-risk PCa-group, the Retzius-sparing technique should be investigated in further studies.

For oncological reasons, preservation of erectile function is not highly propagated in men confronted with the diagnosis of high-risk disease [33]. Nonetheless, of the preoperatively potent men with a strong wish for neurovascular bundle preservation and an IIEF-5 score > 17 who underwent unilateral or bilateral nerve-sparing, 41% had had sexual intercourse in the year following rsRARP. Abdollah et al. performed nerve-sparing in 88% of patients with high-risk PCa undergoing conventional RARP and reported that 26% of preoperatively potent men were able to have intercourse 12 months after surgery [12].

Since recovery of sexual function in general continues beyond 12–24 months post surgery [12], it is too early to estimate the full percentage of men that can expect to recover sexual function after rsRARP in high-risk PCa. Neurovascular bundle preservation should, nonetheless, be reserved to highly informed men consenting to nerve-sparing despite increased risk of PSMs in aggressive and locally advanced PCa.

A limitation of this study was that it is non-randomized, non-comparative and retrospective in nature. However, this represents a natural step during the exploration of a new surgical technique. In light of the results of the current study, we initiated a prospective randomized clinical trial at our institution that compares the outcomes of conventional and rsRARP in low-, intermediate and high-risk PCa.

Another limitation was that a single, highly experienced team performed RARP at an academic institution and that the results may not be generalizable.

In addition, it is premature to foresee long-term oncological outcomes in this cohort, since results regarding oncologic efficacy and probability of biochemical failure > 12 months after RARP are pending.

Lastly, the promising first results of sexual function recovery after rsRARP in a purely aggressive PCa-collective need to be confirmed in larger cohorts and over a longer period of time.

Conclusions

With the increasing role of RARP in the management of aggressive and locally advanced PCa, we present the 1-year functional and oncological outcomes in a cohort of

50 men with high-risk PCa treated with rsRARP. RsRARP is feasible, safe and associated with few peri-operative complications. We demonstrate (very) good results regarding the recovery of urinary continence in patients with high-risk PCa. Continence results following rsRARP and postoperative radiotherapy are promising. Potency rates appear encouraging but need further clarification in larger cohorts. Longterm oncological outcomes are awaited.

Supplementary information

Additional file 1. Demographic, preoperative and pathologic features.
Additional file 2. Sexual function recovery.

Abbreviations

ADT: Androgen deprivation therapy; EAU: European Association of Urology; IIEF-5 : International Index of Erectile Function-5; IPSS: International Prostate Symptom Score; IQR: Interquartile range; PCa: Prostate cancer; PSA: Prostate-specific antigen; PSM: Positive surgical margin; RARP: Robot-assisted laparoscopic radical prostatectomy; RP: Radical prostatectomy; rsRARP: Retzius-sparing robot-assisted laparoscopic radical prostatectomy

Acknowledgements

Not applicable.

Authors' contributions

JN: Protocol development, Data analysis, Manuscript writing. MG: Protocol development, Data collection, Data analysis, Manuscript writing. GG: Data collection. LH: Data collection, Manuscript editing. VS: Data collection, Manuscript editing. CG: Manuscript editing. JR: Manuscript editing. MH: Protocol development, Manuscript editing. All authors read and approved the final manuscript.

Author details

[1]Department of Urology, University Hospital Heidelberg, Im Neuenheimer Feld 110, 69120 Heidelberg, Germany. [2]Ruprecht-Karls University of Heidelberg, Medical Faculty, Heidelberg, Germany.

References

1. Binder J, Kramer W. Robotically-assisted laparoscopic radical prostatectomy. BJU Int. 2001;87(4):408–10.
2. Yaxley JW, Coughlin GD, Chambers SK, Occhipinti S, Samaratunga H, Zajdlewicz L, et al. Robot-assisted laparoscopic prostatectomy versus open radical retropubic prostatectomy: early outcomes from a randomised controlled phase 3 study. Lancet. 2016;388(10049):1057–66.
3. Bianco FJ Jr, Scardino PT, Eastham JA. Radical prostatectomy: long-term cancer control and recovery of sexual and urinary function ("trifecta"). Urology. 2005;66(5 Suppl):83–94.
4. Paparel P, Akin O, Sandhu JS, Otero JR, Serio AM, Scardino PT, et al. Recovery of urinary continence after radical prostatectomy: association with urethral length and urethral fibrosis measured by preoperative and postoperative endorectal magnetic resonance imaging. Eur Urol. 2009;55(3): 629–37.
5. Rocco B, Cozzi G, Spinelli MG, Coelho RF, Patel VR, Tewari A, et al. Posterior musculofascial reconstruction after radical prostatectomy: a systematic review of the literature. Eur Urol. 2012;62(5):779–90.
6. Nyarangi-Dix JN, Tichy D, Hatiboglu G, Pahernik S, Tosev G, Hohenfellner M. Complete bladder neck preservation promotes long-term post-prostatectomy continence without compromising midterm oncological outcome: analysis of a randomised controlled cohort. World J Urol. 2018; 36(3):349 55.
7. Galfano A, Ascione A, Grimaldi S, Petralia G, Strada E, Bocciardi AM. A new anatomic approach for robot-assisted laparoscopic prostatectomy: a feasibility study for completely intrafascial surgery. Eur Urol. 2010;58(3):457–61.
8. Galfano A, Di Trapani D, Sozzi F, Strada E, Petralia G, Bramerio M, et al. Beyond the learning curve of the Retzius-sparing approach for robot-assisted laparoscopic radical prostatectomy: oncologic and functional results of the first 200 patients with >/= 1 year of follow-up. Eur Urol. 2013;64(6): 974–80.
9. Dalela D, Jeong W, Prasad MA, Sood A, Abdollah F, Diaz M, et al. A pragmatic randomized controlled trial examining the impact of the Retzius-sparing approach on early urinary continence recovery after robot-assisted radical prostatectomy. Eur Urol. 2017;72(5):677–85.
10. Stonier T, Simson N, Davis J, Challacombe B. Retzius-sparing robot-assisted radical prostatectomy (RS-RARP) vs standard RARP: it's time for critical appraisal. BJU Int. 2019;123(1):5–7.
11. Mottet N, Bellmunt J, Bolla M, Briers E, Cumberbatch MG, De Santis M, et al. EAU-ESTRO-SIOG guidelines on prostate Cancer. Part 1: screening, diagnosis, and local treatment with curative intent. Eur Urol. 2017;71(4):618–29.
12. Abdollah F, Dalela D, Sood A, Sammon J, Cho R, Nocera L, et al. Functional outcomes of clinically high-risk prostate cancer patients treated with robot-assisted radical prostatectomy: a multi-institutional analysis. Prostate Cancer Prostatic Dis. 2017;20(4):395–400.
13. Stewart SB, Boorjian SA. Radical prostatectomy in high-risk and locally advanced prostate cancer: Mayo Clinic perspective. Urol Oncol. 2015;33(5): 235–44.
14. Hager B, Kraywinkel K, Keck B, Katalinic A, Meyer M, Zeissig SR, et al. Increasing use of radical prostatectomy for locally advanced prostate cancer in the USA and Germany: a comparative population-based study. Prostate Cancer Prostatic Dis. 2017;20(1):61–6.
15. Jang TL, Patel N, Faiena I, Radadia KD, Moore DF, Elsamra SE, et al. Comparative effectiveness of radical prostatectomy with adjuvant radiotherapy versus radiotherapy plus androgen deprivation therapy for men with advanced prostate cancer. Cancer. 2018;124(20):4010–22.
16. Dindo D, Demartines N, Clavien PA. Classification of surgical complications: a new proposal with evaluation in a cohort of 6336 patients and results of a survey. Ann Surg. 2004;240(2):205–13.
17. Phukan C, McLean A, Nambiar A, Mukherjee A, Somani B, Krishnamoorthy R, et al. Retzius sparing robotic assisted radical prostatectomy vs. conventional robotic assisted radical prostatectomy: a systematic review and meta-analysis. World J Urol. 2019; https://doi.org/10.1007/s00345-019-02798-4. [Epub ahead of print].
18. Cadeddu JA. Re: a pragmatic randomized controlled trial examining the impact of the Retzius-sparing approach on early urinary continence recovery after robot-assisted radical prostatectomy. J Urol. 2018;199(4): 875–6.
19. Yuh B, Artibani W, Heidenreich A, Kimm S, Menon M, Novara G, et al. The role of robot-assisted radical prostatectomy and pelvic lymph node dissection in the management of high-risk prostate cancer: a systematic review. Eur Urol. 2014;65(5):918–27.
20. Choo MS, Kim M, Ku JH, Kwak C, Kim HH, Jeong CW. Extended versus standard pelvic lymph node dissection in radical prostatectomy on oncological and functional outcomes: a systematic review and meta-analysis. Ann Surg Oncol. 2017;24(7):2047–54.
21. Briganti A, Chun FK, Salonia A, Suardi N, Gallina A, Da Pozzo LF, et al. Complications and other surgical outcomes associated with extended pelvic lymphadenectomy in men with localized prostate cancer. Eur Urol. 2006;50(5):1006–13.
22. Saika T, Miura N, Fukumoto T, Yanagihara Y, Miyauchi Y, Kikugawa T. Role of robot-assisted radical prostatectomy in locally advanced prostate cancer. Int J Urol. 2018;25(1):30–5.
23. Harty NJ, Kozinn SI, Canes D, Sorcini A, Moinzadeh A. Comparison of positive surgical margin rates in high risk prostate cancer: open versus minimally invasive radical prostatectomy. Int Braz J Urol. 2013;39(5):639–46 discussion 47-8.
24. Lightfoot AJ, Su YK, Sehgal SS, Lee Z, Greaves GH, Yu SJ, et al. Positive surgical margin trends in patients with pathologic T3 prostate Cancer treated with robot-assisted radical prostatectomy. J Endourol. 2015;29(6): 634–9.
25. Hwang WL, Tendulkar RD, Niemierko A, Agrawal S, Stephans KL, Spratt DE, et al. Comparison between adjuvant and early-salvage Postprostatectomy radiotherapy for prostate Cancer with adverse pathological features. JAMA Oncol. 2018;4(5):e175230.

26. Abdollah F, Sood A, Sammon JD, Hsu L, Beyer B, Moschini M, et al. Long-term cancer control outcomes in patients with clinically high-risk prostate cancer treated with robot-assisted radical prostatectomy: results from a multi-institutional study of 1100 patients. Eur Urol. 2015;68(3):497–505.
27. Gandaglia G, De Lorenzis E, Novara G, Fossati N, De Groote R, Dovey Z, et al. Robot-assisted radical prostatectomy and extended pelvic lymph node dissection in patients with locally-advanced prostate Cancer. Eur Urol. 2017; 71(2):249–56.
28. Michl U, Tennstedt P, Feldmeier L, Mandel P, Oh SJ, Ahyai S, et al. Nerve-sparing surgery technique, not the preservation of the neurovascular bundles, leads to improved long-term continence rates after radical prostatectomy. Eur Urol. 2016;69(4):584–9.
29. Seikkula H, Janssen P, Tutolo M, Tosco L, Battaglia A, Moris L, et al. Comparison of functional outcome after extended versus super-extended pelvic lymph node dissection during radical prostatectomy in high-risk localized prostate Cancer. Front Oncol. 2017;7:280.
30. Adam M, Tennstedt P, Lanwehr D, Tilki D, Steuber T, Beyer B, et al. Functional outcomes and quality of life after radical prostatectomy only versus a combination of prostatectomy with radiation and hormonal therapy. Eur Urol. 2017;71(3):330–6.
31. Nyarangi-Dix JN, Steimer J, Bruckner T, Jakobi H, Koerber SA, Hadaschik B, et al. Post-prostatectomy radiotherapy adversely affects urinary continence irrespective of radiotherapy regime. World J Urol. 2017;35(12):1841–7.
32. Chang LW, Hung SC, Hu JC, Chiu KY. Retzius-sparing robotic-assisted radical prostatectomy associated with less bladder neck descent and better early continence outcome. Anticancer Res. 2018;38(1):345–51.
33. Imbimbo C, Creta M, Gacci M, Simonato A, Gontero P, de Cobelli O, et al. Patients' desire to preserve sexual activity and final decision for a nerve-sparing approach: results from the MIRROR (multicenter Italian report on radical prostatectomy outcomes and research) study. J Sex Med. 2011;8(5): 1495–502.

20

Staged male genital reconstruction with a local flap and free oral graft

Da-chao Zheng[†], Min-kai Xie[†], Shi-bo Fu, Jian-hua Guo, Wen-ji Li, Hai-jun Yao[*] and Zhong Wang[*]

Abstract

Background: Male genital skin loss is a common disease in urology. However, male genital skin loss accompanying a penile urethra defect is rarely reported. Herein, we describe a novel surgical technique using a composite local flap and oral mucosal graft to reconstruct the penis, which may provide a new solution for patients with similar conditions.

Case presentation: A 36-year-old male with a penile urethra defect and a large area of genital skin loss required urethral reconstruction. The meatus had descended to the penoscrotal junction. This procedure was divided into three stages. The first stage of the surgery involved burying the nude penile shaft beneath the skin of the left anteromedial thigh for coverage of the skin defect. The second stage consisted of releasing the penis and expanding the size of the urethral plate for further urethroplasty. The third stage consisted of reconstruction of the anterior urethra 6 months later. Postoperatively, the patient reported satisfactory voiding. The maximal flow rate (MFR) was 22.2 ml/s with no postvoiding residual urine at the 24-month follow-up visit. No edema, infection, hemorrhage, or cicatricial retraction were observed. The patient's erectile function was satisfactory, and his international index of erectile function-5 score (IIEF-5 score) was 23 at the 24-month follow-up visit. Additionally, the presence of nocturnal penile tumescence demonstrated that he had normal erectile function.

Conclusions: This procedure is an effective surgical option for men with complete foreskin and penile urethra defects. It could also be extended as a treatment strategy when composite local or pedicle transposition flaps and free grafts are needed for specific patients.

Keywords: Genital reconstruction, Penile urethra defect, Local flap, Free oral graft

Background

Male genital skin loss following severe infections such as Fournier's gangrene or injuries is a common condition in urology. Reconstruction with local pedicled penile flaps. Scrotal flaps, split-thickness skin grafting (STSG) and/or pedicle flaps is an effective technique when the urethra is completely preserved [1, 2]. The use of several materials such as genital or extragenital skin or mucosa has also been described to repair pure urethral defects [3, 4]. However, reports describing a solution for male genital skin loss accompanying a penile urethra defect are rare.

This paper aimed to report a unique case of complete genital skin loss and a penile urethral defect due to a severe traffic accident. We designed a novel staged procedure and successfully treated this patient.

Case presentation

Patient information and clinical findings

A 36-year-old male survived a severe traffic accident but lost his right leg, bilateral testicles and a large area of genital skin, including the foreskin and scrotal skin. Additionally, the penile urethra was damaged, resulting in a urethral defect 6 cm in length, and the meatus had descended to the penoscrotal junction.

* Correspondence: dryaohj@163.com; zhongwang2000@sina.com
[†]Da-chao Zheng and Min-kai Xie contributed equally to this work.
Department of Urology, Shanghai 9th People's Hospital, Shanghai JiaoTong University School of Medicine, NO.369, ZhiZaoJu Road, HuangPu District, Shanghai 200011, China

Therapeutic focus and assessment

The patient strongly desired to perform standing urination; therefore, we performed a three-stage procedure to repair his penis. In the first stage, skin saving measures and coverage of the skin loss were the most important treatments. Free skin grafts and pedicle flaps were transposed to repair the skin defects. The nude penile shaft was buried beneath the skin of the left anteromedial thigh (Fig. 1a).

Twelve months later, the patient underwent the second-stage procedure for penile release and urethral plate expansion (Fig. 1b). In this stage, the penis was released from the left thigh and was fully covered with skin and subcutaneous fat. The size of the penile dorsal skin was designed to be large enough to wrap the corpus cavernosum and residual urethral plate. Considering the shrinkage of the residual urethral plate, a lingual mucosal graft [5] was harvested to expand the urethral plate. The neourethral plate was designed to be as large as possible due to the expected 20% shrinkage of the oral graft [6]. A protective tie-over dressing was placed to reduce the chance of hematoma collecting under the graft. No focal graft contracture occurred requiring an additional operation to patch the graft, and no donor site complications were observed at the follow-up evaluation (Additional file 1).

At 6 months after the second-stage surgery, a third stage was performed for urethroplasty. In this stage, the patient underwent a urethroplasty procedure utilizing the preset flap and the neourethral plate with a standard Thiersch-Duplay technique (Fig. 1c) (Additional file 2). The neourethra was tabularized with 2-layer running subepithelial 6–0 Vicryl sutures. Adequate dissection of the new foreskin, excision of a part of the subcutaneous adipose tissue and Z-plasty led to tension free coverage of the corpus cavernosum and neourethra (Fig. 1d) (Additional file 3). The 12-Fr catheter was removed on postoperative day (POD) 21, and no fistula was observed after the urethral catheter was removed.

At the 2-year follow-up evaluation after the repair, the patient voided satisfactorily (Additional files 4 and 5). The maximal flow rates (MFRs) were 27.8 ml/s, 23.3 ml/s, and 22.2 ml/s with no postvoiding residual urine after the third-stage operation and at the 12-month and 24-month follow-up evaluations, respectively. No edema, infection, hemorrhage, or cicatricial retraction were observed. The patient reported penile erectile function and the ability to perform intercourse without penile curvature. A mild reduction of penile hardness and sensitivity were reported during the 2-year follow-up visit. However, his IIEF-5 scores were 22 and 23 at the 12-month

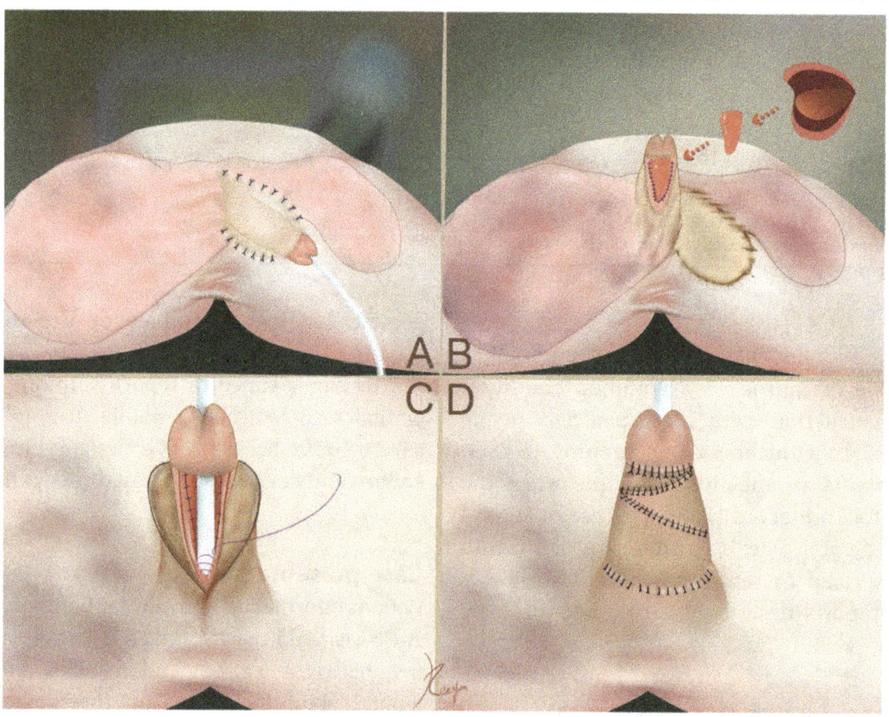

Fig. 1 a. Penile protection and flap preparation: The nude penile shaft was buried beneath the skin of the left anteromedial thigh; **b**. Penile release and urethral plate expansion: The penis was released, and a free lingual mucosal graft was harvested to expand the size of the urethral plate; **c**. Penile and urethral reconstruction: A standard Thiersch-Duplay technique was performed on the preset neourethral plate. **d**. The preset flap was utilized for tension free coverage of the corpus cavernosum and neourethra

and 24-month follow-up evaluations, respectively, as demonstrated by nocturnal penile tumescence (NPT) during postoperative year 2.

Discussion and conclusions

Genital skin loss is usually caused by Fournier's gangrene, trauma, lymphedema, tumors and other diseases [2, 7, 8]. Reconstruction of the urethra and penile or scrotal skin defects with good functional and cosmetic results presents challenges for surgeons. The selection of proper techniques depends on the size of the defect, condition of the local tissue and status of the wound [9].

STSG is a viable treatment option for patients without urethral injuries. The free skin graft can be harvested rapidly to cover large defects [10] and provide a resurfacing solution for the genital region and perineum. However, for this patient, STSG was not feasible. The main disadvantages were as follows. First, the free grafts commonly undergo contraction when they survive. According to our preoperative design, the new foreskin was prepared for coverage of the cavernous bodies and neourethra during the urethroplasty stage. This disadvantages would cause the new foreskin to have an insufficient size and lead to a poor expansive ability for wrapping the neourethra in the final stage. Second, the lack of subcutaneous tissue and abundant blood is another disadvantage for the survived free skin grafts that leads to a poor healing capacity and a high probability of fistula or necrosis in the urethroplasty stage.

To overcome the disadvantages of STSG, fasciocutaneous or musculocutaneous flaps, including the scrotal skin flap, gracilis myocutaneous flap [11], pedicle anterolateral thigh flap [12], and anteromedial thigh fasciocutaneous flap [13], were used, which produced excellent cosmetic outcomes. These flaps had reliable circulation and provided sufficient size, good flexibility and subcutaneous tissues for the penile shaft. However, there were two contradictions. One was that our patient needed a rapid resurfacing for his penis, but these flap techniques would require a long time. The other was the need for STSG for skin defects, which required healthy skin for a donor site. Therefore, burying the nude penile shaft beneath the skin of the left anteromedial thigh was adopted. This technique had been mentioned in a classic textbook describing the treatment of pure penile skin loss using scrotal skin [14]. The skin of the left anteromedial thigh was the nearest healthy skin that could provide similar characteristics to other flaps that were transferred from other donor sites. The greatest advantage of our method was the ability to prefabricate chimeric flaps.

Various techniques for urethral reconstruction have been described [4, 15, 16]. Flaps and grafts, and even the appendix and intestinal segments, have been used as alternative techniques [17–21], and most of these techniques were staged procedures. Yazar [9] and colleagues reported a one-stage technique to repair a complex penile defect with composite anterolateral thigh and vascularized fascia lata flaps. In that case, the vascularized fascia lata flap was utilized to repair the lateral and ventral semicircular wall defect of the urethra. They chose this technique because the patient lacked a well-vascularized recipient bed for the surviving free graft. In this situation, the vascularized fascia lata flap could provide reliable circulation for urethroplasty. In contrast, our patient had a vascularized recipient bed for grafts, and the grafts could be easily harvested. Thus, transforming the penis into a penoscrotal hypospadias for an easier operation was a better choice. Moreover, we had no time to harvest such a composite anterolateral thigh and vascularized fascia lata flap in the first stage. Our method was not as creative as Yazar's, but it was much safer for the repair of the urethral defect. If the graft developed local contracture and necrosis, an additional operation could be performed to patch the graft. Furthermore, an additional operation could be performed to harvest a vascularized fascia lata flap from the other leg when Yazar's patient experienced operative failure, but we had no room for failure because our patient had only one leg.

In the second stage, the lingual mucosa was utilized to expand the urethral plate for urethroplasty. Oral mucosal grafts have been demonstrated to be an effective technique for urethroplasty [22, 23]. Buccal mucosa grafting is another choice, and the selection depends on the surgeon's preference. We did not choose an onlay graft technique or a tubed graft technique because of the high breakdown rates, which may be related to the lack of an adequately vascularized graft bed [24]. The dorsal inlay grafting technique that we selected could provide a large, hairless and well-vascularized neourethral plate for urethroplasty. This was the one of the reasons why we performed three operations.

In a standard hypospadias repair, fistula is a major complication, and meatal stenosis, strictures, infection, and chordee are other common complications [25]. Barrier flap coverage with scrotal dartos flaps or tunica vaginalis flaps is a routine procedure in the treatment of hypospadias and decreases the incidence of fistulas [26, 27]. This patient had lost his genital skin and testicles. Fortunately, the preset flap with reliable circulation and a large amount of subcutaneous tissue provided a good wound healing, and no fistula was observed. Stricture is another major complication of urethroplasty. For this patient, a semi-circular anastomosis was performed to prevent stricture. The satisfactory wound healing and anti-infective ability of the preset flap played an important role in the prevention of stricture. Finally, multiple Z-patterns were designed to reduce the tension of the wounds and the risk of chordee.

In this case, penile erection and subsequent sexual intercourse were preserved postoperatively. Although the final outcomes including the function and cosmetic appearance were satisfactory, the patient still had a binding sensation. This may be associated with a large area of scar tissue on the abdominal, perineal and penile skin. The patient also experienced a mild reduction of penile hardness and sensitivity after the operations, although rigiscan testing indicated that he still had satisfactory erectile function. We suspected that the lack of a penile urethra and foreskin were the contributing factors.

Our result showed that this staged procedure was a simple, effective and safe technique. Furthermore, this approach is also practicable for surgeons who have not mastered complicated flap techniques. Although this procedure was time consuming, we still recommend it for cases with complete genital skin loss and penile urethra defects. Moreover, this staged technique can be improved as a treatment strategy by using proper composite local or pedicle transferred flaps and free grafts for repair of complete genital skin and urethra defects. However, longer follow-up and additional cases are needed to further evaluate the continued use of this technique.

Supplementary information

Additional file 1. Preoperative status: The penis was released, and a free lingual mucosal graft was preset as new urethral plate for the urethraplasty.

Additional file 2. Urethroplasty: A standard Thiersch-Duplay technique was performed on the preset neourethral plate.

Additional file 3. Postoperative status: The figure showed the cosmetic outcome of operation.

Additional file 4. Postoperative status 2 yrs.: The postoperative cosmetic appearance of penis after 2 years.

Additional file 5. Urination:The video demonstrate a normal voiding without any complications.

Abbreviations

IIEF-5: International index of erectile function-5 score; MFR: Maximal flow rate; NPT: Nocturnal penile tumescence; POD: Postoperative day; STSG: Split-thickness skin grafting

Acknowledgements

We thank the staff of the Department of Urology, Shanghai 9th People's Hospital for their help in data collection for publication.

Authors' contributions

DCZ and HJY conceived of the study, participated in its design and coordination, drafted the manuscript and performed the surgeries. MKX and SBF conducted the outpatient care. MKX, JHG and WJL participated in the data acquisition. DCZ and ZW made critical revisions to the manuscript for important intellectual content. All authors read and approved the final manuscript.

References

1. Yao H, Zheng D, Wen J, et al. Reconstruction of Major Scrotal Defects by Anterolateral Thigh Flap. Cell Biochem Biophys. 2014;70(2):1331–5.
2. Alwaal A, McAninch JW, Harris CR, et al. Utilities of Split-Thickness Skin Grafting for male genital reconstruction. Urology. 2015;86(4):835–9.
3. Eppley BL, Keating M, Rink R. A buccal mucosal harvestin technique for urethral reconstruction. J Urol. 1997;157:1268.
4. Bracka A. Hypospadias repair: the two-stage alternative. Br J Urol. 1995; 76(Suppl 3):31–41.
5. Barbagli G, De Angelis M, Romano G, et al. The use of lingual mucosal graft in adult anterior urethroplasty: surgical steps and short-term outcome. Eur Urol. 2008;54(3):671e6.
6. Fichtner J, Filipas D, Fisch M, et al. Long term follow up of buccal mucosa onlay graft for hypospadias repair: analysis of complications. J Urol. 2004;172:1970.
7. Zhao JC, Xian CJ, Yu JA, et al. Reconstruction of infected and denuded scrotum and penis by combined application of negative pressure wound therapy and split-thickness skin grafting. Int Wound J. 2013;10(4):407–10.
8. Black PC, Friedrich JB, Engrav LH, et al. Meshed unexpanded split-thickness skin grafting for reconstruction of penile skin loss. J Urol. 2004;172(3):976–9.
9. Yazar Ş, Eroğlu M, Gökkaya A, et al. The repair of complex penile defect with composite anterolateral thigh and vascularized fascia lata flap. Ulus Travma Acil Cerrahi Derg. 2015;21(3):223–7.
10. Maguiña P, Palmieri TL, Greenhalgh DG. Split thickness skin grafting for recreation of the scrotum following Fournier's gangrene.[J]. Burns J Int Soc Burn Injuries. 2003;29(8):857–62.
11. Ramos RR, Andrews JM, Ferreira LM. A gracilis myocutaneous flap for reconstruction of the scrotum. Br J Plast Surg. 1984;37(2):171–4.
12. Chen SY, Fu JP, Chen TM, et al. Reconstruction of scrotal and perineal defects in Fournier's gangrene. J Plast Reconstr Aesthet Surg. 2011;64(4): 528–34.
13. El-Mageed MA. Evaluation of the anteromedial thigh fasciocutaneous flap for scrotal reconstruction. Plast Reconstr Surg. 2007;31(2):149–55.
14. Yachia D. Penile Injuries. In: Yachia D, editor. Text atlas of penile surgery. London: Informa Healthcare; 2007. p. 136–8.
15. Jeong JH, Shin HJ, Woo SH, et al. A new repair technique for penile para noma: bilateral scrotal aps. Ann Plast Surg. 1996;37:386–93.
16. Gravvanis AI, Tsoutsos DA, Iconomou TG, et al. Penile resurfacing with vascularized fascia lata. J Urol. 2010;25(6):462–8.
17. Cheng KX, Hwang WY, Eid AE, et al. Analysis of 136 cases of reconstructed penis using various methods. Plast Reconstr Surg. 1995;95:1070–84.
18. Dabernig J, Shelley OP, Cuccia G, et al. Urethral reconstruction using the radial forearm free flap: experience in oncologic cases and gender reassignment. Eur Urol. 2007;52(2):547–53.
19. Snodgrass WT, Bush N, Cost N. Algorithm for comprehensive approach to hypospadias reoperation using 3 techniques. J Urol. 2009;182(6):2885–91.
20. Bales GT, Kuznetsov DD, Kim HL, et al. Urethral substitution using an intestinal free flap: a novel approach. J Urol. 2002;168:182–4.
21. Xu YM, Fu Q, Sa YL, et al. Outcome of small intestinal submucosa graft for repair of anterior urethral strictures. Int J Urol. 2013;20(6):622–9.
22. Johal NS, Nitkunan T, O'Malley K, et al. The two-stage repair for severe primary hypospadias. Eur Urol. 2006;50:366–71.
23. Simonato A, Gregori A, Lissiani A, et al. The tongue as an alternative donor site for graftnurethroplasty: a pilot study. J Urol. 2006;175:589e92.
24. Maarouf AM, Elsayed ER, Ragab A, et al. Buccal versus lingual mucosal graft urethroplasty for complex hypospadias repair. J Pediatr Urol. 2013;9(6 Pt A): 754–8.
25. Zheng DC, Wang H, Lu MJ, et al. A comparative study of the use of a transverse preputial island flap (the Duckett technique) to treat primary andsecondary hypospadias in older Chinese patients with severe chordee. World J Urol. 2013;31(4):965–9.
26. Nguyen MT, Snodgrass WT. Tubularized incised plate hypospadias reoperation. J Urol. 2004;171:2404.
27. Babu R, Hariharasudhan S. Tunica vaginalis flap is superior to inner preputial dartos flap as a waterproofing layer for primary TIP repair in midshaft hypospadias. J Pediatr Urol. 2013;9(6 Pt A):804–807.

21

Robot-assisted laparoscopic antegrade versus open inguinal lymphadenectomy: A retrospective controlled study

Hualiang Yu[1†], Yongliang Lu[1†], Yi Xiao[1], Jiaxiang Guo[1], Xiaotao Yin[1], Yu Yang[1], Hongwei Wang[2] and Jiangping Gao[1*]

Abstract

Background: To investigate the surgical methods and clinical results of robot-assisted laparoscopic antegrade inguinal lymphadenectomy.

Methods: A retrospective study was performed on clinical data from 19 patients with penile cancer admitted from March 2013 to October 2017. Among them, nine patients underwent robot-assisted laparoscopic antegrade inguinal lymphadenectomy (robot-assisted group) and 10 patients underwent open inguinal lymphadenectomy (open group). In the robot-assisted group, preoperative preparation, patient position, robot placement, design of operating channel and establishment of operating space are described. Key surgical procedures and techniques are also summarized. In addition, the number of lymph nodes removed, postoperative complications and follow-up in both groups were statistically analyzed.

Results: For the 9 patients in the robot-assisted group, surgery was successfully accomplished at 17 sides without intraoperative conversion to open surgery. The surgery time for each side was 45~90 min using laparoscope with an average of 68.5 ± 13.69 min/side. The intraoperative blood loss was estimated to be < 10 ml/side, and the number of removed lymph nodes was not significantly different from that of the open group (12 ± 4.2/side vs.11 ± 5.8/side, P = 0.84). There were no postoperative complications such as skin necrosis, delayed wound healing and cellulitis in the robot-assisted group. Skin-related complications occurred in 9 (45%) of the 20 sides in the open group. During a median follow-up of 25 months in robot-assisted group and 52.5 mouths in open group, was not significantly different there were no statistical differences in recurrence-free survival between the groups (75% vs 60%, $p = 0.536$).

Conclusion: Robot-assisted laparoscopic antegrade inguinal lymphadenectomy achieved the desired surgical outcomes with fewer intraoperative and postoperative complications. The robotic arms of the surgical system were placed between the lower limbs of each patient. There was no need to re-position the robotic arms during bilateral inguinal lymphadenectomy. This simplified the procedure and reduced the use of trocars. If necessary, pelvic lymphadenectomy could be performed simultaneously using the original trocar position.

Keywords: Robot-assisted surgery, Penile cancer, Antegrade, Inguinal lymphadenectomy

* Correspondence: jpgao@163.com; jiangping_gao@126.com
†Hualiang Yu and Yongliang Lu contributed equally to this work.
[1]Department of Urology, The Fourth Medical Center of Chinese PLA General Hospital, 51th Fucheng Street, Haidian District, Beijing 100048, China
Full list of author information is available at the end of the article

Background

Penile cancer is a relatively rare genitourinary malignancy. Regional lymph node metastasis is considered to associate closely with the patient prognosis. Patient 5-year survival rate without regional lymph node metastasis is 95 to 100%, and drops to 50% for patients with multiple inguinal lymph node metastasis [1]. Hence, inguinal lymphadenectomy is an important treatment strategy for penile cancer. The efficacy of open inguinal lymphadenectomy is definite, however the incidence rates of postoperative complications such as skin necrosis and delayed wound healing are about 50% [2, 3]. The use of laparoscopic technology is compromised due to its own operational limitations [4, 5]. The da Vinci robotic system can provide stable three-dimensional images for surgeons, with high precision and excellent flexibility. Many of the shortcomings of simple laparoscopic surgery are addressed using the da Vinci robotic system. Da Vinci robot-assisted laparoscopic antegrade inguinal lymphadenectomy was successfully performed in nine patients from August 2016 to October 2017, obtaining satisfactory efficacy, which we report in this study.

Methods

General characteristics

The robot-assisted group had nine patients with penile cancer with an average age of (50.0 ± 7.17) years old, ranging from 40 to 62 years old. Their body mass index was (27.3 ± 3.93) kg/m^2, ranging from 21.67 kg/m^2 to 33.21 kg/m^2. The open surgery group had ten patients with an average age of (54.9 ± 13.12) years old, ranging from 24 to 68 years old. Their body mass index was (27.0 ± 2.53) kg/m^2, ranging from 22.03 to 30.03 kg/m^2. All nine patients in the robot-assisted group underwent treatment for penile cancer with pathological diagnosis of primary lesions being all squamous cell carcinoma. This included three patients with well-differentiated squamous cell carcinoma, four with moderately differentiated squamous cell carcinoma, and two with poorly differentiated squamous cell carcinoma. Of the nine patients, six had subcutaneous connective tissue invasion (T1 stage) and three had corpus spongiosum urethrae infiltrate (T3 stage). Preoperative and assistant trocar examinations suggested that there were inguinal lymphadenectasis, but no pelvic lymphadenectasis. One patient was cN1 stage, five were cN2 stage, and three were cN3 stage. None of the patients had distant metastasis (M0 stage). All patients had surgical indicators for inguinal lymphadenectomy. Based on preoperative evaluation and intraoperative pathology of frozen sections, six patients simultaneously underwent robot-assisted laparoscopic pelvic lymphadenectomy using the original trocar position. In the open group, eight of the ten patients were T1 stage, one was T2 stage and one was T3 stage. The preoperative clinical N stage were as follows, cN1 in two patients, cN2 in seven and cN3 in one (Table 1).

Surgical procedure

The open inguinal lymphadenectomy was performed via the (inverse) S-shaped inguinal incision. While the robot-assisted surgical procedure was as follows.

Patient and trocar position

General anesthesia was administered to patients. Patients were in the supine position with the head 15° lower compared to the hip. Both lower extremities were straightened and abducted by about 45° (scissor position). Both of the knee joints were slightly flexed and rotated externally, with the catheter indwelled. The bedside robotic arm of the da Vinci robot was pushed between the two legs of the patient. A 2 cm longitudinal incision was made at the lower margin of the umbilicus. The skin, adipose layer of superficial fascia (Camper fascia) and membranous layer of superficial fascia (Scarpa fascia) were incised. Blunt dissection was performed using the index finger on the surface of the external oblique aponeurosis, and subcutaneous space was established by expansion of self-made balloon. A 12 mm trocar was placed via the incision to be used as a lens hole. Subcutaneous pneumoperitoneum space was created using CO_2, with pressure maintained at 12 mmHg (1 mmHg = 0.133 kPa). During right inguinal lymphadenectomy, a metal trocar of arm-2 was placed at the midpoint between the umbilical cord and pubis, subsequently a metal trocar of arm-1 was placed at the midpoint between the umbilical cord and right anterior superior iliac spine. A 12 mm trocar was then placed under arm-1 outside the metal trocar as an assistant trocar (Fig. 1). During left inguinal lymphadenectomy, the lens hole was unchanged, and the original trocar of arm-2 was used as the trocar of arm-1. Afterwards, a metal trocar of arm-2 was placed at the midpoint between the umbilical cord and the right anterior superior iliac spine.

Surgical procedure

1) *Inguinal lymphadenectomy:* The range of inguinal lymphadenectomy was 2 cm above the inguinal ligament as the upper boundary, apex of the femoral triangle as the lower boundary, medialis sartorius muscle as the outer boundary, and lateralis of the long adductor muscle as the inner boundary. First, dissociation was performed from the surface of the external oblique aponeurosis to the superficial layer in order to remove adipose tissues and superficial lymph nodes in the superficial fascia. Then pressure was applied to the inguinal ligaments by hand and surface projection of the femoral blood vessel was performed. The spermatic cord was pulled to help localization during surgery. The fascia lata under the inguinal ligament was exposed and the cribriform fascia was

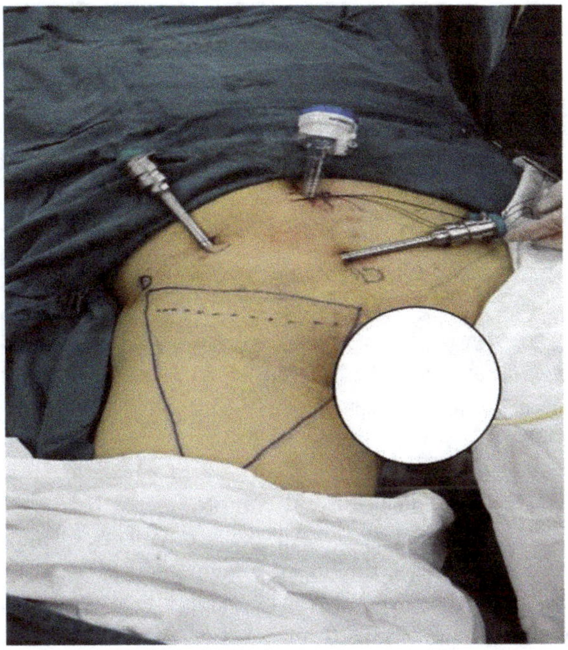

Fig. 1 Position of the Trocar during robot-assisted laparoscopic antegrade inguinal lymphadenectomy

cut open while the femoral artery and vein were exposed to let the surface skeletonize. The femoral vein was dissociated downward to expose the great saphenous vein and its branches, which were retained. The dissociation was continued until the apex of the femoral triangle. Then, the lateralis of the long adductor muscle was exposed on the medial side of the femoral vein. The medialis sartorius muscle was then exposed on the lateral side of the femoral artery. The femoral nerves were protected, and adipose tissue as well as deep lymph nodes in the femoral canal were removed from the assistant trocar and placed in a specimen bag for pathological examination (Fig. 2). After completing the surgery, hemostasis was performed thoroughly on the wound and a negative-pressure drainage tube was placed via the assistant trocar. Puncture holes were then sutured. The opposite side was treated in the same way.

Table 1 Demographic and Clinical Characteristics of Patients

	robotic group($n = 9$)	open group($n = 10$)
Age	50.0 ± 7.17 (40–62)	54.9 ± 13.12 (24–68)
BMI (kg/m^2)	27.3 ± 3.93 (21.67–33.21)	27.0 ± 2.53 (22.03–30.03)
pT stage pT1/ pT2/ pT3	6/0/3	8/1/1
cN stage cN0/cN1/cN2/cN3	0/1/5/3	0/2/7/1

Pathology examination of frozen sections was performed for the nine patients during surgery. Results from five patients showed that the number of positive lymph nodes in the unilateral groin was ≥2. Preoperative examination of one patient showed that there was recurrence of lymph node metastasis in the right groin and fused nodular enlargement of about 4.5 cm × 4.3 cm × 3.0 cm. Hence, pelvic lymphadenectomy was performed via the original trocar position for the above six patients.

2) *Pelvic lymphadenectomy:* Lymph nodes in the bilateral iliac crests, external iliac, internal iliac and obturator were removed. After bilateral inguinal lymphadenectomy, the docking of the robotic arm and the corresponding trocar were released and the arms were temporarily closed. However, the entire system was not moved. At the position of the original lens hole, a veress needle or a 12 mm trocar was punctured into the abdominal cavity to establish pneumoperitoneum with pressure maintained at 14 mmHg. The trocar position of arm-1 in the right inguinal lymphadenectomy and trocar position of arm-2 in the left inguinal lymphadenectomy was used as the positions of arm-1 and arm-2 for pelvic lymphadenectomy. 8 mm trocars were placed at the corresponding puncture points. 12 mm trocars were placed under arm-1 or arm-2 as the assistant trocar to dock robotic arms. Subsequently, monopolar electrosurgical and bipolar electrosurgical scissors were used to remove pelvic lymph nodes, respectively.

Postoperative treatment

After surgery, the groin area was bandaged with elastic. Patients were asked to lie in bed with limited movement and have a low-fat high-protein diet. The drainage tube was removed if drainage volume at 24 h was less than 40 ml. Patients were regularly followed-up at the outpatient department after discharge or continued follow-up treatment.

Results

For the nine patients in the robot-assisted group, surgeries for all the 17 sides were successful without intraoperative conversion to open surgery. The operation time was (68.5 ± 13.69) min/side under laparoscope; the intraoperative blood loss was < 10 ml/side, and (12 ± 4.0) lymph nodes in the left side were removed, ranging from 7 to 18. A total of (12 ± 4.0) lymph nodes in the right side were removed, ranging from 5 to 21, with the average of (12 ± 4.2) node/side. For the ten patients in the open-surgery group, surgeries were successful for all the 20 sides. The average number of lymph nodes removed was (11 ± 5.8) per side, ranging from 2 to 27, which was not statistically different compared to the robot-assisted group ($P = 0.84$).

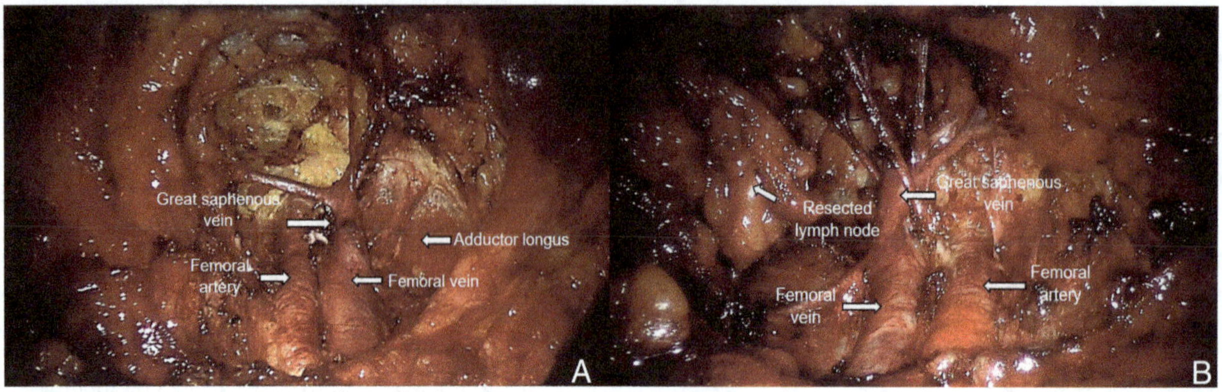

Fig. 2 Robot-assisted laparoscopic antegrade inguinal lymphadenectomy. **a**. Resection of inguinal lymph nodes on the left side. **b**. Resection of inguinal lymph nodes on the right side

The postoperative pathological N staging of the robotic-assisted group were pN0, pN1, pN2, pN3 in 2, 2, 4 and 1 patients, and the open group were pN0, pN1, pN2 in 1, 1, and 8 patients. For the 20 sides in the open surgery group, 9 sides (45%) had skin-related complications., including skin necrosis, wound inflammatory exudation and cellulitis with different severity. When necessary, the negative pressure suction or flap transplantation were conducted for the infected or non-healing wound. In the robot-assisted group, stitches were removed for all nine patients around 7 days post-surgery. There were no complications such as skin necrosis, delayed wound healing and cellulitis. The lymphatic complications of two groups occurred slightly, which had a good outcome after proper treatment. In the open group, lymphorrhagia occurred in 4 cases, and lower limbs edema occurred occasionally in 1case after too much physical work. In the robot-assisted group five patients had lymphatic leakage in the inguinal region, which resolved after appropriate treatments such as pressurization and drainage. Lymphocoele occurred in one post-discharge patient, which was cured by puncture and continuous drainage. No genitalia lymphedema was observed in both groups. In the robot-assisted group, nine patients were followed up for 15–29 months with a median follow-up time of 25 months. However, one patient was lost for follow-up. Two patients developed recurrence and metastasis of the pelvic and abdominal cavities at five to 6 months post-surgery and died of tumor progression. The remaining six patients had no recurrence and metastasis. The recurrence-free survival rate was 75%. In the open surgery group, ten patients were followed up for 25–70 months with a median time of 52.5 months. Of them, four patients died of tumor recurrence and metastasis and the remaining 6 patients had no recurrence and metastasis. The recurrence-free survival rate was 60%, and there were no statistical differences between the groups ($P =$ 0.536) (Fig. 3) (Table 2). Of the two groups, all the six cases with recurrence or metastasis had a staging of pN2 or pN3, while other 14 cases with pN0 or pN1 had no recurrence and metastasis. All the six patients, dying of tumor progression, developed inguinal and pelvic lymph nodes recurrence or metastasis, leading to extensive abdominal metastasis with cancer cachexia. In summary, from the number of lymph nodes removed by surgery and the follow-up status, robotic-assisted laparoscopic antegrade inguinal lymphadenectomy was a safe and effective surgical method and was superior to traditional open surgery in terms of postoperative complications.

Discussion

Penile cancer is a relatively rare malignancy. Due to differences in religious beliefs and health habits, the incidence of penile cancer varies significantly, with incidences of 0.1–0.9/100,000 in Europe and the United States and 19/100, 000 in some economically underdeveloped regions in Asia, Africa and South America [6, 7]. Penile cancer spreads via lymph node metastasis, and first occurs in the inguinal lymph nodes. Lymph node metastasis is considered to be closely associated with the prognosis of penile cancer. Hence, the prognosis of penile cancer is not only associated to the stage and grade of the primary tumor, but also the presence of metastasis, degree of metastasis, lymph node dissection and timing of lymph node dissection [8]. The 5-year survival rate of patients after preventive lymph node dissection can reach 80 to 90%, while the 5-year survival rate is only 30 to 40% for patients who undergo surgery after lymph node metastasis [9]. For patients with inguinal lymphadenectasis, antibiotic treatment is usually recommended to eliminate inflammatory lesions. However, since the European Association of Urology Guidelines 2014 edition, the recommendation is as follows: With uni- or bilateral palpable inguinal lymph nodes (cN1/cN2), metastatic lymph node disease is highly likely. The notion that these may be inflammatory and that antibiotic treatment should first be used is unfounded and dangerous as it delays curative treatment. Palpably enlarged groin lymph nodes should

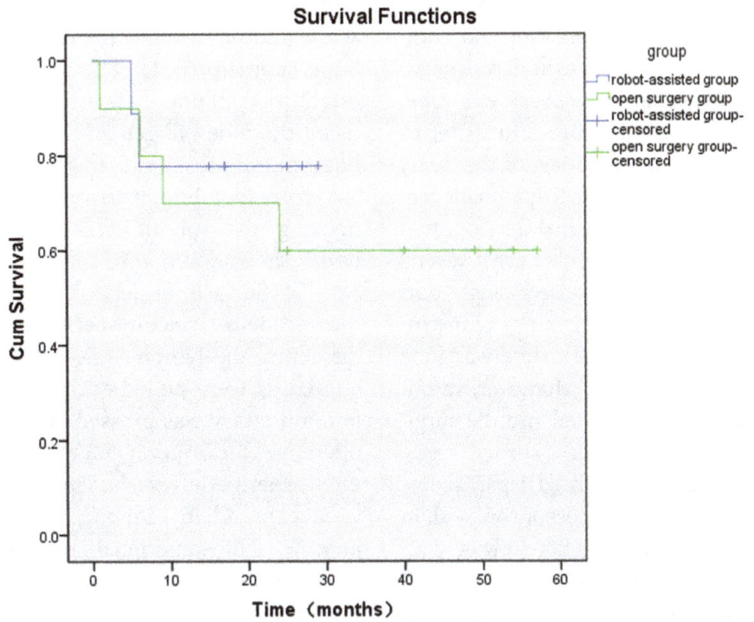

Fig. 3 Kaplan-Meier survival curve of two groups

be surgically removed, pathologically assessed (by frozen section) and, if positive, a radical inguinal lymphadenectomy should be performed. In clinically doubtful cases, US-guided fine needle aspiration cytology is an option. For patients with cN0 primary tumor stage >T1G2, bilateral modified inguinal lymphadenectomy (mILND) or dynamic sentinel node biopsy (DSNB) is recommended [10].

The range of the inguinal lymphadenectomy was constituted as 2 cm above the inguinal ligament as the upper boundary, apex of the femoral triangle as the lower boundary, medialis sartorius muscle as the outer boundary, and lateralis of long adductor muscle as the inner boundary [8]. Open surgery can completely resect regional lymph nodes, however the subcutaneous exfoliation surface is wide, the blood supply to the skin margin is poor, and the incidence of postoperative skin flap necrosis as well as delayed healing are as high as 50% [11, 12]. Extended hospitalization stay and wound care are required after open surgery. In 2006, Tobias-Machado et al. reported on laparoscopic inguinal lymphadenectomy for the first time. Its feasibility was primarily proved by comparison with open surgery. Laparoscopic inguinal lymphadenectomy had the same efficacy for tumor control compared to traditional open surgery.

Table 2 Intra- and Post-Operative Characteristics of Robotic and Open Groups

	robotic group (N = 9,17 sides)	open group (N = 10, 20 sides)	p
Operation time/side (min)	68.5 ± 13.69	Null	
Blood loss /side (ml)	< 10	Null	
Lymph nodes/side	12 ± 4.2(5–21)	11 ± 5.8 (2–27)	0.84
pN stage pN0/pN1/pN2/pN3	2/2/4/1	1/1/8/0	
Complication	0/17	9/20	
Skin-related (side)	5/9	4/10	
Lymphorrhagia (case number)	1/9	0/10	
Lymphocoele (case number)	I, 8	I, 5	
Clavien classification	IIIa,1	IIIa, 4 IIIb, 1	
Follow up			0.536
No recurrence	6	6	
Recurrence	2	4	
Loss to follow-up	1	0	

However, the overall incidence rate of postoperative complications decreased significantly, and there were no complications related to skin incision, such as skin flap necrosis and non-healing wound. Postoperative recovery was rapid compared to open surgery [11–13]. In 2015, Liu CE et al. obtained similar results in a systematic review of the safety and feasibility of video endoscopic inguinal lymphadenectomy for vulvar cancer [12]. With the gradual development of video endoscopic inguinal lymphadenectomy, several surgeons tried to perform the surgery under a single-port laparoscope. However, due to limitations in surgical instruments and operation methods, the surgery time was long and required extensive surgical expertise. Moreover, vascular complications were difficult to be treated and the surgical technique had a high learning curve [14].

In the first reported case of robot-assisted laparoscopic inguinal lymphadenectomy (RAVEIL) by Josephson et al. in 2009, as well as surgical cases reported by Sotelo R et al. in 2013 and Ma Jiajia in 2014, the great saphenous vein and its branches were precisely separated and retained, which reduced vascular injury and had a more thorough dissection. The flexibility and precision of robots can better handle the possible complications during surgery [15–17]. In previous RAVEIL, the robotic arms are usually pushed from the side of the body, and retrograde dissection was conducted from the apex of the femoral triangle [18]. In addition, during surgery, the robotic arms had to be moved to clear inguinal lymph nodes in the opposite side or in pelvic lymph nodes. In this study, the robotic arms were placed between the legs of the patients and antegrade dissection was performed from the top of the inguinal ligament downward. The advantages of this method are summarized as follows: ① There was no need to move the robotic arm during bilateral inguinal lymphadenectomy because the robotic arm were placed between the lower limbs, which simplified the surgical steps, reduced the number of trocars and decreased surgery time. ② During surgery, based on pathological results of frozen sections, pelvic lymphadenectomy could be performed simultaneously using the original skin incision with the patient's position and position of the robotic arm not shifting. ③ During surgery, inguinal ligament, spermatic cord, femoral artery and vein were used as markers for antegrade separation of the great saphenous vein and its branches. This reduced intraoperative vascular injury and postoperative complications. ④ Space between the robotic arms was larger, hence a greater degree of freedom and flexibility, which was conducive to intraoperative surgeries.

With regards to the nine patients in the robot-assisted group, robotic assisted endoscopic antegrade inguinal lymphadenectomy was performed for 17 sides. The experience gathered is summarized as follows: ① Layers were selected correctly to establish pneumoperitoneum. Various layers of the skin and the superficial fascia (adipose layer, membranous layer) were cut open. Then, sharp and blunt dissections were used until external oblique aponeurosis. ② The initial surgical space was fully established. Blunt dissection was performed exclusively using the index finger on the surface of the external oblique muscle to ensure that arm-1 and arm-2, as well as the corresponding instruments could be placed. After docking the robotic arms, separation was continued under the endoscope to the position of the assistant trocar. ③ Surface projection of the femoral artery was marked before pneumoperitoneum was achieved. Before dissecting the lymph nodes, the testicle and the spermatic cords were pulled and the surface projection of the femoral artery was pressed. This was conducive to intraoperative localization for the surgeons. Inguinal ligament, spermatic vessels, femoral artery and femoral vein were exposed in sequence, which avoided vascular injury. ④ The superficial and deep lymph nodes were resected and boundary markers were exposed. Complying the principle of en bloc resection, ligation was preferred for disconnected lymphatic vessels, while electrocoagulation was the second option.

Conclusions

In summary, compared with traditional open surgery, robot-assisted laparoscopic antegrade inguinal lymphadenectomy had the same efficacy on tumor control for the treatment of penile cancer. However, it was safer and had fewer postoperative wound complications. Currently only a few patients undergo this type of surgery and its efficacy and safety needs to be evaluated with more clinical data and longer-term follow-ups.

Abbreviations

CO2: carbon dioxide; DSNB: dynamic sentinel node biopsy; mILND: modified inguinal lymphadenectomy; RAVEIL: robot-assisted laparoscopic inguinal lymphadenectomy

Acknowledgements

I also would like to express my graduate to all anesthetists and nurses for the surgery cooperation.

Authors' contributions

JPG designed the study. JPG, HLY, YLL and YX performed the research. HLY, YLL, JXG and YY contributed the essential cases. HLY, YLL and XTY analysed the data and wrote the paper. HWW provided the intraoperative pathology results of frozen-examination. All authors read and approved the final manuscript.

Author details

[1]Department of Urology, The Fourth Medical Center of Chinese PLA General Hospital, 51th Fucheng Street, Haidian District, Beijing 100048, China. [2]Department of Pathology, The Fourth Medical Center of Chinese PLA General Hospital, 51th Fucheng Street, Haidian District, Beijing 100048, China.

References

1. Mohs FE, Snow SN, Larson PO. Mohs micrographic surgery for penile tumors. Urol Clin North Am. 1992;19(2):291–304.
2. Stuiver MM, Djajadiningrat RS, Graafland NM, et al. Early wound complications after inguinal lymphadenectomy in penile cancer: a historical cohort study and risk-factor analysis. Eur Urol. 2013;64(3):486–92.

3. Koifman L, Hampl D, Koifman N, et al. Radical open inguinal lymphadenectomy for penile carcinoma: surgical technique, early complications and late outcomes. J Urol. 2013;190(6):2086–92.
4. Zhou XL, Zhang JF, Zhang JF, et al. Endoscopic inguinal lymphadenectomy for penile carcinoma and genital malignancy: a preliminary report. J Endourol. 2013;27(5):657–61.
5. Matin SF, Cormier JN, Ward JF, et al. Phase 1 prospective evaluation of the oncological adequacy of robotic assisted video-endoscopic inguinal lymphadenectomy in patients with penile carcinoma. BJU Int. 2013;111(7):1068–74.
6. Chaux A, Netto GJ, Rodriguez IM, et al. Epidemiologic profile, sexual history, pathologic features, and human papillomavirus status of 103 patients with penile carcinoma. World J Urol. 2013;31(4):861–7.
7. Backes DM, Kurman RJ, Pimenta JM, et al. Systematic review of human papillomavirus prevalence in invasive penile cancer. Cancer Causes Control. 2009;20(4):449–57.
8. Protzel C, Alcaraz A, Horenblas S, et al. Lymphadenectomy in the surgical management of penile cancer. Eur Urol. 2009;55(5):1075–88.
9. Kroon BK, Horenblas S, Lont AP, et al. Patients with penile carcinoma benefit from immediate resection of clinically occult lymph node metastases. J Urol. 2005;173(3):816–9.
10. EAU Guidelines. Edn. presented at the EAU Annual Congress Copenhagen 2018. ISBN 978-94-92671-01-1.
11. Tobias-Machado M, Tavares A, Molina WR Jr, et al. Video endoscopic inguinal lymphadenectomy (VEIL): minimally invasive resection of inguinal lymph nodes. Int Braz J Urol. 2006;32(3):316–21.
12. Liu CE, Lu Y, Yao DS. Feasibility and Safety of Video Endoscopic Inguinal Lymphadenectomy in Vulvar Cancer: A Systematic Review. PLoS One. 2015; 10(10):e0140873.
13. Tobias-Machado M, Tavares A, Ornellas AA, et al. Video endoscopic inguinal lymphadenectomy: a new minimally invasive procedure for radical management of inguinal nodes in patients with penile squamous cell carcinoma. J Urol. 2007;177(3):953–7.
14. Tobias-Machado M, Correa WF, Reis LO, et al. Single-site video endoscopic inguinal lymphadenectomy: initial report. J Endourol. 2011;25(4):607–10.
15. Josephson DY, Jacobsohn KM, Link BA, et al. Robotic-assisted Endoscopic Inguinal Lymphadenectomy. J. Urol. 2009;73(1):167–70.
16. Sotelo R, Cabrera M, Carmona O, et al. Robotic bilateral inguinal lymphadenectomy in penile cancer,development ofa technique without robot repositioning: a case report. J Ecancer. 2013;7:356.
17. Ma J, Chen B. The clinical effect and surgical strategy of robot-assisted video endoscopic inguinal lymphadenectomy for vulvar cancer. Chin J Laparoscopic Surgery (Electronic Edition). 2014;3:172–6.
18. Alexis Sánchez, Rene Sotelo, Omaira Rodriguez, et al. Robot-assisted video endoscopic inguinal lymphadenectomy for melanoma J. J Robotic Surg Published online: 2016.

Is it safe to use a ureteral access sheath in an unstented ureter?

Asaf Shvero[1*], Haim Herzberg[2], Dorit Zilberman[1], Yoram Mor[1], Harry Winkler[1] and Nir Kleinmann[1]

Abstract

Background: The aim of this study was to examine ureteral stricture rate after the use of UAS in an unstented ureter and compare complications of smaller vs. larger-caliber UAS.

Methods: We conducted a retrospective analysis of consecutive RIRS for renal stones, with the use of UAS in unstented ureters. We excluded cases with previous ureteroscopies, who carried ureteral stent or nephrostomy, had impacted stones, underwent radiation treatment, or had urinary tract malignancies. The primary outcome was formation of ureteral strictures diagnosed by hydronephrosis in ultrasound test and late secretion in dynamic renal scan. Secondary outcome was stone-free-rate (SFR) and complications. In addition, we compared safety and efficacy of smaller (9.5/11.5Fr) vs. larger-caliber (12/14Fr) UAS.

Results: The cohort included 165 patients with a median follow-up time of 115 days. There was no case of ureteral stricture formation after the use us UAS, despite using a larger-caliber UAS in nearly half the cases. Larger-caliber UAS was not associated with more complications compared to the smaller-caliber one ($p = 0.780$). SFR was non-significantly higher in the larger-caliber UAS group ($p = 0.056$), despite having a larger stone burden, and only stone number was associated with SFR ($p = 0.003$).

Conclusions: These data suggest that the use of UAS during RIRS in an unstented ureter is safe and does not involve ureteral stricture formation after one procedure. Furthermore, the use of wider sheaths was not found to be associated with higher complications rate.

Keywords: Ureteroscopy, Ureter, Stricture, Lithotripsy, Ureteral access sheath

Background

The role of retrograde intra-renal surgery (RIRS) in stone disease is continuously increasing due to improved surgical outcomes compared to extracorporal shockwave lithotripsy [1] and lower complication rates compared to percutaneous nephrolithotomy [2].

Ureteral access sheaths (UASs) are being commonly used during RIRS in order to decrease intra-renal pressure, improve visibility, and provide easy access to the renal pelvico-calyceal system; consequently, reducing the risk of bleeding and infections. Larger-diameter UASs provide improved visibility and facilitates the removal of larger stone fragments [3–6].

However, several studies report that the use of UAS might cause severe damage to the ureteral wall, tissue ischemia with subsequent reperfusion damage, and benign ureteral strictures [5, 7, 8]. The clinical significance of this damage to the ureter still remains controversial [9]. Nonetheless, these reports have still led many urologists to avoid the use of UAS in unstented ureters due to fear of associated ureteral strictures. Furthermore, even when they eventually use UAS in a virgin ureter, some urologists avoid using large-caliber UAS. Ureteral strictures following ureteroscopy were reported to develop in a short period of time after surgery, mostly during 4 weeks of follow-up [10].

The objective of this study was to determine the rate of clinically significant ureteral strictures following the use of ureteral access sheaths in an unstented ureter during RIRS, and to compare complications of smaller and larger-diameter UASs.

* Correspondence: asaf.shvero@sheba.health.gov.il
[1]Department of Urology, The "Chaim Sheba" Medical Center, Ramat-Gan, Israel. Affiliated to Sackler School of Medicine, Tel-Aviv University, Tel-Aviv, Israel
Full list of author information is available at the end of the article

Methods

The study was approved by the Ethics committee at the "Chaim Sheba" Medical Center, Israel (reference no. 4478-17). Medical files of patients undergoing ureteronephroscopy between 2013 and 2016 at our medical center were reviewed. During that period, 2601 endourologic procedures were overall performed. Patients undergoing RIRS for kidney stones with the use of UAS in an unstented ureter were included. Exclusion criteria included: prior impacted ureteral stones, presence of ureteral stones during surgery, prior ureteroscopies, prior ureteral drainage (double-J ureteral stent or PCN), documented ureteral strictures, prior radiation treatment, presence of renal or ureteral malignancy.

The pre-operative evaluation was done using NCCT or RUS. RIRSs were performed under general anesthesia by 3 fellowship-trained endourologists. Irrigation was done using 0.9% saline solution via a pressure-infusing system. After cystoscopy, a working guide-wire (hydrophilic 0.038-in. wire) is advanced up to the level of the renal pelvis. A semi-rigid 6.5/8.5fr URS is then carried out in order to inspect the ureter. After ruling out the presence of ureteral stones, a UAS is gently inserted up to the level of the proximal ureter under fluoroscopic guidance. If there is difficulty advancing the access sheath, ureteral dilation using serial dilators is carried out. Two sizes of UAS were used: COOK Medical Flexor 12/14Fr (wider) and 9.5/11.5Fr (narrower). The size of the UAS was determined at the surgeons' discretion. We then perform a flexible ureteroscopy (using Storz Flex X2 7.5fr flexible ureteroscope) to inspect the proximal ureter, renal pelvis, and calyces for the presence of stones. Next, Holmium laser lithotripsy is carried out and/or stone extraction with a basket device. At the end of the procedure, a double pigtail ureteral stent is left for 5-14 days.

Follow-up includes laboratory tests (CBC, SMAC) and imaging (RUS after hydration), performed 2 months after stent removal and in each follow-up visit thereafter (follow-up regimen is tailored according to patient and stone characteristics). Hydronephrosis without ureteral stones was further evaluated by dynamic renal scan. Stone-free status was defined as no residual fragments, or the presence of residual fragments up to 3 mm, on renal ultrasound.

Demographic data (age, gender, BMI, systemic conditions), operative time, intra-operative complications (bleeding, perforation, incompletion of procedure) and clinical follow-up were collected.

The primary outcome of the study was to evaluate stricture formation rates. Strictures were suspected following a demonstration of new ipsilateral hydronephrosis with delayed secretion in a renal scan. Secondary outcomes included stone-free rates and development of flank pain, elevated serum creatinine level, and UTIs in the follow-up period. To evaluate the safety and efficacy of wider-caliber UAS, patients were stratified to 2 groups: wider (12/14Fr) and narrower (9.5/11.5Fr), in order to compare primary and secondary outcomes between the 2 groups.

Statistical analysis was performed using a chi-square test for nominal variables and student t-test for continuous variables. Multivariate analysis was performed using Binary logistic regression analysis for discrete dependent variables, and Linear regression analysis for continuous ones. The follow-up period was calculated from URS to an event, or to last follow-up visit.

Statistical significance was defined as $p = 0.05$. All reported P values are two-sided. Statistical analyses were performed using Statistical Package for Social Sciences (SPSS version 23.0, SPSS Inc.).

Results

Demographic data, stone characteristics data and pre-operative evaluation are given in Table 1. Of the 165 patients included, on 86 a wide UAS was used, and on 79 a narrow one. The median age was 57 years with 62% males. The average number of stones treated was 1.5 and 1.6, while stone burden was 2.3 and 3.4 cm3, in the narrow and wide groups, respectively. The stone burden was significantly higher in the wider UAS group ($p = 0.031$). Pre-operative hydronephrosis was found to be a predictor of improvement in serum creatinine levels after surgery [0.02 vs. 0.09, $\beta = -0.09$, 95% CI -0.17- (− 0.2), $p = 0.039$].

A comparison of operative and post-operative complications between narrow and wide UASs is provided in Table 2. Length of stay was 0-1 day, depending on the time surgery was undertaken - when performed in the morning till noon, patients were discharged the same day. The rest were discharged the morning after surgery. Out of the 86 cases where a narrower UAS was used, in 13 (15%) a prior attempt of insertion of the wider UAS had failed. In 5 cases, serial ureteral dilators have been used before the introduction of a narrower UAS. There were no cases of failed insertion of UAS and no conversion to other methods of surgery. During a median follow-up period of 115 days, we did not observe any clinically significant stricture formation. Overall complication rate was 18.2%, including: flank pain (9%), UTI (2.4%), referrals to ER (12.1%). We did not observe any difference in complication rates comparing the two groups.

Factors associated with SFR are presented in Table 3. The only factor which was significantly different between stone-free and non-stone-free patients was the number of stones treated ($p = 0.003$), and noteworthy is the fact that SFR was not affected by the total stone burden ($p = 0.194$).

Table 1 Demographic and pre-operative data

UAS size	9.5/11.5fr	12/14fr	Total	*p*-value
N	86	79	165	
Gender (%male)	69.7	54.4	62.4	0.121
Median age (range)	53.5 (18-81)	58 (24-83)	57 (18-83)	**0.042**
BMI (median, IQR)	28.4 (24.5-32.3)	28.6 (25-31.2)	28.4 (24.7-31.8)	0.821
Systemic conditions				
Diabetes mellitus (%)	25.6	39.2	32.1	0.061
Hypertension (%)	41.9	48.1	44.8	0.424
Chronic renal failure (%)	7.0	3.8	5.5	0.299
Peripheral vascular disease (%)	1.2	0	0.6	0.339
Ischemic heart disease (%)	7.0	3.8	5.5	0.372
Hyperlipidemia (%)	30.2	40.5	35.2	0.169
Average number of conditions	1.4	1.52	1.45	0.534
Stone disease				
Number of stones (average, range)	1.5 (1-5)	1.6 (1-7)	1.6 (1-7)	0.506
Largest stone diameter (mm) (median, IQR)	13 (9-16)	15 (11-20)	15 (10-19)	**0.019**
Total stone burden (cm^3) (median, IQR)	2.3 (1.0-5.4)	3.4 (1.6-8.0)	3.4 (1-7.4)	**0.031**
Lower pole stone (%)	39	38	38.7	0.907
Pre-operative hydronephrosis				0.461
No (%)	57.0	64.9	60.7	
Mild (%)	25.6	19.5	22.7	
Intermediate (%)	15.1	13	14.1	
Severe (%)	2.3	2.6	2.4	

p-value is for univariate analysis. Statistical significance was defined as $p \leq 0.05$ and is shown in bold

Table 2 Operative and post-operative complications and SFR

UAS size	9.5/11.5fr	12/14fr	Total	*p*-value
N	86	79	165	
Operative Time (median, minutes)	39.5	61	46.5	**0.002**
Intra-operative complications				
Bleeding	1	0	1	
Ureteral perforation	0	0	0	
Other	0	0	0	
Peri-operative complications				
Fever	1	5	6	0.077
Pain requiring IV/IM analgesics	4	6	10	0.429
Follow-up period (days) (median, IQR)	112 (88-187)	125 (82-237)	115 (82-216)	
Post-operative				
Flank pain (%)	8 (9.3%)	7 (8.8%)	15 (9.0%)	0.864
Creatinine change (mg/dl, median, IQR)	−0.03 (−0.18-0.03)	0.00 (−0.09-0.05)	−0.02(−0.12-0.05)	0.228
UTI (%)	3 (3.6%)	4 (5.1%)	7 (4.3%)	0.650
Referrals to ER	10 (11.6%)	10 (12.7%)	20 (12.1%)	0.906
Hydronephrosis (%)	0 (0%)	2 (2.5%)	2 (1.2%)	–
New hydronephrosis	0 (0%)	0 (0%)	0 (0%)	–
Stone-free-rate (%)	73.5%	85.7%	79.4%	0.056

p-value is for univariate analysis. Statistical significance was defined as $p \leq 0.05$ and is shown in bold

Table 3 Comparison of Stone-Free and non-Stone-Free patients

Stone free status	Yes	No	Total	Univariate analysis	Multivariate analysis		
				p-value	p-value	OR	95% CI
N	127	33	160				
Male gender (%)	77 (60.6%)	23 (69.7%)	100 (62.5%)	0.338	0.761	1.15	0.45-2.96
Age (median, range)	58 (18-83)	56 (24-74)	57 (18-83)	0.407	0.188	1.02	0.98-1.05
Number of stones (median, range, mean, SD)	1 (1-7) 1.4 ± 0.9	2 (1-5) 2.0 ± 1.2	1 (1-7) 1.5 ± 1.0	**0.003**	**0.010**	**0.60**	**0.41-0.88**
Stone Burden (cm^3) (median, IQR)	3.3 (1.0-6.3)	4.4 (1.2-8.0)	3.3 (1.0-7.2)	0.194	0.993	1.00	0.92-1.08
Pre-operative hydronephrosis (%)	47 (37%)	15 (45.4%)	62 (38.7%)	0.411	0.182	1.88	0.74-4.78
UAS size (% wide)	66 (51.9%)	11 (33.3%)	77 (48.1%)	0.056	0.191	1.87	0.73-4.78

Statistical significance was defined as $p \leq 0.05$ and is shown in bold

When comparing the 2 sizes of UAS, wider UASs were used in cases of significantly larger stone burden, older patients and in those with more co-morbidities. In addition, there was a trend towards higher SFR with the use of wider UAS compared to the narrower one (85.7% vs. 73.5% respectively, $p = 0.056$). Moreover, wider UASs were not associated with higher rates of stricture formation or other complications (Table 4).

Discussion

Our study demonstrated two important issues regarding the use of UAS in unstented patients. First, wider UASs are safe, even among patients with virgin-ureters. In the whole series, we did not observe any case of post-operative ureteral stricture formation. Complication rates were low in the large-diameter UAS group, similar to the small-diameter UAS group. Second, despite handling larger stone burden, we found a trend towards higher SFR in the large-diameter UAS group.

There are several advantages to the use of UAS including improved visibility, easier removal of stone fragments, and decreased intra-renal pressures during the procedure. Large-diameter UASs emphasize these advantages [3–6]. Alongside these advantages of UAS, ureteral strictures may presumably complicate its use [5, 7, 8]. Earlier reports demonstrated ureteral injuries after UAS use, with a total incidence of up to 46%, including 13.4% of severe ureteral injuries [7].

Traxer et al. [7] evaluated the ureter endoscopically at the end of the procedure. At that time, the ureter does not have enough time to recover from the procedure. Accordingly, the rate of the observed injury has not been shown to predict future ureteral strictures. In a later report in an experimental animal model showed that after 2 weeks, only minimal inflammatory changes are evident [11], which can explain the absence of long-term effects of UAS.

Recent studies report lower rates of ureteral strictures after ureteroscopy. Tracy et al. [12] reported no long-term post-operative hydronephrosis after the use of UAS in 168 cases, and no difference in SFR and complication rates comparing between different UAS sizes. However, in 49% of the cases, a pre-operative stent has been placed. Similarly, Delvecchio et al. [9] reported post-operative stricture rate of 1.4% after 71 ureteroscopies, but with 32% of cases bearing a pre-operative ureteral stent. The presence of a ureteral stent prior to surgery can potentially prevent stricture formation by leaving a wider ureter for the UAS to enter and by that reducing wall ischemia. Therefore, it constitutes a significant bias when evaluating the post-operative stricture formation rates following the use of UASs.

There are several technical factors which are important to consider during URS in order to prevent ureteral damage. Unlike earlier reports [9], we do not use UAS for stones in the distal or mid-ureter. In addition, before introducing the UAS, we inspect the ureter endoscopically

Table 4 Predictors of post-operative outcome after RIRS with the use of UAS

	Post-operative complications)Yes/No)			Creatinine change (mg/dL)		
	p-value	OR	95% CI	p-value	β	95% CI
Gender (Male/Female)	0.658	1.21	0.51-2.89	0.198	−0.04	−0.11 − 0.03
Age	0.217	0.98	0.94-1.01	0.161	− 0.002	− 0.005 − 0.001
No. of stones	**0.044**	**1.47**	**1.01-2.16**	0.741	−0.008	−0.04-0.02
Stone burden	0.171	1.04	0.98-1.10	0.165	0.004	−0.002 − 0.01
Pre-operative hydronephrosis (Yes/No)	0.138	0.51	0.21-1.23	**0.039**	**−0.09**	**− 0.17-(− 0.02)**
UAS size (Narrow/Wide)	0.780	1.13	0.47-2.69	0.380	−0.03	−0.10 - 0.40

p-value is for univariate analysis. Statistical significance was defined as $p \leq 0.05$ and is shown in bold

for the presence of ureteral stones. In cases that stones are identified, we treat them prior to the introduction of UAS to prevent ureteral trauma. Using these techniques, we demonstrated it is safe to use wider UAS even in virgin ureters.

In our study, we found a trend towards higher SFR in the wider UAS group even despite treating larger baseline stone burden. Stone-free patients compared to non-stone-free patients did not differ in age or gender but did differ in the number of stones (mean ± SD of 1.4 ± 0.9 Vs. 2.0 ± 1.2 respectively, $p = 0.003$) (Table 3). Interestingly, stone burden itself (summation of stone volumes) did not differ significantly ($p = 0.194$). Berquet G et al. [13] assessed SFR with and without the use of a UAS in 280 patients and reported that the use of UAS itself does not improve SFR.

Change in serum creatinine levels (before and after treatment) did not significantly differ between the two UAS groups, as the wider UAS did not compromise renal function. The change was found to be associated with pre-operative hydronephrosis ($p = 0.039$), which reflects the efficacy of the procedure in cases of pre-operative obstruction.

Intra-operative complications were very rare in our study: only 1 procedure in the narrower UAS group was stopped due to bleeding which impaired visualization. In the wider UAS group, no intra-operative complications were recorded. We also assessed post-operative complications for a median of 115 days after surgery: UTIs were very rare and occurred in only 4.3% of cases (3 patients in the small and 4 patients in the large-caliber groups, for a total of 7 patients), 3 of them had positive pre-operative cultures taken the day before surgery. In each UAS group, there were 10 ER visits mainly due to LUTS and stent pain (11.6% and 12.7% in the narrow and wide UAS groups, respectively), and there was no statistically significant difference between the two groups ($p = 0.716$). Operative time was significantly longer in the wider UAS group (39.5 Vs. 61 minutes, $p = 0.002$), which can be explained by the higher stone burden in that group. Despite the longer operative time (and the longer duration of UAS use), the rate of ureteral strictures was still low.

Limitations

Our study is one of the first to assess stricture formation in previously unstented and unmanipulated ureters, though it is not without limitations. The series is retrospective in nature which may lead to selection bias. We tried to overcome this limitation by including all cases operated for kidney stones during the study period. The size of the cohort is relatively small and the follow-up periods are somewhat short, giving the rarity of the complication. The procedures were performed by 3 different surgeons, which may cause variation in technique, but on the other hand focuses on the method itself and not the skill of a specific surgeon. In addition, the choice of the size of the UAS was at the surgeons' discretion and not randomly determined. This represents personal preferences of sheath size, but does not change the outcome – that UAS use is safe in unstented ureters. Ureteral dilation was carried out in 5 cases in which the ureter was thought to be tight, which by itself may possibly prevent stricture and cause bias. Nonetheless, we see ureteral dilation (if needed) to be an integral part of UAS use and should not be considered as an auxiliary procedure. Another drawback is the diagnosis or exclusion of stricture formation being indirect and based upon the appearance of new post-operative hydronephrosis with delayed ipsilateral drainage in renal scans, as we are interested in clinical significance. Indirect signs like hydronephrosis or hydroureter are accurately visible on RUS, although it is likely that estimated SFR is higher when using ultrasound in comparison to NCCT [10]. Nonetheless, in order to focus on the effect of UAS and prevent bias, many other factors that can influence ureteral strictures were excluded: pre-stenting, pre-nephrostomy, previous surgical manipulations, previous ESWL, and impacted ureteral stones. After excluding these factors, our results show that the clinical significance of injuries resulting from the use of UAS is very low, and ureteral strictures after the use of UAS in unstented patients are extremely rare, despite the usage of a wider UAS in 47.8% of cases. Therefore, when a more extensive lithotripsy is planned, it is safe in our opinion to use a large-caliber UAS to improve visualization and enable extraction of larger fragments.

Conclusions

To conclude, these data suggest that the use of UAS during RIRS in an unstented ureter is safe and is not associated with increased risk for ureteral stricture formation. Furthermore, the use of a wider UAS was not found to be associated with higher complications rate. Due to its observed rarity, large scale randomized prospective trials should be conducted to elucidate the real magnitude of ureteral strictures after the use of UAS and the effect of different sizes of UAS.

Abbreviations

ER: Emergency room; ESWL: Extra-corporal shock wave lithotripsy; NCCT: Non-contrast computerized tomography; RIRS: Retrograde intra-renal surgery; SFR: Stone-free rate; UAS: Ureteral access sheath; URS: Ureteroscopy; RUS: Renal Ultrasound; UTI: Urinary tract infection

Acknowledgements

Not applicable.

Authors' contributions

AS, NK, HW contributed to study conception and design. AS, HH contributed to data acquisition. AS, NK, DZ contributed to analysis and interpretation of data. AS, NK contributed to drafting the manuscript. DZ, YM, HW were involved in revising the manuscript. All authors have read and approved the manuscript.

Author details
[1]Department of Urology, The "Chaim Sheba" Medical Center, Ramat-Gan, Israel. Affiliated to Sackler School of Medicine, Tel-Aviv University, Tel-Aviv, Israel. [2]Department Of Urology, Sourasky Medical Center, Tel-Aviv, Israel. Affiliated to Sackler School of Medicine, Tel-Aviv University, Tel-Aviv, Israel.

References

1. Donaldson JF, Lardas M, Scrimgeour D, Stewart F, MacLennan S, Lam TB, et al. Systematic review and meta-analysis of the clinical effectiveness of shock wave lithotripsy, retrograde intrarenal surgery, and percutaneous nephrolithotomy for lower-pole renal stones. Eur Urol. 2015;67:612–6.
2. Bozkurt OF, Resorlu B, Yildiz Y, Can CE, Unsal A. Retrograde intrarenal surgery versus percutaneous nephrolithotomy in the management of lower-pole renal stones with a diameter of 15 to 20 mm. J Endourol. 2011; 25:1131–5.
3. Auge BK, Pietrow PK, Lallas CD, Raj GV, Santa-Cruz RW, Preminger GM. Ureteral access sheath provides protection against elevated renal pressures during routine flexible ureteroscopic stone manipulation. J Endourol. 2004; 18:33–6.
4. Kourambas J, Byrne RR, Preminger GM. Does a ureteral access sheath facilitate ureteroscopy? J Urol. 2001;165:789–93.
5. Kaplan AG, Lipkin ME, Scales CDJ, Preminger GM. Use of ureteral access sheaths in ureteroscopy. Nat Rev Urol. 2016;13:135–40.
6. Monga M, Bhayani S, Landman J, Conradie M, Sundaram CP, Clayman RV. Ureteral access for upper urinary tract disease: the access sheath. J Endourol. 2001;15:831–4.
7. Traxer O, Thomas A. Prospective evaluation and classification of ureteral wall injuries resulting from the insertion of a ureteral access sheath during retrograde intra-renal surgery (RIRS). J Urol. 2012;189:580–4.
8. Lallas CD, Auge BK, Raj GV, Santa-Cruz R, Madden JF, Preminger GM. Laser Doppler flowmetric determination of ureteral blood flow after ureteral access sheath placement. J Endourol. 2002;16:583–90.
9. Delvecchio FC, Auge BK, Brizuela RM, Weizer AZ, Silverstein AD, Lallas CD, et al. Assessment of stricture formation with the ureteral access sheath. Urology. 2003;61:518–22.
10. Manger JP, Mendoza PJ, Babayan RK, Wang DS. Use of renal ultrasound to detect hydronephrosis after ureteroscopy. J Endourol. 2009;23:1399–402.
11. Özsoy M, Kyriazis I, Vrettos T, Kotsiris D, Ntasiotis P, Seitz C, et al. Histological changes caused by the prolonged placement of ureteral access sheaths: an experimental study in porcine model. Urolithiasis. 2018;46:397–404.
12. Tracy CR, Ghareeb GM, Paul CJ, Brooks NA. Increasing the size of ureteral access sheath during retrograde intrarenal surgery improves surgical efficiency without increasing complications. World J Urol. 2018;36:971–8.
13. Berquet G, Prunel P, Verhoest G, Mathieu R, Bensalah K. The use of a ureteral access sheath does not improve stone-free rate after ureteroscopy for upper urinary tract stones. World J Urol. 2014;32:229–32.

23

Robot-assisted laparoendoscopic single-site surgery for the simultaneous management of multiple urinary tract calculi: A case report and experience sharing

Fan Zhang[1,2], Lisong Shan[2], Jiahui Yin[2], Luyang Liu[2], Pengchao Wang[2], Shengkun Sun[1,2], Xu Zhang[1], Hongzhao Li[1], Xin Ma[1], Gang Guo[1] and Qiming Liu[2*]

Abstract

Background: Urolithiasis is a clinically common benign disease in urology. Surgical treatments that are widely used in urolithiasis are percutaneous nephrolithotomy, rigid/flexible ureteroscopy, laparoscopic surgery, and endoscopic combined intrarenal surgery. The da Vinci surgical system is rarely used in the treatment of urolithiasis. In the current study, we report a case of multiple urinary tract calculi treated by robot-assisted laparoendoscopic single-site (RA-LESS) surgery.

Case presentation: A 49-year-old male patient was admitted to our hospital and diagnosed with multiple urinary tract calculi. He previously underwent right ureterolithotomy, laparoscopic cholecystectomy, and extracorporeal shockwave lithotripsy. Computed tomography (CT) scan and three-dimensional reconstruction CT image showed that multiple calculi were located in the right kidney, right upper ureter, and bladder. The preoperative glomerular filtration rate (GFR) were 17.81 ml/min (right kidney) and 53.11 ml/min (left kidney). We utilized the da Vinci system docking with a single-site port to perform pyelolithotomy, ureterolithotomy, and cystolithotomy, simultaneously. The operative time was 135 min and estimated blood loss was 30 ml. The postoperative hospital stay was 5 days. Three months after surgery, the serum creatinine and urea nitrogen levels dropped to a normal range, and no residual fragments were found in the CT scan. The postoperative GFR were 26.33 ml/min (right kidney) and 55.25 ml/min (left kidney).

Conclusions: RA-LESS surgery is a safe and effective surgical procedure in the treatment of multiple urinary tract calculi; however, further investigation is needed to validate its long-term therapeutic effect.

Keywords: Urolithiasis, Urinary calculi, Robotic surgery, Laparoendoscopic single-site, Case report

Background

Urolithiasis is the most common urological benign disease [1], and its prevalence rate has increased worldwide in the past decades. At present, the prevalence rate of urolithiasis varies from 1 to 20% [2–4]. The common surgical procedures for multiple calculi and/or complicated calculi are percutaneous nephrolithotomy (PCNL), rigid/flexible ureteroscopy (URS), laparoscopic surgery, and endoscopic combined intrarenal surgery (ECIRS) [5–7]. However, two or more operations may be needed for patients with a heavy stone burden to achieve an ideal stone-free rate (SFR). In recent years, the surgical management of urinary tract calculi becomes increasingly efficient and minimally invasive due to new technologies and developments in equipment [8]. The da Vinci surgical system has garnered extensive interest from urologists and is widely used in tumor resection and urinary reconstruction due to its improved 3D visualization with magnification of operating field and endo-wrist technology with seven degrees of freedom

* Correspondence: lqm1199@163.com
[2]Department of Urology, Hainan Hospital of Chinese PLA General Hospital, Sanya, China
Full list of author information is available at the end of the article

that improves surgical precision [9]. Presently, robot-assisted laparoscopic surgery is rarely used in the treatment of urolithiasis. In the current study, we present a case of multiple urinary tract calculi treated by robot-assisted laparoendoscopic single-site (RA-LESS) surgery at our center.

Case presentation

Patient

A 49-year-old male patient with the diagnosis of multiple urinary tract calculi at the right side was admitted to our hospital for regular operation. He had surgical histories of right ureterolithotomy in 1992 and laparoscopic cholecystectomy in 2005 and underwent extracorporeal shock wave lithotripsy (SWL) several times. No history of hypertension, heart disease, diabetes, or metabolic diseases was recorded. The body mass index (BMI) was 21.9 kg/m^2. No other positive sign was observed during the abdominal examination except mild percussion pain in the right renal area. Laboratory tests revealed elevated serum creatinine level of 111 μmol/L (normal range: 30–110 μmol/L) and elevated urea nitrogen level of 9.3 mmol/L (normal range: 1.8–7.5 mmol/L). The result of the urine sediment analysis was within the normal range. The isotope renogram result showed that the glomerular filtration rate (GFR) were 17.81 ml/min (right kidney) and 53.11 ml/min (left kidney). Computed tomography (CT) (Fig. 1) and three-dimensional reconstruction CT image (Fig. 2) showed that three calculi were located in the right kidney, one calculi was located in the right upper ureter, and three calculi were located in the bladder. The size and hounsfield unit for the renal calculi were 3.2 cm × 1.9 cm (1174 Hu), 2.0 cm × 1.3 cm (1036 Hu), and 1.4 cm × 1.1 cm (1052 Hu), respectively (Fig. 1a and d); for the ureter calculi were 2.1 cm × 1.7 cm (1098 Hu) (Fig. 1b and e); for the bladder calculi were 2.5 cm × 1.6 cm (529 Hu), 2.3 cm × 1.5 cm (558 Hu), and 2.1 cm × 1.3 cm (564 Hu), respectively (Fig. 1c and f).

Position and port placement

The whole operation was performed through a transperitoneal approach by using the da Vinci Si system (INTUITIVE SURGICAL) and LAGIPORT™ single-site port (LAGIS ENTERPRISE CO.) (Fig. 3a). After endotracheal intubation under general anesthesia, the patient was first placed in a modified left lateral decubitus position with a 60°–70° bump (Fig. 3b). A 4 cm longitudinal incision was made around the umbilicus, and the single-site port was placed to establish the abdominal operative access. On the upper and lower symmetrical position of the port, two 12 mm trocars were placed for robot camera and assistant. On the left and right symmetrical position, two 8 mm robotic trocars were placed for the first and second robot arm (Fig. 3c). After taking out the calculi of the kidney and upper ureter, the patient was adjusted to a Trendelenburg position. The same port was used for docking robot to deal with bladder calculi. No additional incision was added during the whole procedure.

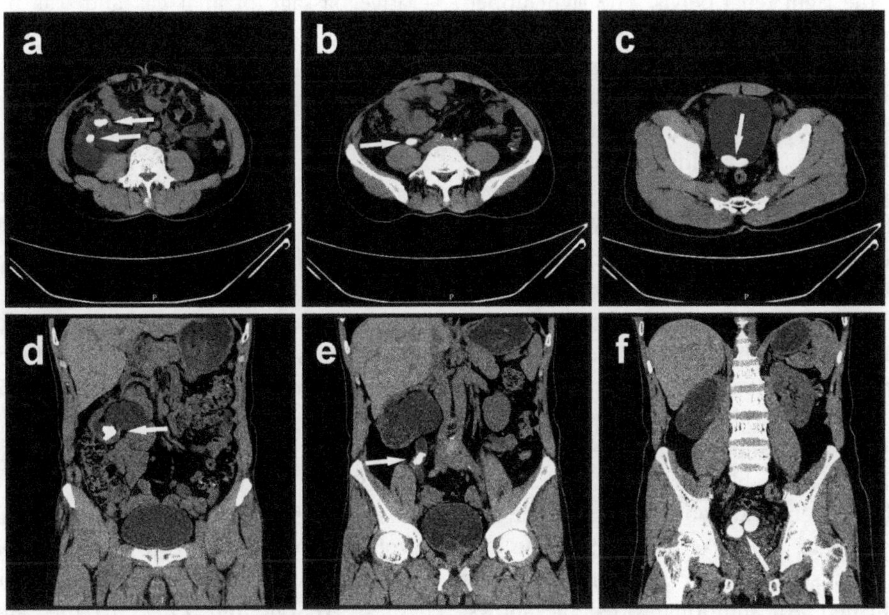

Fig. 1 Axial and coronal images of computed tomography showing multiple urinary tract calculi (white arrows). **a** and **d** Calculi in the right kidney. **b** and **e** Calculi in the right upper ureter. **c** and **f** Calculi in the bladder

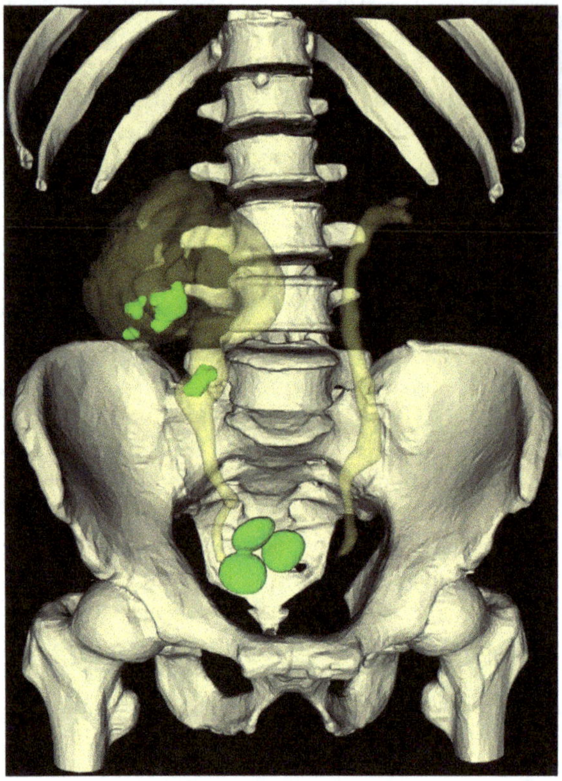

Fig. 2 Three-dimensional reconstruction CT image showing the multiple urinary tract calculi and the morphology of the urinary tract

Surgical procedure

After entering the abdominal cavity, the hepatocolic ligament was incised, and the lateral peritoneum was incised along the paracolic sulcus. Next, the Gerota's fascia was incised to expose the right renal pelvis. The right upper ureter was tortuous seriously due to the previous ureterolithotomy related tissue adhesion. The upper ureter, was firstly isolated from the adhesion tissue, and then was dissociated carefully to expose the calculi location. Next, the ureterolithotomy and pyelolithotomy were performed according to the standard procedures (Fig. 4a and Fig. 4b). After the ureter calculi and renal calculi were all removed, the double-J stent was indwelled into the ureter (Fig. 4c), and the incisions on the ureter and renal pelvis were closed with a 4–0 absorbable suture (Fig. 4d). The Trendelenburg position was adjusted, and a Foley catheter was inserted. Then, the robot was docked with the same single-site port to perform the cystolithotomy. After the bladder calculi were removed (Fig. 4e), the incision on the bladder was closed with a Quill™ self-retaining system (SRS) absorbable surgical suture (Fig. 4f). A drainage tube was placed, and the abdominal incision was sutured after no leakage of the bladder was confirmed. An additional video file shows the surgical procedure with more details (see Additional file 1: Video clip).

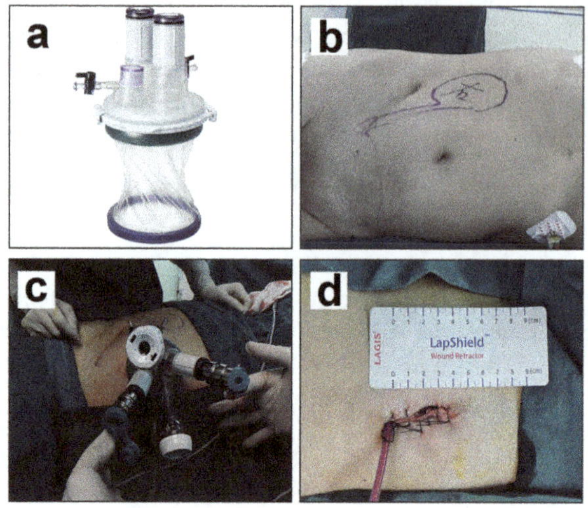

Fig. 3 The patient position and port placement for robot-assisted laparoendoscopic single-site surgery. **a** Single-site port used for docking with da Vinci Si system. **b** Modified left lateral decubitus position with a 60°–70° bump. **c** Two 12 mm trocars are placed on the upper and lower symmetrical position, and two 8 mm trocars are placed on the left and right symmetrical position. **d** The abdominal incision after operation

Results

All the urinary tract calculi were totally removed by the procedure. No blood transfusion was required, and no intraoperative complication occurred. The length of the abdominal incision was 4 cm (Fig. 3d), the operative time was 135 min, and the estimated blood loss was 30 ml. The patient started off-bed activity 1 day after surgery. Three days after surgery, the patient had smooth postoperative passage of anal gas and was prescribed an oral diet. Four days after surgery, the drainage tube was removed. The total postoperative hospital stay was 5 days. No perioperative complications, such as fever, urinary leakage, bleeding, and hematuria were observed. The initial follow-up was performed 3 months after surgery. No residual fragments were found in the CT scan (Fig. 5a to c). The double-J stent was removed after finishing the CT scan, and no calculi was attached on the stent wall. The laboratory test revealed that the serum creatinine (86 μmol/L) and urea nitrogen (3.6 mmol/L) levels dropped to normal ranges. The isotope renogram result showed that the postoperative GFR were 26.33 ml/min (right kidney) and 55.25 ml/min (left kidney).

Discussion and conclusions

Robotic surgery has brought the surgical operation third revolutionary change [10], along with laparoscopic surgery, which changed the concept of surgery. From the earliest AESOP and ZEUS to the latest da Vinci Xi, robot-assisted surgeries have been increasingly used in clinical practice. In the field of urology, da Vinci system

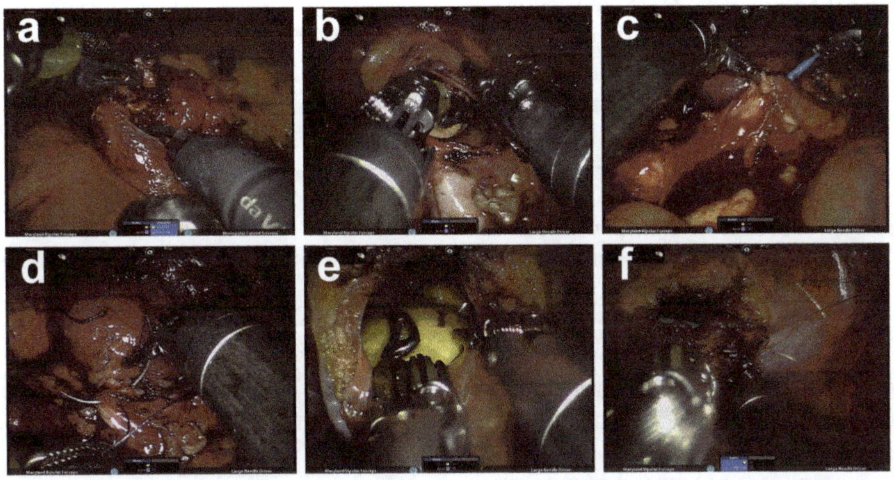

Fig. 4 Intraoperative images of the surgical procedure. **a** The ureter calculi is removed by performing ureterolithotomy. **b** The renal calculi are removed by performing pyelolithotomy. **c** A double-J stent is indwelled into the ureter. **d** The incisions on the ureter and renal pelvis are closed with 4–0 absorbable suture. **e** The bladder calculi are removed by performing cystolithotomy. **f** The bladder incision is closed continuously with Quill™ self-retaining system absorbable surgical suture

offer advantages to tumor resection and urinary reconstruction [11, 12]. However, in the treatment of urinary calculi, da Vinci system is often used in performing nephrolithotomy [13, 14] or ureteroscopy lithotripsy during the robot-assisted pyeloplasty for ureteropelvic junction obstruction [15, 16]. No report of simultaneous treatment of calculi in the kidney, ureter, and bladder by using the da Vinci system has been found.

ECIRS is a combination of traditional PCNL and retrograde ureteroscopy. It was initially used in the year of 2008 [5], and became more and more popular in recent years. ECIRS can be utilized to remove kidney and ureter calculi simultaneously. It has been demonstrated that ECIRS is feasible and safe for patients with large and/or complex urolithiasis [6].

For the present patient, both ECIRS and RA-LESS surgery can be used as surgical methods. We finally chose RA-LESS surgery mainly based on the following considerations: first, the patient had an open ureterolithotomy history, the condition of the ureteral cavity was unclear. The preoperative CT scan showed a tortuous upper ureter, and the retrograde ureteroscopy may not be succeed in approaching the calculi location. Second, the calculi were distributed in the different renal calices, more than one working channel may be needed during the ECIRS. The potential bleeding risk may be increased during the operation. Third, pure endoscopic surgery may extend operative time and raise the chance of infection and potential perioperative complication and may thus prolong hospital stay. Lastly, the previous open ureterolithotomy may add risks and difficulties for traditional surgical methods such as ECIRS and laparoscopic surgery. Robotic surgery has more advantages in suturing and dissociating, and may avoid these unfavorable factors. We selected RA-LESS surgery instead of the traditional robot-assisted laparoendoscopic surgery in dealing with multiple urinary tract calculi because by docking with robot parked in different positions, a single-site port can be used in handling all the calculi without additional trocar, while the traditional surgery needs more than four trocars.

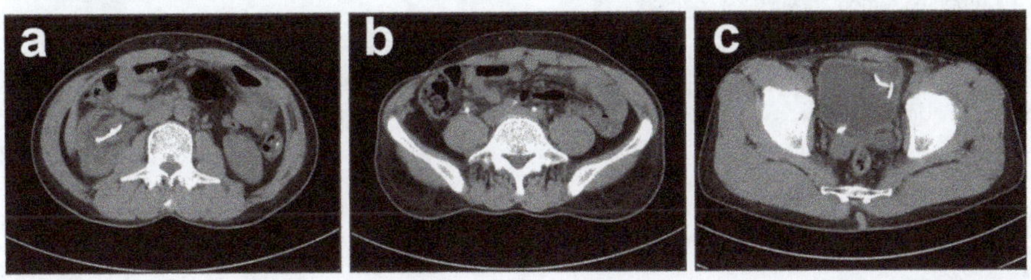

Fig. 5 The computed tomography scan is performed 3 months after surgery. **a**, **b**, and **c** Axial images showing that no residual fragments are found

We found that RA-LESS surgery offers the following advantages to the treatment of multiple urinary tract calculi. First, by adjusting the robot position to dock with the same single-site port, calculi in the upper and lower urinary tracts can be removed in a single surgery. No additional trocar is required. This feature is suitable for patients with unknown ureteral conditions or urinary tract surgery histories. Second, a transperitoneal approach provides surgeons with extensive working space and prevents operative complications, such as bleeding, ureteral injuries, and infection, which are caused by PCNL and URS. Lastly, RA-LESS surgery provides surgeons with a clearer surgical field of view and more stable controllability and comfortable feeling during the operation than endoscopic or laparoscopic surgery. In addition, RA-LESS surgery does not extend hospital stay.

Meanwhile, certain disadvantages were found. First, only two robot arms can be used in the operation; the third arm cannot fully exert its advantages in exposing surgical sites and grabbing tissues. Second, with the use of single-site port and conventional da Vinci instruments, external collision of robot arms and internal collision of instruments occurred more frequently than we expected. Lastly, the indications were relatively narrow, and the cost of a single operation is expensive compared with that of endoscopic surgery.

In summary, RA-LESS surgery is safe and effective for patients with multiple urinary tract calculi and shows certain advantages for selected patients. In spite of these advantages, RA-LESS surgery only provides surgeons with another option and still cannot replace the traditional surgical methods. Furthermore, more technical details need to be optimized in the future. The long-term therapeutic effect of RA-LESS surgery requires further investigation due to the relatively few patient and short follow-up time.

Supplementary information

Additional file 1. Video Clip. A short video clip of the surgical procedure.

Abbreviations

BMI: Body mass index; CT: Computed tomography; ECIRS: Endoscopic combined intrarenal surgery; GFR: Glomerular filtration rate; PCNL: Percutaneous nephrolithotomy; RA-LESS: Robot-assisted laparoendoscopic single-site; SFR: Stone-free rate; SRS: Self-retaining system; SWL: Shock wave lithotripsy; URS: Ureteroscopy

Acknowledgements

The authors thank the patient for allowing us to publish this case report.

Authors' contributions

QML, HZL, and XM participated in the design of this study. FZ drafted the manuscript. QML, FZ, LSS, and JHY performed the surgery. FZ, LSS, JHY, LYL, PCW, and SKS cared for the patient and collected the data. GG collected background information. XZ and QML critically revised the manuscript. All authors have read and approved the final manuscript.

Author details

[1]Department of Urology, The First Medical Center of Chinese PLA General Hospital, Beijing, China. [2]Department of Urology, Hainan Hospital of Chinese PLA General Hospital, Sanya, China.

References

1. De Coninck V, Antonelli J, Chew B, Patterson JM, Skolarikos A, Bultitude M. Medical expulsive therapy for urinary stones: future trends and knowledge gaps. Eur Urol. 2019;76(5):658–66.
2. Turk C, Petrik A, Sarica K, Seitz C, Skolarikos A, Straub M, Knoll T. EAU guidelines on diagnosis and conservative Management of Urolithiasis. Eur Urol. 2016;69(3):468–74.
3. Knoll T, Schubert AB, Fahlenkamp D, Leusmann DB, Wendt-Nordahl G, Schubert G. Urolithiasis through the ages: data on more than 200,000 urinary stone analyses. J Urol. 2011;185(4):1304–11.
4. Kittanamongkolchai W, Vaughan LE, Enders FT, Dhondup T, Mehta RA, Krambeck AE, McCollough CH, Vrtiska TJ, Lieske JC, Rule AD. The changing incidence and presentation of urinary stones over 3 decades. Mayo Clin Proc. 2018;93(3):291–9.
5. Scoffone CM, Cracco CM, Cossu M, Grande S, Poggio M, Scarpa RM. Endoscopic combined intrarenal surgery in Galdakao-modified supine Valdivia position: a new standard for percutaneous nephrolithotomy? Eur Urol. 2008;54(6):1393–403.
6. Scoffone CM, Cracco CM. Invited review: the tale of ECIRS (endoscopic combined IntraRenal surgery) in the Galdakao-modified supine Valdivia position. Urolithiasis. 2018;46(1):115–23.
7. Pradere B, Doizi S, Proietti S, Brachlow J, Traxer O. Evaluation of guidelines for surgical Management of Urolithiasis. J Urol. 2018;199(5):1267–71.
8. Matlaga BR. What is the future of kidney stone management? Eur Urol. 2014;66(6):1052–3.
9. Merseburger AS, Herrmann TR, Shariat SF, Kyriazis I, Nagele U, Traxer O, Liatsikos EN. European Association of U: EAU guidelines on robotic and single-site surgery in urology. Eur Urol. 2013;64(2):277–91.
10. Leal Ghezzi T, Campos Corleta O. 30 years of robotic surgery. World J Surg. 2016;40(10):2550–7.
11. Wei HB, Qi XL, Liu F, Wang J, Ni XF, Zhang Q, Li EH, Chen XY, Zhang DH. Robot-assisted laparoscopic reconstructed management of multiple aneurysms in renal artery primary bifurcations: a case report and literature review. BMC Urol. 2017;17(1):96.
12. Asimakopoulos AD, Miano R, Annino F, Micali S, Spera E, Iorio B, Vespasiani G, Gaston R. Robotic radical nephrectomy for renal cell carcinoma: a systematic review. BMC Urol. 2014;14:75.
13. King SA, Klaassen Z, Madi R. Robot-assisted anatrophic nephrolithotomy: description of technique and early results. J Endourol. 2014;28(3):325–9.
14. Ghani KR, Rogers CG, Sood A, Kumar R, Ehlert M, Jeong W, Ganpule A, Bhandari M, Desai M, Menon M. Robot-assisted anatrophic nephrolithotomy with renal hypothermia for managing staghorn calculi. J Endourol. 2013; 27(11):1393–8.
15. Yang C, Zhou J, Lu ZX, Hao Z, Wang J, Zhang L, Liang C. Simultaneous treatment of ureteropelvic junction obstruction complicated by renal calculi with robotic laparoscopic surgery and flexible cystoscope. World J Urol. 2019;37(10):2217–23.
16. Zheng J, Yan J, Zhou Z, Chen Z, Li X, Pan J, Li W. Concomitant treatment of ureteropelvic junction obstruction and renal calculi with robotic laparoscopic surgery and rigid nephroscopy. Urology. 2014;83(1):237–42.

24

Outcome of staged buccal mucosal graft for repair of long segment anterior urethral stricture

Mohamed Selim[1], Shady Salem[1], Eid Elsherif[1], Atef Badawy[1], Mohamed Elshazely[1] and Maher Gawish[2*]

Abstract

Background: Long anterior urethral stricture due to variable etiological factors constitutes a challenge for reconstruction.
We evaluated our centers experience with cases of long anterior urethral stricture due to different etiologies that were managed by 2-stage substitution urethroplasty using buccal mucosal graft procedure.

Methods: During the period between November 2009 and November 2016. All cases with long anterior urethral stricture that were planned for substitution urethroplasty in our department were enrolled in this study. The first stage was excision of most fibrotic areas of the urethral plate, the remaining of the urethra is laid open and augmented with buccal mucosal graft for second stage closure after 6–9 months.

Results: The study included 123 patients who underwent first stage, 105 patients of them underwent second stage urethroplasty. Eighteen cases were missed after first stage. The mean (range) age was 38.4 (17–60 years). The mean (range) stricture length was 8.3 (4–13 cm). The cause of stricture was idiopathic in 47, inflammatory in 15, lichen sclerosus in 26 and post failed hypospadias repair in 35 patients. First stage was complicated by graft contracture in 11 (8.9%) patients that needed re-grafting, 5(4.1%) patient had bleeding from the buccal mucosa site that needed haemostatic sutures, oral numbness was reported in 7 (5.7%) patients. Second stage was complicated by wound dehiscence in 2(1.9%) patients, restricture in 11 (10.5%), fistula in 6 (5.7%) patients, meatal stenosis in 3 (2.9%). The overall success rate was 79.1% (83 cases out of 105) with a mean (range) follow-up of 34.7 (10–58 months).

Conclusions: Staged urethroplasty using buccal mucosal graft procedure is an effective surgical option for patients with long anterior urethral strictures especially for patients with lichen sclerosus and those with failed previous surgical repair.

Keywords: Urethra, Stricture, Anterior, Staged

Background

Urethral stricture is a process of progressing spongiofibrosis that leads to subsequent urethral narrowing and persistent lower urinary tract symptoms (LUTS) [1]. The management of long anterior urethral stricture remains an issue of controversy and continuing challenge, especially if it is lengthy or recurrent [2]. The treatment options has been modified form visual internal urethrotomy (VIU) and dilatation to urethroplasty, either anastomotic or augmentation, using buccal mucosal grafts or penile skin flaps [3–5].

The widespread application of buccal mucosal graft is partly due to its favourable characteristics, including a thick epithelium, highly vascularized lamina propria, availability, strength and resistance to infection [6].

Single stage augmentation urethroplasty is recommended for most of penile urethral stricture. Penile skin flaps was the main modality of management of penile urethral strictures [7, 8].

Barbagli and colleagues reported the dorsal free graft urethroplasty initially using skin, but subsequently buccal mucosa, which was a modification of the Monseur

* Correspondence: mahergawish2002@yahoo.com
[2]Department of Urology, Faculty of Medicine, Alazhar University, Governorate, Assiut, Egypt
Full list of author information is available at the end of the article

technique [9, 10]. Asopa and colleagues described a ventral sagittal urethrotomy approach and dorsally placed BM graft with good success rates [11]. Kulkarni and Barbagli used a technique to preserve the nerve and blood supply to the urethra by one sided dissection of anterior dorsal aspect of the bulbospongiosus muscle [12]. Two-staged reconstruction should be utilized without hesitation on cases of prior failed hypospadias management or those with severe urethral LS [13, 14].

Kulkarni and Barbagli, have suggested that it may be possible to do a one stage procedure with buccal mucosa in patients with LS where there is an adequate roof strip 20F [15]. It is of note though, looking at this series of patients a relatively small number of patients out of the total with LS were suitable for this approach.

Other reasons for the staged procedure are in recurrent complicated cases after previous failed procedures. The two stage skin reconstruction is very appropriate for patients with failed hypospadias, but in case of LS, skin should be avoided and buccal mucosa substitution is recommended. There is a small literature researches relating to this [16] and it is recognized that there is a 22.5% revision for the first stage urethroplasty [17]. These authors concluded that two stage urethroplasty of complex penile urethral stricture had lower restricture rate than one stage, and clearly there is a significant rate of revision of the first (22.5%).

Andrich and Mundy reported that the presence of LS complicating the urethral stricture compromises the rate of success of one stage approach, also there is tendency of recurrence in the marsupialised urethra and dictated perineal urethrostomy as an option for panurethral stricture and elder patients [18].

In this study, we report our experience of the feasibility of staged urethroplasty using buccal mucosal grafting to repair all long penile urethral strictures. We tried to identify the predictors of success. We analysed outcome and complications in relation to the site of stricture (bulpopenile versus penile), length of stricture and etiology.

Methods

This was an observational study conducted over seven years, from November 2009 to November 2016, at Menoufia and Al Azhar University teaching hospitals. Cases with recurrent anterior urethral stricture, who were subjected to augmentation urethroplasty, were evaluated. The study included all patients with long urethral stricture with previous history of failed attempts to repair including several dilatations or internal uerthrotomy or previous urethroplasty and those with obliterative strictures who are on suprapubic catheters also we included cases with susbected LS based on clinical criteria without histological examination and adult patient with previous failed repeated attempts of repair of penile and penoscrotal hypospadias. We excluded all cases with minimal fibrosis and short strictures with patent urethra that are feasible for single stage management.

Detailed urological and medical histories were obtained. History of trauma to the pelvis, the perineum and/or the genitalia, as well as urethral infections and previous urological procedures (dilatation, DVIU, previous surgical repair of urethral stricture or hypospadias) were recorded. General and complete genitourological examinations were done.

All patients had previous urethral instrumentation in the form of several dilatations or internal uerthrotomy. In addition, thirty-one patients underwent previous urethroplasty elsewhere. Forty-seven patients had suprapubic cystostomy for urinary retention. The patients were treated by the two-stage augmentation urethroplasty using buccal mucosal grafts. All patients signed a detailed formal consent. The study was approved by our institutional ethical committee.

Preoperative evaluation

New urine culture done for all cases to detect urinary tract infection. Patients with positive cultures were treated with the proper antibiotic before surgery.

The patients were evaluated regarding stricture etiology, length and site. Preoperative retrograde urethrography, previous surgical or endoscopic treatment, surgical findings, postoperative complications, follow up, outcome and success rate were also recorded.

Uroflowmetry, retrograde urethrography and voiding cystourethrography were performed for all patients. Urethroscopy with semirigid cystoscopy was conducted for every case on the day of surgery to confirm the presence of the stricture before proceeding with urethroplasty and to assess the patency and calibre of the urethra.

Operative details

All surgical procedures were done under general anaesthesia with nasotracheal intubation. All patients were placed in the lithotomy position. A ring retractor was used for retraction and exposure of perineal approaches and hanging up the penis during penile approaches.

Harvesting the buccal mucosal graft The buccal graft was harvested by the assistant surgeon using the technique described by Barbagli and his colleagues [19].

Urethroplasty using buccal mucosa graft

The reconstruction of the urethra was done in two stages. The buccal mucosal was engrafted to the neourethra alongside the native urethra that was laid open and observed for 6 to 9 months according to the healing of the graft and absence of fibrosis. Then, the second stage closure of the urethra was done.

First stage buccal mucosal augmentation urethroplasty

For penile urethral stricture, an incision was made longitudinally and dorsolaterally to the healthy urethra. Areas with extensive spongiofibrosis were excised, leaving the healthy portions that were laid open.

Neourethrostomy of the proximal end of the urethra and marsupialization of the opened urethra were conducted. Buccal mucosal graft was laid to the side of the opened urethra and fixed to it. An incision was made on the edge of the skin, which was then fenestrated and quilted. The 16F silicon urethral catheter was fixed for 5 days (Fig. 1a, b).

For bulbopenile strictures, the incision was made on the ventral of proximal penile shaft and extended through the scrotum with separation of the scrotal compartments to expose the urethra according to the extension of the stricture. The urethra was dissected laterally and then incised dorsolaterally without any circular dissection of the urethra. Some cases with stricture reaching the bulbar urethra beneath bulbospongiosus muscle needed dissection and separation of the muscle at the midline so the dorsolateral incision could be extended to this segment. After that, the urethra was marsupialized and laid open; the buccal mucosal graft was fixed alongside the urethra and quilted. Then, the skin penis and scrotum was fixed along the free side of the graft and the urethra leaving the scrotum splitted around the neomeatus. The dressing was removed 5 days post operative for both penile and bulbopenile stricture and patients were taught how to care for the graft by cleaning the wound with antiseptic solution and application of eye ointment (oxytetracycline HCl) together with vaselinated gauze and continued to do this for 6 weeks to prevent the row areas of the graft from sticking together.

Second stage urethroplasty

Second stage urethroplasty was preformed 6 to 9 months after the first stage according to the healing process and the absence of fibrosis.

Operative technique

The neourethral tube was outlined and marked giving urethral plate width of 2.5–3 cm. An incision was done and the roof strip was mobilized by dissecting the skin at the edge of the strip (Fig. 2a, b). The urethral tube was closed over 16F silicone urethral catheter.

Postoperative care

The urethral catheter was left in its place for three weeks and was removed after confirming its healing, by performing peri-catheter urethrogram. Patients were followed up and evaluated regularly till the 6th week from the surgical procedure, then every 3 months in the first year, then every 6 months and then yearly for 5 years. The follow up included clinical observation of the patient, the process of healing of the wound and routine flexible urethrocystoscopy, our defined criteria for success was the patency and prompt healing of the

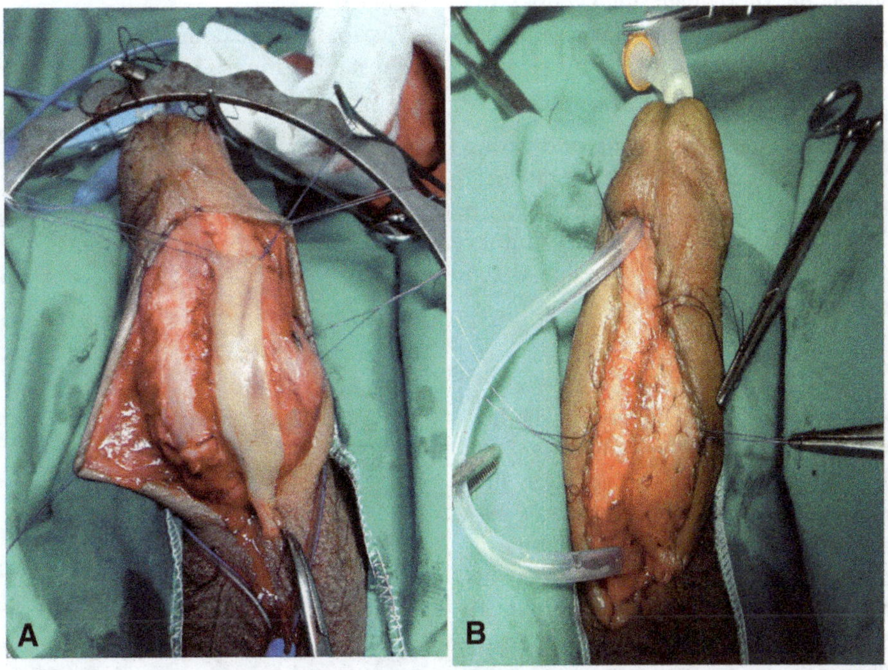

Fig. 1 a, buccal mucosa graft was tailored and placed beside the marsupialized urethra. 1. **b**, buccal mucosa was fixed alongside the urethra, penile skin, fenestrated, quilted and urethral catheter was fixed

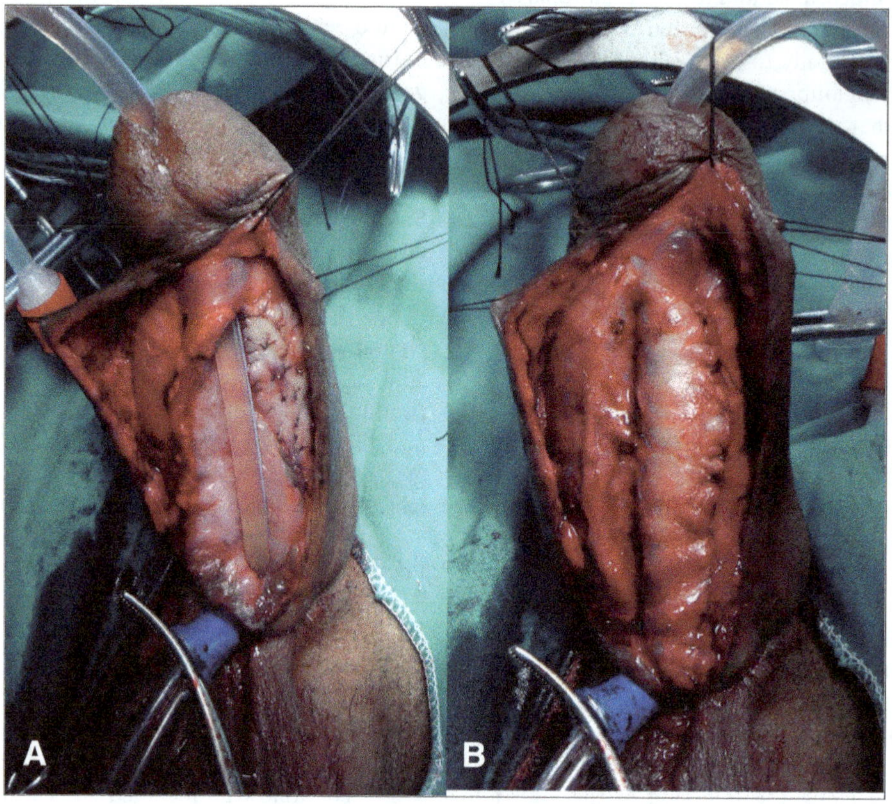

Fig. 2 **a**, Roof strip was mobilized by dissection of the skin at the edge of the strip, one stage buccal mucosal roof strip augmentation of the narrow distal neourethra and urethral catheter.2. **b** tubularization of the neourethra

neourethra confirmed by pericatheter urethrogram and absence of restricture on subsequent follow up visits without need for dilatation or endoscopic management.

Statistical analysis

Data was tabulated and statistically analysed using Stata® software (Stata Corp. 2011. Stata Statistical Software: Release 12. College Station, TX: Stata Corp LP). We used Fisher's exact test and Mann-Whitney U test, wherever appropriate. We used *P*. value < 0.05 as statistically significant.

Results

The study included 123 patients who underwent the first stage urethroplasty, 105 patients of them underwent the second stage. Eighteen cases were missed after first stage. The mean (range) age of the patients was 38.4 (17–60 years). The cause of stricture was idiopathic in 47 patients, inflammatory in 15 patients, lichen sclerosus in 26 patients and post failed hypospadias repair in 35 patients. The stricture was in the penile urethra in 68 patients and bulbopenile in 55 patients. The mean (range) length of the overall stricture was 8.3 (4–13 cm), penile stricture was 7.4 (4–10.5 cm) and bulbopenile 9.3 (5–13 cm) respectively with no statistical significance (Table 1).

Five patients had mucosal site bleeding that needed hemostatic sutures. Seven patients had oral numbness and were referred to the dentist. Graft contracture was encountered in 11 patients and they needed surgical re-adjustment before the second stage.

Table 1 Patients' demography and stricture characteristics (site and length) (*N* = number of cases)

variable	*N* (%)
Total patient, *N*	123
Stricture etiology, *N* (%)	
Idiopathic	47 (38%)
Inflammatory	15 (12%)
Lichen sclerosus	26 (21%)
Post failed hypospadias repair	35 (29%)
Stricture site, *N* (%)	
Bulbopenile	55 (44.7%)
Penile	68 (55.3%)
Length of stricture cm, mean (range)	
Penile	7.4 (4–10.5)
Bulbopenile	9.3 (5–13)

The second stage was done after a mean (range) of 6.7 (6–9 months) after the first stage. Second stage augmentation urethroplasty using buccal mucosa was done for 105 patients. During follow up, early postoperative leakage in the pericatheter urethrogram complicated 9 patients who needed prolonged urethral catheterization up to 4 weeks. Spontaneous healing occurred in 3 patients. Urethrocutaneous fistula developed in 6 patients. Meatal stenosis developed in 3 patients.

Failed cases include wound dehiscence and restricture. Wound dehiscence complicated 2 patients due to wound infection.

Recurrence of stricture occurred in 11 patients. All of these cases had a long history of stricture disease and had previously undergone multiple procedures. Two of them had changes of lichen sclerosus (LS), 4 had multiple failed hypospadias repair attempt and others shared the remaining numbers. The recurrence was distal to the graft site in two patients, multiple in two patients (patchy), and a diffuse narrowing in 7 patients (two penile and 5 bulbopenile).

The overall success rate was 79.1% (83 cases out of 105) with a mean follow-up of 34.7 (10–58 months). (Table 2).

Correlating the site of stricture with success rates showed a significantly statistical outcome with higher success rates for penile urethral strictures. Correlating the site with the complications was statistically insignificant. (Table 3).

When comparing the size of stricture to the outcome and complications. The results showed statistical significance: the shorter the stricture length, the higher the success rate. The correlation of the size of stricture and complications showed statistical significance with less fistula occurrence and restricture with shorter stricture length. Other complications were insignificant in correlation to the size of stricture (Table 4).

Analysis of outcome in relation to the etiology showed no statistical significance. There was no significant relation between the etiology of stricture and the rate of complication (Table 5).

Table 2 Complications of 1st and 2nd stage substitution urethroplasty using buccal mucosal graft (*N* = number)

Variable	No
1st stage patients, *N* (%)	123
Mucosal site bleeding	5 (4.1%)
Oral numbness	7 (5.7%)
Graft contracture	11 (8.9%)
Mean time elapsed between 1st and 2nd stage (range) months	6.7 (6–10)
2nd stage patients, *N* (%)	105
Wound dehiscence	2 (1.9%)
Restricture	11 (10.5%)
Fistula	6 (5.7%)
Meatal stenosis	3 (2.7%)
Mean follow-up (range) months	34.7 (10–58)
Failure rate	22 (21%)
Success rate	83 (79%)

Table 3 Analysis of the site of stricture in relation to outcome and complications (*N* = number)

Variable	Bulbopenile (46)	Penile (59)	*P.* value
Success rate *N* (%)	32 (69.57%)	51 (86.44%)	0.036
Fistula *N* (%)	4 (8.7%)	2 (3.39%)	0.148
Meatal stenosis *N* (%)	1 (2.1%)	2 (3.4%)	0.711
Restricture *N* (%)	7 (15.2%)	4 (6.7%)	0.161
Dehiscence *N* (%)	2 (4.3%)	0 (0%)	0.106

Discussion

The first preliminary report for successful use of buccal mucosa for the urethral reconstruction in adults was in 1992 [20]. El-Kasaby et al., in 1993, reported 90% success rate with buccal mucosa urethroplasty in 20 patients [21]. The buccal mucosa is a preferred substitute of the urethra. It is accustomed to wet condition, resilient to infection, easy to harvest and handle with good take after engraftment [6].

The preferred technique for pendulous urethral stricture reconstruction is urethroplasty using penile

Table 4 Analysis of the size of stricture in relation to outcome and complications (N = number)

	N (%)	Length of stricture (Mean ± SD)	*P.* value
Outcome			
Successful	83 (79.05%)	7.6 ± 1.7	0.0000
Failed	22 (20.95%)	9.7 ± 1.9	
Fistula formation			
Yes	6 (5.71%)	10.1 ± 1.8	0.0009
No	99 (94.29%)	7.9 ±	
Meatalstenosis			
Yes	3 (2.8%)	8 ± 0.87	0.93
No	102 (97.2%)	8.1 ± 1.99	
Restricture			
Yes	11 (10.4%)	9.8 ± 2.19	0.0018
No	94 (89.6%)	7.89 ± 1.84	
Dehisence			
Yes	2 (1.9%)	9.5 ± .7	0.3113
No	103 (98.1%)	8.1 ± 1.97	

Table 5 Analysis of the etiology of stricture in relation to outcome and complications

	Idiopathic	LS	Failed hypospadias	Inflammatory	total	*P* – value
Outcome						
Successful	37	17	18	11	83	0.06
Failed	5	6	9	2	22	
Fistula						
Yes	2	2	2	0	6	0.8
No	40	20	25	13	98	
Dehiscence						
Yes	0	1	1	0	2	0.7
No	42	22	26	13	103	
Meatal stenosis						
Yes	1	1	1	0	3	0.6
No	41	22	26	13	102	
Restricture						
Yes	2	2	5	2	11	0.5
No	40	21	22	11	94	

skin flap, after the description of the Orandi procedure [7].

The results reported by Wesseles and McAninch for ventral onlay free graft urethroplasty of the pendulous urethra were poor. They did not advocate the use of free graft on penile urethra as they were cautious about the poor vascularity of the corpus spongiosum at the stricture site [22]. This might be valid when placing the graft ventrally on the spongiosum. With this technique, the spongiosum does not contribute significantly to graft support or graft take.

The other concern is detaching a long segment of urethra from the corpora cavernosa, which could compromise its vascularity. However, the distal urethra receives its blood supply in a retrograde way from the glans, which is maintained during dorsal dissection. Also, in dorsal onlay grafting, the graft take depends posteriorly on the corpora cavernosa [23].

Stricture recurrence after bulbar or penile augmentation onlay urethroplasty showed extensive fibrosis involving the whole grafted site and fibrotic ring stricture at proximal or distal ends of the anastomosis with the urethral plate [24, 25].

Reconstructive urologists reported cosmetic problems with pedicled flaps such as scars, webbing and curvature [26].

Two-stage buccal mucosal graft urethroplasty avoids these problems. It has only a scar in the midline of the penis. There is no torsion of the penis due to limited mobilization of the dartos fascia. Also the fixation of the graft to the under lying spongiosum, fixes the neo-urethra and prevents it from "bow-stringing".

The criteria for successful management was determined, as described by Barbagli et al., as no need for postoperative procedure, including urethral dilation, no urinary retention, no fistula nor chordee [26, 27].

The most common complications following second stage tubularization are urethrocutaneous fistula, dehiscence and recurrent stricture. In our series, the over- all complications rate was 21% (22 cases out of 105 cases). Restricture was the most common complication in our series (11 cases), that could be due prior surgeries with extensive spongiofibrosis that could not be removed totally due deficient of the tissue of ventral aspect of the penis with subsequent incorporation of such segments in the tubularization stage. Urethrocutaneous fistula (6 cases) came in the second place and could be explained due to deficiency of the tunica dartos that were used as second reinforcement layer at the other cases and meatal stenosis (3 cases). This is in agreement with the other series which was reported by Mori and Angermier having complications rate of 19% [14].

Our success rate (79%) after a mean follow up of approximately 3 years (34 months) is comparable to other reported series [13]. Most authors believe that LS adds surgical challenge and increases the chance of restructure [28]. Our results show no significant differences in the overall complications, or failure rate (restricture) between strictures related to LS and those related to other causes. This may be manifest with longer term follow-up beyond 3 years in further reports. Revision rate after repair of complex cases of anterior urethral stricture ranges from 6.7 to 59% as reported by different series [12, 13, 29, 30]. As suggested by Mori and Angermier, to use the term multistage instead of 2 staged urethroplasty [14], we believe that higher success rate could be achieved with further revisions, especially for complex cases.

Limitation of the study is heterogeneity of cases due to different etiologies and being retrospective.

Conclusions

Staged urethroplasty using buccal mucosal graft is an effective surgical option for patients with long anterior urethral strictures, especially for those with lichen sclerosus or failed previous surgical repair.

Abbreviations

BXO: Balanitis xerotica obliterans; DVIU: Dilatation and Visual internal urethrotomy; LS: Lichen sclerosus; LUTS: Lower urinary tract symptoms.; VIU: Visual internal urethrotomy

Acknowledgements

None.

Authors' contributions

All authors have made substantial contributions to conception and design; analysis and interpretation of data and manuscript writing.

Author details

[1]Department of Urology, Faculty of Medicine, Menoufia University, Governorate, Menoufia, Egypt. [2]Department of Urology, Faculty of Medicine, Alazhar University, Governorate, Assiut, Egypt.

References

1. Fenton AS, Morey AF, Aviles R, Garcia CR. Anterior urethral strictures: etiology and characteristics. Urology. 2005;65(6):1055–8.
2. Andrich DE, Mundy AR. What is the best technique for urethroplasty? Eur Urol. 2008;54(5):1031–41.
3. Anger JT, Buckley JC, Santucci RA, Elliott SP, Saigal CS. Trends in stricture management among male Medicare beneficiaries: underuse of urethroplasty? Urology. 2010;77(2):481–5.
4. Barbagli G, Palminteri E, Balo S, Vallasciani S, Mearini E, Costantini E, Mearini L, Zucchi A, Vivacqua C, Porena M. Lichen sclerosus of the male genitalia and urethral stricture diseases. Urol Int. 2004;73(1):1–5.
5. Dubey D, Vijjan V, Kapoor R, Srivastava A, Mandhani A, Kumar A, Ansari MS. Dorsal onlay buccal mucosa versus penile skin flap urethroplasty for anterior urethral strictures: results from a randomized prospective trial. J Urol. 2007; 178(6):2466–9.
6. Levine LA, Strom KH, Lux MM. Buccal mucosa graft urethroplasty for anterior urethral stricture repair: evaluation of the impact of stricture location and lichen sclerosus on surgical outcome. J Urol. 2007;178(5): 2011–5.
7. Orandi A. One-stage urethroplasty: 4-year followup. J Urol. 1972;107(6): 977–80.
8. McAninch JW, Morey AF. Penile circular fasciocutaneous skin flap in 1-stage reconstruction of complex anterior urethral strictures. J Urol. 1998;159(4): 1209–13.
9. Barbagli G, De Stefani S, Sighinolfi MC, Annino F, Micali S, Bianchi G. Bulbar urethroplasty with dorsal onlay buccal mucosal graft and fibrin glue. Eur Urol. 2006;50(3):467–74.
10. Monseur J. Widening of the urethra using the supra-urethral layer (author's transl). J Urol (Paris). 1980;86(6):439–49.
11. Asopa HS, Garg M, Singhal GG, Singh L, Asopa J, Nischal A. Dorsal free graft urethroplasty for urethral stricture by ventral sagittal urethrotomy approach. Urology. 2001;58(5):657–9.
12. Kulkarni S, Barbagli G, Sansalone S, Lazzeri M. One-sided anterior urethroplasty: a new dorsal onlay graft technique. BJU Int. 2009;104(8):1150–5.
13. Kozinn SI, Harty NJ, Zinman L, Buckley JC. Management of complex anterior urethral strictures with multistage buccal mucosa graft reconstruction. Urology. 2013;82(3):718 22.
14. Mori RL, Angermeier KW. Staged urethroplasty in the management of complex anterior urethral stricture disease. Transl Androl Urol. 2016;4(1): 29–34.
15. Kulkarni S, Barbagli G, Kirpekar D, Mirri F, Lazzeri M. Lichen sclerosus of the male genitalia and urethra: surgical options and results in a multicenter international experience with 215 patients. EurUrol. 2009; 55(4):945–54.
16. Patterson JM, Chapple CR. Surgical techniques in substitution urethroplasty using buccal mucosa for the treatment of anterior urethral strictures. EurUrol. 2008;53(6):1162–71.
17. Andrich DE, Greenwell TJ, Mundy AR. The problems of penile urethroplasty with particular reference to 2-stage reconstructions. J Urol. 2003;170(1):87–9.
18. Andrich DE. Outcome of different management options for full length antreior urethral strictures. J Urol Supplement. 2009;181(4):13.
19. Barbagli G, Palminteri E, De Stefani S, Lazzeri M. Harvesting buccal mucosal grafts. Keys to success. Contemp Urol. 2006;18:17–245.
20. Burger RA, Muller SC, el-Damanhoury H, Tschakaloff A, Riedmiller H, Hohenfellner R. The buccal mucosal graft for urethral reconstruction: a preliminary report. J Urol. 1992;147(3):662–4.
21. el-Kasaby AW, Fath-Alla M, Noweir AM, el-Halaby MR, Zakaria W, el-Beialy MH. The use of buccal mucosa patch graft in the management of anterior urethral strictures. J Urol. 1993;149(2):276–8.
22. Wessells H, McAninch JW. Use of free grafts in urethral stricture reconstruction. J Urol. 1996;155(6):1912–5.
23. Dubey D, Sehgal A, Srivastava A, Mandhani A, Kapoor R, Kumar A. Buccal mucosal urethroplasty for balanitis xerotica obliterans related urethral strictures: the outcome of 1 and 2-stage techniques. J Urol. 2005;173(2):463–6.
24. Greenwell TJ, Venn SN, Mundy AR. Changing practice in anterior urethroplasty. BJU Int. 1999;83(6):631–5.
25. Barbagli G, Palminteri E, Lazzeri M, Turini D. Interim outcomes of dorsal skin graft bulbar urethroplasty. J Urol. 2004;172(4 Pt 1):1365–7; discussion 1367.
26. Barbagli G, Guazzoni G, Palminteri E, Lazzeri M. Anastomotic fibrous ring as cause of stricture recurrence after bulbar onlay graft urethroplasty. J Urol. 2006;176(2):614–9.
27. Hick EJ, Morey AF. Initial experience with fibrin sealant in pendulous urethral reconstruction. Is early catheter removal possible? J Urol. 2004; 171(4):1547–9.
28. Hudak SJ, Lubahn JD, Kulkarni S, Morey AF. Single-stage reconstruction of complex anterior urethral strictures using overlapping dorsal and ventral buccal mucosal grafts. BJU Int. 1111;110(4):592–6.
29. Hudak SJ, Lubahn JD, Kulkarni S, Morey AF. Single-stage reconstruction of complex anterior urethral strictures using overlapping dorsal and ventral buccal mucosal grafts. BJU Int. 2012;110(4):592–6.
30. Mori R, Wood H, Angermeier K. PD3-01 multistage buccal mucosa graft Urethroplasty for complex anterior urethral strictures. J Urol. 2014;191(4): e19–20.

25

Oncologic outcomes comparison of partial ureterectomy and radical nephroureterectomy for urothelial carcinoma

Shengxian Li[1,2], Yuchen Pan[3] and Jinghai Hu[1*]

Abstract

Background: The appropriate application of various treatment for upper tract urothelial carcinomas (UTUCs) is the key to prolong the survival of UTUC patients. Herein, we used data in our database to assess the oncological outcomes between partial ureterectomy (PU) and radical nephroureterectomy (RNU).

Methods: From 2007 to 2014, 255 patients with UTUC undergoing PU or RNU in our hospital database were investigated. Perioperative, postoperative data, and pathologic outcomes were obtained from our database. Cancer-specific survival (CSS) was assessed through the Kaplan-Meier method with Cox regression models to test the effect of these two surgery types.

Results: The mean length of follow-up was 35.8 months (interquartile range 10–47 months). Patients with high pT stage (pT2–4) suffered shorter survival span (HR: 9.370, 95% CI: 2.956–29.697, $P < 0.001$). There were no significant differences in CSS between PU and RNU ($P = 0.964$). In the sub-analysis, CSS for RNU and PU showed no significant difference for pTa–1 or pT2–4 tumor patients ($P = 0.516$, $P = 0.475$, respectively).

Conclusions: PU is not inferior to RNU in oncologic outcomes. Furthermore, PU is generally recognized with less invasive and better renal function preservation compared with RNU. Thus, PU would be rational for specific patients with UTUCs.

Keywords: Urothelial carcinoma, Partial ureterectomy, Radical nephroureterectomy, Caner specific survival

Background

Upper tract urothelial carcinomas (UTUCs), as a kind of urothelial carcinomas (UCs), accounting for only 5–10% [1]. Generally, 60% of UTUCs are invasive [2]. Seventy to Ninety years old showed the highest morbid risk among all age groups and are three times more ordinary in men [2]. UTUC with pure nonurothelial histology is quite rare, but about 25% of cases have variants. Computed tomography (CT) is an available imaging technique with high diagnostic accuracy [3]. In about 90% of cases, the tumor grade can be determined with a low false negative rate [4]. Ureteroscopic biopsy combining with urinary cytology, and imaging findings such as hydronephrosis may contribute for the decision of surgical type like partial ureterectomy (PU) and radical nephroureterectomy (RNU) [5]. Tumor stage and grade, lymph node involvement, lymphovascular invasion, surgical margins, and pathological factors could be used to estimate prognosis [2]. Nowadays, the concept for preservation of renal function has been emphasized. For low-risk UTUC, kidney-sparing surgery (KSS) unlike radical surgery could preserve kidney function without compromising oncological outcomes. KSS such as PU are performed for the patients with solitary kidney, renal insufficiency, or low-risk tumors. RNU is still the standard treatment for high-risk UTUCs, no matter where the tumor location is [2, 6]. Herein, we used data in our database to assess the oncological outcomes between PU and RNU.

* Correspondence: jinghai_hu@126.com
[1]Department of Urology, First Hospital of Jilin University, Changchun 130021, People's Republic of China
Full list of author information is available at the end of the article

Methods

Study population and treatment

The research protocol was approved by the ethics committee of Jilin University's Institutional Ethical Review Board, and written informed consent was obtained. Three hundred thirty two patients with UTUC from January 2007 to December 2014 in our database were included in First Hospital of Jilin University. Of them, 52 patients were excluded for suspected multifocal tumors in the upper urinary tract preoperatively. Another 25 patients were excluded for distant metastases (n = 14), no surgical treatment (n = 3), suffering previous or concurrent radical cystectomy (n = 8). Among the remaining 255 patients, 182 of them underwent RUN, 73 of them underwent PU. All Patients were evaluated disease progression by CT preoperatively. During the study period, ureteroscopy with biopsy was not routinely performed. The choice and surgical technique of RNU and PU could not be standardized. Surgeon preferences have a significant impact on the selection and surgical technique of RNU and PU. For RNU, the kidney and entire ureter with a bladder cuff were excised. PU was performed along with the excision of ureteral segment. There were no statistically differences between age at surgery, sex, tumor side, presence of hematuria, and presence of hydronephrosis. Clinical and pathological staging was in accordance with TNM classification 2002 [7, 8].

Statistical analysis

Outcomes were measured by survival time (from the time of surgery to cancer specific mortality). Continuous variables were described as the median (interquartile range). T tests or nonparametric tests were carried out to assess the differences in variables with a continuous distribution. Categorical variables were described as the frequency (percentage) and analyzed by the Chi-square

Table 1 Clinical and pathologic characteristics of the two groups

Variables	RNU	PU	t/χ^2	*P*
Age	66.74 ± 8.41	67.62 ± 10.09	−0.709	0.479
Sex				
Male	90 (49.5%)	30 (41.4%)	1.460	0.227
Female	92 (50.5%)	43 (58.9%)		
Smoking				
No	47 (61.8%)	27 (84.4%)	5.300	0.021
Yes	29 (38.2%)	5 (15.6%)		
Tumor side				
Left	98 (54.1%)	29 (39.7%)	4.325	0.038
Right	83 (45.9%)	44 (60.3%)		
Hydronephrosis				
No	18 (10.3%)	11 (16.4%)	1.727	0.189
Yes	157 (89.7%)	56 (83.6%)		
Hematuria				
No	59 (33.7%)	30 (44.1%)	2.283	0.131
Yes	116 (66.3%)	38 (55.9%)		
Renal function				
Normal	48 (43.6%)	20 (47.6%)	0.195	0.659
Abnormal	63 (56.4%)	22 (52.4%)		
Operation time	157.50 (116.25–180.00)	95.00 (76.25–126.25)	−4.476	< 0.001
pT stage			8.287	0.067
pTa	9 (5.2%)	2 (3.0%)		
pT 1	73 (42.0%)	33 (49.3%)		
pT 2	48 (27.6%)	25 (37.3%)		
pT 3	41 (23.6%)	6 (9.0%)		
pT 4	3 (1.7%)	1 (1.5%)		
Lymphovascular invasion	4 (2.2%)	0 (0%)	1.630	0.202

RUN Radical nephroureterectomy, *PU* Partial ureterectomy

or Fisher exact test. The Cox proportional hazard models were employed for univariate and multivariate analyses to determine whether surgery type (RNU vs PU) and other variables was associated with CSS. The survival curves of each stratified variablewere plotted by the Kaplan-Meier method and compared by log-rank test. SPSS version 18.0 (SPSS Inc., Chicago, IL) was used for statistical analyses. All *P* values were two-tailed, and P value < 0.05 indicated statistical significance.

Results

Clinicopathological characteristics

The mean length of follow-up was 35.8 months (interquartile range 10–47 months). The baseline characteristics of the patients are shown in Table 1. The mean age and percent of male in RNU group were 66.74 ± 8.41 and 49.5%, respectively; 67.62 ± 10.09 and 41.4% in PU group, respectively. Smokers in RNU group were much more than in PU group (38.2% vs 15.6%, $P = 0.021$). In RNU group, half of the patients had tumor in the left kidney (54.1%). PU group is contrary to it (39.7%). The proportion of patients with hydronephrosis, hematuria or abnormal renal function in RNU group were close to PU group ($P > 0.05$). Compared with PU group,operation time of patients in RNU group was much longer (157.50 (116.25–180.00) vs 95.00 (76.25–126.25), $P < 0.001$). In RNU group, nearly half (42.0%) were diagnosed at pT stage1, 5.2% at pT stage a, 27.6% at pT stage 2, 23.6% at pT stage 3, and only 1.7% at pT stage4. In PU group, the proportion is 49.3, 3, 37.3, 9, and 1.5%, respectively.

Oncological outcome

Univariable and multivariable analyses for CSS after surgery were shown in Table 2. On multivariable analysis, pT stage

Table 2 Cox regression analysis of factors associated with CSS

Variables	Univariate			Multivariate		
	HR	95% CI	*P*	HR	95% CI	*P*
Age (years)						
≤ 70	1.000			1.000		
> 70	0.885	0.581–1.348	0.569	1.240	0.488–3.150	0.652
Sex						
Male	1.000			1.000		
Female	0.713	0.478–1.062	0.096	1.328	0.477–3.693	0.587
Smoking						
No	1.000			1.000		
Yes	1.095	0.548–2.190	0.797	0.695	0.225–2.147	0.527
Tumor side						
Left	1.000			1.000		
Right	0.726	0.486–1.084	0.117	1.136	0.451–2.861	0.787
Hydronephrosis						
No	1.000			1.000		
Yes	1.134	0.588–2.188	0.707	0.742	0.149–3.698	0.716
Hematuria						
No	1.000			1.000		
Yes	1.307	0.842–2.029	0.233	2.405	0.820–7.048	0.110
Renal function						
Normal	1.000			1.000		
Abnormal	1.130	0.688–1.911	0.650	1.503	0.613–3.686	0.374
pT stage						
pTa–1	1.000			1.000		
pT2–4	6.907	4.028–11.845	< 0.001	9.370	2.956–29.697	< 0.001
Surgical intervention						
RNU	1.000			1.000		
PU	1.010	0.651–1.567	0.964	1.705	0.608–4.778	0.310

RUN Radical nephroureterectomy, *PU* Partial ureterectomy

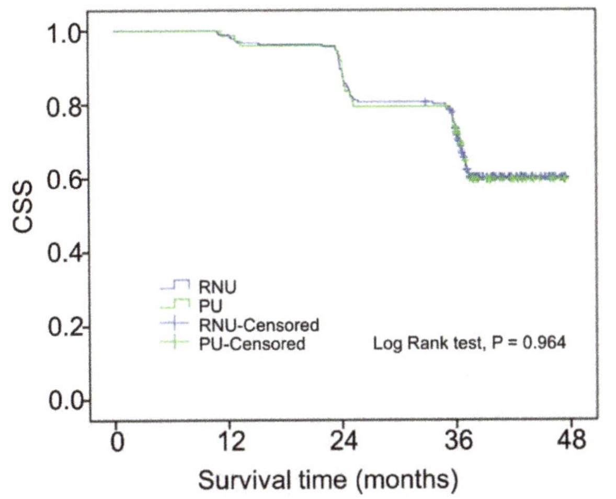

Fig. 1 Kaplan–Meier estimates of CSS according to surgery type in patients with UTUC

was significantly associated with CSS. The results showed that patients with high pT stage (pT2–4) suffered shorter survival span (HR: 9.370, 95% CI: 2.956–29.697, $P <$ 0.001). The independent predictors of CSS were higher pT ($P < 0.001$; Table 2). The specific results are exhibited in Table 2. Furthermore, there were no significant differences in CSS between PU and RNU ($P = 0.964$) (Fig. 1). In the sub-analysis, there was no significant difference in 3-year CSS probability between pTa–1 tumor patients treated with RNU (87.7%) and PU (82.9%) ($P = 0.516$). Similarly, for patients with pT2–4 tumors, 3-year CSS for RNU and PU showed no significant difference (38.0% vs 31.3%, $P = 0.475$, respectively) (Fig. 2).

Discussion

UTUC is a kind of rare malignancy. The main treatments for URUC are RNU and KSS like PU. Recent data indicated that patients with low grade UTUC could be treated by PU effectively. The guidelines of the European Association of Urology suggested that PU is a legitimate therapy for small, unifocal, low grade UTUC with no signs of infiltration [2, 7, 9], and indicated that RNU is still the standard treatment for high-risk UTUCs [2, 10]. However, Bagrodia et al. compared the prognosis of UTUC patients who suffered either RNU or PU. They suggested that PU seemed to possess oncologic efficacy equal to RNU. Meanwhile, PU could preserve the renal function to the maximum extent [9]. Similar results were also demonstrated in the investigation from Fukushima et al. [11]. Colin et al. conducted a multicenter cohort study of UTUC which suggested that surgical interventions was not the independent prognostic factor for recurrence-free survival (RFS) and CSS [6]. The investigation from Hung et al. indicated that the local recurrences, bladder recurrences, distant metastasis, and CSS showed no significant differences between RNU and PU [12]. These findings mentioned above would show the ability of PU to maximize the preservation of renal function in carefully selected patients.

In the current study, we noticed that pathological stage remained the most important predictor for the CSS of patients with UTUCs. The results also revealed that CSS showed no significant differences between RNU and PU in both low pT stage (pTa–1) and high pT stage (pT2–4) UTUCs. The probable reason is that the number of patients involved in our study is not large enough, thus this study may not be powerful enough to

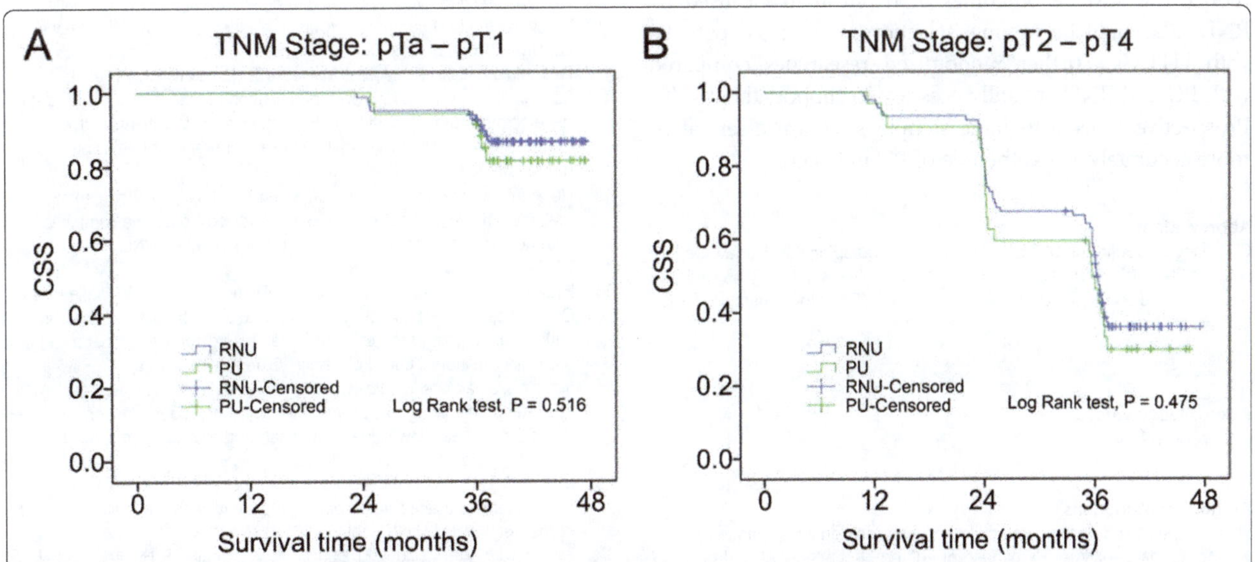

Fig. 2 Kaplan–Meier estimates of CSS according to surgery type in patients with pTa – pT2 (**a**) and pT2 – pT4 (**b**) UTUC

show significance [6]. Furthermore, there were some selection biases that RNU group seemed to have more aggressive pathological features compared with PU group, because there was not the standardized indication for PU and surgeon preferred PU for lower stage UTUCs [13, 14]. Selection biases can lead to better survival in PU group compared with RNU group, though the difference was not significant in our analysis. Our findings, and similar findings from other researchers, indicated that PU could act as a selectable treatment for selected UTUC patients [15]. In addition, pathologists with expertise rechecked all the pathologic specimens, and all pathologic results were collected standardly.

This study is retrospective study, and the number of involved patients is relatively small. These two characteristics are the main limitations of this study. Because a prospective randomized controlled study of PU compared with RNU is difficult due to the rarity of UTUC. Secondly, we could not ascertain whether PU was done imperatively or electively. Furthermore, surgeon preferences have a great impact on the surgical technique and indication for RNU and PU, which could not be determined standardly. Nor can we assess which cases are suitable for endoscopic treatment when receiving RNU therapy [16, 17].. Multiple surgeons were employed to operate on the investigated patients. This situation might lead to a selection bias and variable surgical techniques. Finally, another limitation of our research is that we could not provide the information about tumor grade and metastases due to the sample problem.

Conclusion

In conclusion, PU and RNU might possess equivalent long-term oncologic outcomes. Furthermore, PU could reduce the adverse outcomes of nephron loss caused by RNU. PU could be rational selection for selected patients with UTUCs. Further randomized researches compared with PU and RNU are still necessary to support the results. Prospective trials with large sample sizes are essential to more accurately assess the role of PU in UTUC.

Abbreviations

CSS: Cancer-specific survival; CT: Computed tomography; KSS: Kidney-sparing surgery; PU: Partial ureterectomy; RFS: Recurrence-free survival; RNU: Radical nephroureterectomy; UC: Urothelial carcinomas; UTUC: Upper tract urothelial carcinoma

Acknowledgments

Not applicable.

Authors' contributions

SL: conception and design, data collection, statistical analysis, manuscript writing. YP: data analysis. JH: manuscript editing, supervision. All authors read and approved the final manuscript.

Author details

[1]Department of Urology, First Hospital of Jilin University, Changchun 130021, People's Republic of China. [2]Key Laboratory of Polymer Ecomaterials, Changchun Institute of Apllied Chemistry, Chinese Academy of Sciences, Changchun 130022, People's Republic of China. [3]Department of Clinical Epidemiology, First Hospital of Jilin University, Changchun 130021, People's Republic of China.

References

1. Siegel RL, Miller KD, Jemal A. Cancer statistics, 2018. CA Cancer J Clin. 2018;68(1):7–30.
2. Roupret M, Babjuk M, Comperat E, Zigeuner R, Sylvester RJ, Burger M, et al. European Association of Urology guidelines on upper urinary tract urothelial carcinoma: 2017 update. Eur Urol. 2018;73(1):111–22.
3. Zigeuner R, Shariat SF, Margulis V, Karakiewicz PI, Roscigno M, Weizer A, et al. Tumour necrosis is an indicator of aggressive biology in patients with urothelial carcinoma of the upper urinary tract. Eur Urol. 2010; 57(4):575–81.
4. Rojas CP, Castle SM, Llanos CA, Cortes JAS, Bird V, Rodriguez S, et al. Low biopsy volume in ureteroscopy does not affect tumor biopsy grading in upper tract urothelial carcinoma. Urol Oncol: Semin Orig Invest. 2013:1696–700. https://doi.org/10.1016/j.urolonc.2012.05.010.
5. Clements T, Messer JC, Terrell JD, Herman MP, Ng CK, Scherr DS, et al. High-grade ureteroscopic biopsy is associated with advanced pathology of upper-tract urothelial carcinoma tumors at definitive surgical resection. J Endourol. 2012;26(4):398–402.
6. Colin P, Ouzzane A, Pignot G, Ravier E, Crouzet S, Ariane MM, et al. Comparison of oncological outcomes after segmental ureterectomy or radical nephroureterectomy in urothelial carcinomas of the upper urinary tract: results from a large French multicentre study. BJU Int. 2012;110(8):1134–41.
7. Amin MB, Greene FL, Edge SB, Compton CC, Gershenwald JE, Brookland RK, et al. The eighth edition AJCC cancer staging manual: continuing to build a bridge from a population-based to a more "personalized" approach to cancer staging. CA Cancer J Clin. 2017;67(2):93–9.
8. Mostofi FK, Sobin LH, Torloni H, Organization WH. Histological typing of urinary bladder tumours; 1973.
9. Bagrodia A, Kuehhas FE, Gayed BA, Wood CG, Raman JD, Kapur P, et al. Comparative analysis of oncologic outcomes of partial ureterectomy vs radical nephroureterectomy in upper tract urothelial carcinoma. Urology. 2013;81(5):972–7.
10. Seisen T, Peyronnet B, Dominguez-Escrig JL, Bruins HM, Yuan CY, Babjuk M, et al. Oncologic outcomes of kidney-sparing surgery versus radical Nephroureterectomy for upper tract urothelial carcinoma: a systematic review by the EAU non-muscle invasive bladder cancer guidelines panel. Eur Urol. 2016;70(6):1052–68.
11. Fukushima H, Saito K, Ishioka J, Matsuoka Y, Numao N, Koga F, et al. Equivalent survival and improved preservation of renal function after distal ureterectomy compared with nephroureterectomy in patients with urothelial carcinoma of the distal ureter: a propensity score-matched multicenter study. Int J Urol. 2014;21(11):1098–104.
12. Hung SY, Yang WC, Luo HL, Hsu CC, Chen YT, Chuang YC. Segmental ureterectomy does not compromise the oncologic outcome compared with nephroureterectomy for pure ureter cancer. Int Urol Nephrol. 2014;46(5):921–6.
13. Pedrosa JA, Masterson TA, Rice KR, Kaimakliotis HZ, Monn MF, Bihrle R, et al. Oncologic outcomes and prognostic impact of urothelial recurrences in patients undergoing segmental and total ureterectomy for upper tract urothelial carcinoma. Can Urol Assoc J. 2015;9(3–4):E187–92.
14. Simhan J, Smaldone MC, Egleston BL, Canter D, Sterious SN, Corcoran AT, et al. Nephron-sparing management vs radical nephroureterectomy for low- or moderate-grade, low-stage upper tract urothelial carcinoma. BJU Int. 2014;114(2):216–20.
15. Dalpiaz O, Ehrlich G, Quehenberger F, Pummer K, Zigeuner R. Distal ureterectomy is a safe surgical option in patients with urothelial carcinoma of the distal ureter. Urol Oncol. 2014;32(1):34 e31–8.
16. Fajkovic H, Klatte T, Nagele U, Dunzinger M, Zigeuner R, Hubner W, et al. Results and outcomes after endoscopic treatment of upper urinary tract carcinoma: the Austrian experience. World J Urol. 2013;31(1):37–44.

26

Complications of high volume circumcision: Glans amputation in adolescents

Mmatsie Manentsa, Hilary Mukudu, Nthabiseng Koloane, Ashley Ringane, Eleanor Matta, Neil A. Martinson and Limakatso Lebina*

Abstract

Background: The past four years has seen a rapid roll-out of male medical circumcision services in South Africa in response to clinical trials showing circumcision prevents HIV acquisition in heterosexual men. Clinics conduct substantial numbers of circumcisions per day. We report three cases of glans amputation in adolescents attending high volume clinics where modified Models of Optimising Volume and Efficiency (MOVE) are implemented.

Case presentations: Three cases of glans amputation in young healthy men that presented for voluntary medical male circumcision. The procedures were performed by highly experienced medical officers in two cases. All these cases shared characteristics: younger males with immature genitalia, forceps guided circumcision, and likely operator fatigue. Voluntary male medical circumcision programs should include regular monitoring and evaluation and training of operators to ensure high quality surgical techniques such as working in clean areas and taking frequent breaks.

Conclusion: Circumcision is a relatively simple medical procedure, however regular training and quality control in high volume Male Medical Circumcision sites is essential to prevent rare catastrophic adverse events.

Keywords: MMC, Adverse events, HIV prevention, Surgical circumcision

Background

In 2007 the World Health Organisation (WHO) recommended that countries with low levels of circumcision, high HIV prevalence rates and mainly heterosexual Human Immunodeficiency Virus (HIV) transmission levels should scale-up access to safe male circumcision services [1]. The WHO in its Joint Strategic Action Framework 2012–2016, outlined steps necessary to implement scale-up [2]. The framework made a call for innovative strategies to be employed in the scale-up. These strategies included innovative use of human resources through Models for Optimizing the Volume and Efficiency (MOVE) of male circumcision services [2, 3]. The MOVE model for VMMC services enhances efficiency by coordinating client flow, using multiple surgical beds to one surgical team, task shifting of some (suturing) surgical procedures to non-physicians and use of pre-packed consumables [3].

In 2010 the South African National Department of Health (DoH) began large scale roll-out of Voluntary Medical Male Circumcision (VMMC) [4]. To date approximately 2,84 million circumcisions have been conducted at multiple high-volume VMMC clinics across the country [5]. Since the roll-out began, moderate adverse events have been reported occurring in fewer than 2% of patients circumcised [5, 6]. It is important for the management of male circumcision programs both in South Africa and elsewhere that adverse events be reported as there are rare instances of severe complications, which should be monitored and responded to, thereby preventing future events [7].

Our organisation managed implementation of VMMC in five high volume clinics. Informed consent was obtained from presenting males, and for those under 18,

* Correspondence: lebinal@phru.co.za
Perinatal HIV Research Unit (PHRU), SA MRC Soweto Matlosana Collaborating Centre for HIV/AIDS and TB, University of the Witwatersrand, Johannesburg, South Africa

parental consent was obtained as well. Pre-operation screening and surgical preparation was done as per the WHO's Manual for Male Circumcision under Local Anaesthetic [6].

As part of quality control, we reviewed three glans amputations that occurred at these high volume VMMC clinics and report them as a case series. To obtain the data, a retrospective record review was conducted at the three clinics, together with one-on-one interviews conducted with medical officers and other staff members involved in the cases.

Case presentations

Case 1

The first case occurred in 2016 at a VMMC clinic established in 2010 in an urban township. The clinic staff numbered 26 including, medical officers, clinical associates, nurses, and support staff. On the day of the event, at total of 97 circumcisions were performed at the clinic, 22 of these by the operator involved in the glans amputation prior to the incident. The case was a 10-year-old boy who presented for medical male circumcision. The operator was a medical officer, with experience of over 13,000 circumcisions, assisted by an enrolled nurse. A total of 7 ml local anaesthetic was injected using the penile ring block technique (4,5 ml lignocaine 2% plus 2,5 ml marcaine 0,5%) [5]. As the patient's penis was relatively small, the volume of local anaesthetic applied caused ballooning of the penis from the base to the tip of the foreskin. The forceps guided circumcision technique was used according to then standard protocols [6]. The operative procedure was initiated at 16 h10. After the operator clamped the foreskin with the forceps, the glans was palpated to ensure that it was below the clamp. When the foreskin was excised, it became clear that the glans had been amputated at a level just below the coronal sulcus.

Haemostatic control of the wound was maintained through compression and the amputated glans was placed on ice. The urologist on call was contacted to immediately assess the patient, and within 40 min the patient was taken into theatre for urgent repair and reconstruction. The glans was successfully re-attached during surgery, a catheter was inserted until the wound was healed. Based on patient feedback, he subsequently, developed a fistula and had to undergo further reconstructive surgery.

Case 2

The second case occurred in 2013 involving a 15-year-old boy who presented for medical male circumcision at a VMMC clinic established in 2012. The clinic staff numbered 22 including managers, medical officers, nurses, and support staff. On the day of the incident 58 circumcisions had been performed, 34 of these by the operator prior to the incident. As in the previous case, after informed consent was sought from the boy's guardian, standard guidelines were followed in the screening and surgical preparation. The operator was a medical officer, who had completed 8000 circumcisions, assisted by 2 nurses. The surgical technique used in the procedure was the forceps-guided method. Local anaesthetic, 2 ml Marcaine 0,5% plus 8 ml lignocaine 2%, was injected into the base of the penis via ring block using a syringe and needle with marked swelling of the penis from the base of the penis to the foreskin. The operative procedure was initiated at 15 h19. The operator clamped the foreskin with a forceps and palpated for the position of the glans. As the foreskin was excised the operator noticed that the glans had been partially amputated and the urethra was exposed. The procedure was abandoned and haemostatic control was maintained whilst a urologist was called in to assess the patient. A partial distal glans amputation was diagnosed by the attending urologist and within 3 hrs the patient was taken to theatre for repair and reconstruction. Glans reconstruction was attempted with re-attachment of the transacted part of the glans and catheter inserted. However, post-operatively, a large portion of the reattached glans became necrotic and the patient subsequently developed a urethro-cutaneous fistula. The patient required further reconstruction.

Case 3

The third case was a 10-year-old boy occurred at a VMMC clinic situated in a rural area. The clinic was established in 2012 and has a total staff complement of 22, including medical officers, clinical associates, nurses and other support staff. On the day of the incident, 120 circumcisions were performed at the clinic. The operator involved was a clinical associate (a cadre of staff with four years of medical training and licensed to do circumcisions) with experience of over 1000 circumcisions. He performed 25 circumcisions that day prior to the incident. The patient was consented and screened as in the previous two cases. The procedure started at 12 h30, using a modified forceps guided circumcision as the patient had phimosis. Local anaesthetic was injected by penile ring block using 3 ml lignocaine 2% and 1 ml Marcaine 0,5%. After the dorsal slit was made, preputial adhesions were released and the glans was palpated before the forceps was clamped. After the foreskin was excised the operator noted a partial amputation of the glans on the dorsal aspect, the urethra was not involved. A medical officer was immediately called to assist. A urethral catheter was inserted and haemostatic control of the wound was achieved through cauterisation and sutures. The patient was referred to a hospital for further reconstruction by a urologist. The patient has healed without sequelae.

The total number of men and boys under 15 years, and those 15 years and over circumcised in five high volume male circumcision clinics under the same administration as the three clinics where the glans amputation occurred was 17,551 and 53,782, respectively, yielding rates of glans amputation of 11.3/100000 and 1.8/100000 in those younger than 15 years, and 15 years of age or older, respectively ($p = 0.0126$).

Discussion

Voluntary medical male circumcision is a common and safe medical procedure with frequencies of complications ranging between 1 and 15% [7]. Most adverse events are mild, but severe complications occur occasionally, and include necrosis of the glans, penile amputation, urethral fistulas and preputial fusion [7, 8]. Complications appear to be higher in older children when compared to neonatal circumcision [9]. In two cases we report, anatomy of the penis was underdeveloped. Both cases reported excessive swelling of the penis after injection of local anaesthetic making it difficult for operators to adequately palpate the glans. In such cases the forceps-guided method is not the best choice. A dissection or resection method would be a safer option.

A higher rate of adverse events have been reported with circumcisions performed by providers with less experience [9]. The operators in the first two cases were both medical officers with extensive surgical experience in MMC. However, the operator in the third case was a clinical associate who had considerably less experience. Both the VMMC clinics where these amputations occurred utilised task-shifting and task-sharing, as recommended by the MOVE principles [3, 10]. Studies have reported no difference in adverse event rates when these strategies are implemented [11]. However, the operator does not examine the patient during eligibility screening, and may only see the patient at the time of the procedure. This does not give the operator sufficient time to consider and plan alternative surgical options when presented with potentially difficult circumcisions. In the first two cases the glans amputation occurred after each operator had already completed over 20 circumcisions. All three events occurred in the afternoon when the operators were most likely fatigued.

Our experience suggests that in high volume circumcision clinics, strict rules be applied to prevent catastrophic adverse events like amputation or partial amputation of the glans. We propose that firstly, no young children (younger than 13 years) should be circumcised in the afternoon, by clinical staff that performed MMC procedures that morning. Secondly, frequent breaks (at least every 1–2 hrs) be given to operators when they doff all protective equipment, and leave the operating theatre for at least 15 min. Consideration should be given to setting a maximum daily cap on the number of men circumcised by an individual surgeon. Thirdly, in young adolescents additional care must be taken: the attending surgeon must individually examine the child before a decision to circumcise is made, thereby noting the maturity of the genitals before starting the procedure; local anaesthetic injected subcutaneously should dissipate, allowing restoration of anatomical landmarks before first incision and dissection. Fourthly, MMC guidelines should recommend the use of open surgical techniques (dorsal slit) that ensure visualisation of the glans prior to excising the foreskin and managers of VMMC programs must ensure that this is adhered to. Fifthly, there should be continuous training and retraining of all ranks of MMC providers, with on-going monitoring and evaluation to ensure quality control. Finally, implementation of a neonatal circumcision program would likely prevent such events, as a systematic literature review has shown there are minimal severe adverse events (infection, ulcers) and no glans amputations with neonatal circumcision [9].

Higher rates of adverse events have been reported during mass circumcision campaigns, mainly related to non-sterile conditions and a lack of equipment [12]. The rapid scale-up of VMMC services in South Africa has reportedly led to a decline in quality of services [10]. This decline is related to the distribution of limited resources as the programme expands and is said not to reflect the quality of surgical technique [13]. A worrying aspect of increased adverse events is the rise in medical liability litigation which may act as a barrier to the provision of VMMC [14]. Severe complications during medical male circumcision occur occasionally, and providers of VMMC services must conduct regular introspection, and quality reviews to ensure service quality is improved and adverse events that we have described, are avoided.

Abbreviations

CDC: Centre for Disease Control; DOH: Department of Health; HIV: Human Immunodeficiency Virus; MMC: Male Medical Circumcision; MOVE: Models of Optimising Volume and Efficiency; VMMC: Voluntary Male Medical Circumcision; WHO: World Health Organisation

Acknowledgements

The authors would like to thank the clinics cases were conducted, the nurses that assisted and the individuals that were studied.

Authors' contributions

MM, HM, EA, NAM, and LL conceptualised the idea of the case report manuscript and collated data on the case reports. MM, NK, AR NAM and LL were involved in the drafting and critical review of the manuscript. All authors read and approved the final manuscript.

References

1. World Health Organization. UNAIDS. New data on male circumcision and HIV prevention: policy and programme implications, vol. 2013. Geneva, Switzerland: World Health Organization; 2007.

2. World Health Organization. UNAIDS joint strategic action framework to accelerate the scale-up of voluntary medical male circumcision for HIV prevention in eastern and southern Africa, 2012–2016. Geneva; 2011.
3. World Health Organization. Considerations for implementing models for optimizing the volume and efficiency of male circumcision services. 2010.
4. Rees H. PIC and SANAC end of term review of the NSP 2007–2011 final report 4; 2011.
5. World Health Organization. Progress brief - voluntary medical male circumcision for HIV prevention in 14 priority countries of east and southern Africa, vol. 2017. Geneva; 2017.
6. World Health Organization. Manual for male circumcision under local anaesthesia. Geneva; 2011.
7. Ceylan K, Burhan K, Yılmaz Y, Can Ş, Kuş A, Mustafa G. Severe complications of circumcision: an analysis of 48 cases. J Pediatr Urol. 2007;3(1):32–5.
8. Johnson PRV. Childhood circumcision. Surgery (Oxford). 2005;23(9):338–40.
9. Weiss HA, Larke N, Halperin D, Schenker I. Complications of circumcision in male neonates, infants and children: a systematic review. BMC Urol. 2010;10(1):2.
10. Rech D, Spyrelis A, Frade S, Perry L, Farrell M, Fertziger R, et al. Implications of the fast-evolving scale-up of adult voluntary medical male circumcision for quality of services in South Africa. PLoS One. 2014;9(5):e80577.
11. Ford N, Chu K, Mills EJ. Safety of task-shifting for male medical circumcision: a systematic review and meta-analysis. AIDS. 2012;26(5):559–66. https://doi.org/10.1097/QAD.0b013e32834f3264.
12. Özdemir E. Significantly increased complication risks with mass circumcisions. Br J Urol. 1997;80(1):136–9.
13. Sgaier SK, Reed JB, Thomas A, Njeuhmeli E. Achieving the HIV prevention impact of voluntary medical male circumcision: lessons and challenges for managing programs. PLoS Med. 2014;11(5):e1001641.
14. Evens E, Lanham M, Hart C, Loolpapit M, Oguma I, Obiero W. Identifying and addressing barriers to uptake of voluntary medical male circumcision in Nyanza, Kenya among men 18–35: a qualitative study. PLoS One. 2014;9(6):e98221.

Laparoscopic adrenalectomy - Is it safe in hands of residents in training?

Jadwiga Dworak, Michał Wysocki, Anna Rzepa, Michał Natkaniec, Michał Pędziwiatr, Andrzej Budzyński and Piotr Major*

Abstract

Background: Laparoscopic adrenalectomy (LA) has become the "gold standard" for treating most adrenal tumors in the past decade. However, it is still considered a relatively complicated procedure requiring experience from surgeon. The aim of the study was to evaluate the safety of laparoscopic adrenalectomy performed by residents who are undergoing training in general surgery.

Methods: A prospectively collected database containing all 300 transperitoneal laparoscopic adrenalectomies performed in II Department of General Surgery JU MC, Krakow between January 2013 and March 2018 was retrospectively reviewed. Patients were divided into two groups; patients operated on by residents (group 1, 54 operations) and by attending general surgeons (group 2, 246 operations). We compared the course of the operation and patient hospitalization in these two groups. If the operation was completed by a different person than the one who started the procedure, we refer to this as "operator conversion".

Results: We found no differences in demographic factors or comorbidities between the two groups. The mean operative time was similar in the residents' and the specialists' groups ($p = 0.5761$). Median blood loss did not differ between the groups ($p = 0.4325$). The overall ratio of intraoperative adverse events was similar in both groups ($p = 0.8643$). The difference in the ratio of perioperative complications between the groups was not statistically significant ($p = 0.6442$). The average mean hospital stay after surgery was 2 days for both groups. We identified 25 cases (8.33%) of operator conversion; the difference in operator conversions between two groups was not statistically significant ($p = 0.1741$).

Conclusions: Laparoscopic transperitoneal adrenalectomy performed by a supervised resident is a safe procedure. The course of the operation and patient hospitalization did not differ importantly when comparing procedures performed by residents and attending surgeons. Liberal use of operator conversions from resident to attending surgeon and from a surgeon to a senior surgeon provides reasonable safety and prevents complications. In high-volume centers performing minimally invasive techniques, closed supervision allows residents to safely perform LA.

Keywords: Laparoscopic adrenalectomy, Adrenal gland, Resident, Learning curve, Operator conversion, Intraoperative difficulties, Complications

* Correspondence: piotr.major@uj.edu.pl
2nd Department of General Surgery, Jagiellonian University Medical College, Kopernika 21 St., 31-501 Kraków, Poland

Background

Laparoscopic adrenalectomy (LA) has become the "gold standard" for treating most adrenal tumors in recent years [1]. Nevertheless, LA is considered an advanced procedure with a potential risk of serious complications requiring a high skill level [2–5]. Surgical residents today face the challenge of learning complex skills in a limited time, growing expectations regarding efficiency, quality, and financial viability of health care delivery. Minimally invasive techniques became more popular and available and were therefore included in surgery residents' training programs [6]. However, it remains unclear whether advanced procedures like LA can be performed as safely by residents as by attending surgeons. Previous studies have addressed the interaction between residents' participation in surgical procedures and outcomes such as morbidity and mortality with conflicting results. Differences in the results likely relate to the variability of research questions, study settings, research strategies and outcome measures. Furthermore, most of these studies addressed this issue indirectly and failed to correctly adjust for potential confounders [7–9].

The aim of this study was therefore to assess the safety of LA performed by residents who are undergoing training in general surgery.

Methods

We performed a retrospective analysis of prospectively collected data of patients who underwent surgical treatment of adrenal tumors in our academic teaching hospital and tertiary referral center between January 2013 and March 2018. The inclusion criterion was laparoscopic transperitoneal adrenalectomy for adrenal tumors. The indication for surgery was either a hormonally active tumor, or, in the case of non-secreting incidentaloma, size ≥40 mm, rapid growth in follow-up studies, or a so-called "*radiological malignant phenotype*" of the tumor. Exclusion criteria were patients undergoing open adrenalectomy, adrenalectomy as a part of multiorgan resection, bilateral adrenalectomy, adrenalectomy from a posterior approach.

All patients underwent preoperative imaging studies (ultrasound, computed tomography, magnetic resonance imaging, or, if necessary, positron emission computed tomography). Tumor size was estimated in imaging studies (computed tomography or magnetic resonance imaging). Prior to surgery, a routine panel of laboratory tests was conducted to establish the tumor's hormonal activity. In cases of suspected pheochromocytoma, patients were preoperatively treated with alpha-blockers (doxazosin 20 mg/day and additional beta-blockers in case of co-existing tachycardia). The operative method of choice in our department is laparoscopic transperitoneal lateral total adrenalectomy, which is performed similarly to its description elsewhere [10, 11]. In this paper, we understood the acronym to mean laparoscopic transperitoneal adrenalectomy.

The team that performed the surgeries comprised six operators, including four attending surgeons (five surgeons with 2–5 years of specialization during their inclusion to the study and one senior surgeon who was experienced in laparoscopic procedures) and two surgery residents (in their fourth to sixth years of training). Patients were divided into two groups. The first group (Group 1) was operated on by a resident and the second group (Group 2) by a attending general surgeon. Prior to attempting first adrenalectomy, the residents in training were required to acquire an appropriate theoretical background in endocrine surgery and experience in laparoscopic surgery (including obligatory structured training on simulators at the Department of Medical Education, Jagiellonian University Medical College). Every resident had to assist in at least 15 LAs, after which they could perform procedures supervised and assisted by a surgeon with expertise in adrenal gland surgery.

The study analyzed the following characteristics: operative time, mean blood loss, number of intraoperative adverse events, intraoperative difficulties and operator conversions, conversion rate, perioperative complications, reoperations, readmissions, length of hospital stay and 30-day-mortality rate.

If the operation was completed by a different person than the one who started the procedure, we refer to this as "operator conversion". The reasons for such conversions were lack of progress in the procedure, anatomical difficulties imposing a high risk of complications and intraoperative adverse events. When residents were operating, the supervising surgeon took over the operation. For patients operated on by attending surgeons, operator conversions to the senior surgeon with the highest expertise in laparoscopic adrenalectomy were included in the analysis. The number of and reasons for such operator conversions were assessed.

Directly after each procedure, every main operator was obligated to note down the intraoperative difficulties, which were defined as surgeon-reported obstacles during the operation. The surgeon had to set all reported obstacles into an LA Matrix Table Questionnaire. The table comprised the following groups: difficulty in achieving good and sufficient working space, intra-abdominal adhesions or anatomy obstructing surgery, difficulty in dissection, difficulty in recognizing the anatomy or the proper layers, difficulty in achieving sufficient hemostasis and the need for assistance from a supervisor (operator conversion).

Intraoperative adverse events were defined as any iatrogenic adverse events during the operation that were not derived from the standard LA technique. Perioperative complications were defined as adverse events occurring within 30 days after the procedure. Major complications were defined as grade III or higher in Clavien-Dindo classification [12]. Intraoperative blood loss was measured from the amount of blood aspirated in the suction machine. Excessive intraoperative blood loss was defined as a loss of more than 500 ml. The operative time was measured from the skin incision to its closure. The length of hospital stay (LOS) was defined as the time in days from surgery until discharge from hospital.

All 300 consecutive patient operated on between January 2013 and March 2018 were included in the study [181 (60.33%) females, 119 (39.67%) males, with a mean age of 57.7 years (19–87 years, SD ± 13.1 years)]. The flow of patients through the study is shown in Fig. 1.

There were 150 left-sided and 150 right-sided procedures. The indication for surgery was a hormonally inactive tumor in 144 (48.0%) patients, a catecholamine-secreting tumor in 58 (19.3%) patients, a glucocorticosteroid-secreting tumor in 30 (10.0%) patients, an aldosterone-producing tumor in 21 (7.0%) patients, a virilizing tumor in 3 (1.0%) patients and a cancer or a metastasis to the adrenal gland in 44 (14.7%) patients. The mean size of the removed lesion was 45 mm (6–150 mm, SD ± 21.7 mm).

We found no statistically significant differences in demographic factors or comorbidities between the two groups. Demographic data of the analyzed groups are shown in Table 1.

Statistical analysis was performed using StatSoft Statistica version 12.0 PL (StatSoft Inc., Tulsa, OK, USA). The results are presented as mean ± standard deviation (SD), median and interquartile range and odds ratios (ORs) with 95% confidence intervals when appropriate. Tests were used according to the type of variable. Groups were compared using the χ^2 test for categorical variables. Because of a lack of normal data distribution, continuous variables were assessed using the Mann–Whitney U test. Results were considered statistically significant when the p-value was less than 0.05.

All procedures involving human participants were performed in accordance with the ethical standards of the institutional and national research committee and with the 1964 Helsinki Declaration and its later amendments or comparable ethical standards [13]. Approval by the local ethics review committee - Komisja Bioetyczna Uniwersytetu Jagiellońskiego was obtained (nr 1072.6120.88.2018).

Results

Out of 300 operations included in this analysis 54 were performed by residents and 246 by attending surgeons. The mean operative time was 103.5 min (range 30–350, SD ± 43.5). The mean operative time of LA was similar in the residents' and the specialists' groups. Median blood loss was 50 ml and did not differ between the groups. Intraoperative adverse events were observed in 26 (8.67%) operations (Table 2). There were five events in Group 1 and 21 events in Group 2. We observed more than one intraoperative adverse event in three patients. The overall intraoperative adverse events ratios were similar in both groups.

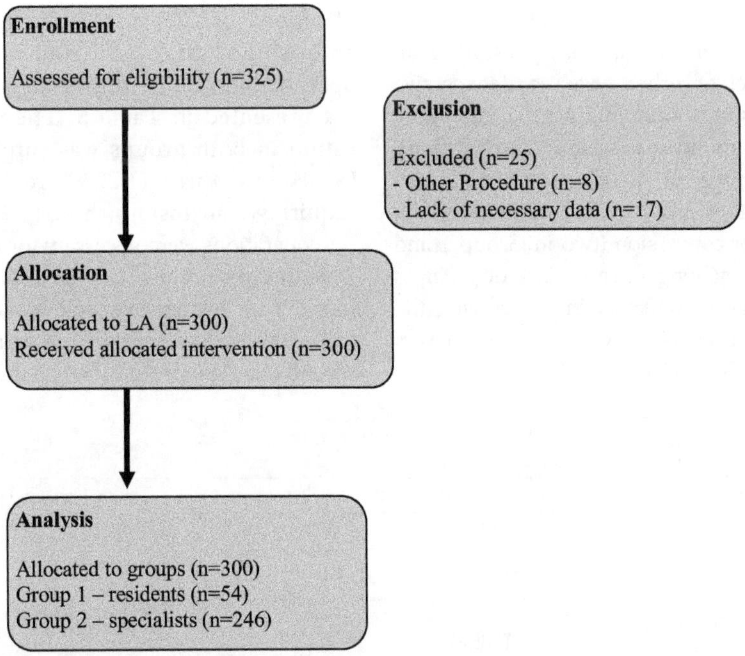

Fig. 1 The flow of patients through the study

Table 1 Characteristics of studied groups

Parameter	All	Group 1 (surgical residents)	Group 2 (attending surgeons)	*p* value
Number of patients, n (%)	300	54	246	–
Females, n (%)	181 (60.33%)	29 (53.70%)	152 (61.79%)	0.2715
males, n (%)	119 (39.67%)	25 (46.30%)	94 (38.21%)	
Mean age (years, ± SD)	57.72 ± 13.10	58.74 ± 12.12	57.50 ± 13.32	0.5352
Mean BMI (kg/m2, ± SD)	28.19 ± 5.44	28.02 ± 4.65	28.23 ± 5.60	0.8062
Mean size (cm, ± SD)	4.50 ± 2.17	4.26 ± 1.96	4.55 ± 2.22	0.3881
Side of the procedure				
-right	150	28	122	0.7638
-left	150	26	124	
Type of the tumor				
-hormonally inactive	144	23	121	0.7238
-catecholamine-secreting	58	11	47	
-glucocorticosteroid-secreting	30	5	25	
-aldosterone-producing	21	6	15	
-virilizing	3	0	3	
-cancer or metastasis	44	9	35	

The incidence of the intraoperative difficulties, which were based on the operators' subjective opinion, were significantly higher in the residents' than the specialists' groups. The intraoperative difficulties required an operator conversion in seven (12.96%) LAs in the residents' group and 18 (7.32%) LAs in the specialists' group. All intraoperative difficulties are shown in Table 3; all intraoperative difficulties requiring an operator conversion are shown in Table 4.

We identified 25 cases (8.33%) of operator conversion, a situation in which the operator could not safely complete LA. Operator conversion was a result of an injury of a major vessel or other organ and excessive blood loss in four cases (one case in Group 1 and three cases in Group 2). We found a description of "difficult or insufficient working space" or "massive intra-abdominal adhesions" in the operation reports of eight cases as the possible cause of operator conversion (two in Group 1 and six in Group 2). In the remaining 13 cases, lack of progress in the procedure was due to difficulty in recognizing the anatomical structures or layers or dissection in those layers (four in Group 1, nine in Group 2).

There were two conversions from laparoscopic to classical "open" surgery in Group 2. The first conversion was due to intraoperative difficulties with recognition of anatomical structures and intense bleeding that was impossible to manage laparoscopically. The second was due to an intense bleeding from inferior vena cava that was repaired after conversion with a vein patch from the saphenous vein.

Perioperative complications were observed in 15 (5.0%) patients. Seven patients had perioperative complications of Clavien–Dindo class I, six had class II and two had class III. Detailed characteristics of perioperative morbidity regarding the Clavien–Dindo scale are presented in Table 5. The most common complication in both groups was surgical site infection [two (3.70%) vs. three (1.22%), respectively] and bleeding requiring transfusion [three (1.22%)] in Group 2.

Reoperations were necessary for two patients from Group 2. Both reoperations were performed because of bleeding. In one case, just laparoscopic hematoma removal and control of bleeding from small vessels was performed. In the second case, splenectomy was required.

Table 2 Intraoperative adverse events

Parameter	Group 1 (residents)	Group 2 (specialists)	*p* –value
Total	5 (9.26%)	21 (8.54%)	0.8643
Tumour capsule rupture	1 (1.85%)	1 (0.41%)	0.7960
Vessel injury	2 (3.70%)	5 (2.03%)	0.8112
Other organ injury	1 (1.85%)	8 (3.25%)	0.9158
Excessive intraoperative blood loss	1 (1.85%)	10 (4.07%)	0.7011

Table 3 Intraoperative difficulties

Parameter	Group 1(residents)	Group 2 (specialists)	p -value
Total	13 (24.07%)	27 (10.98%)	0.0104
Difficulty to achieve good and sufficient working space	4 (7.41%)	4 (1.63%)	0.0547
Intra-abdominal adhesions obstructing performance of the surgery	2 (3.70%)	6 (2.44%)	0.9554
Difficulty in preparation	4 (7.41%)	12 (4.88%)	0.6784
Difficulty in recognizing the anatomy, the layers	2 (3.70%)	2 (0.81%)	0.3068
Difficulty to achieve sufficient hemostasis	1 (1.85%)	3 (1.22%)	0.7732

Five patients (all from Group 2) were readmitted because of complications after discharge. Two of these were readmitted due to pneumonia, two due to a fever of unknown origin, and one due to bleeding from iatrogenic injury of the spleen. The average LOS after surgery for both groups was 2 days. No patients died during the 30-day perioperative period.

All end-points of study for groups 1 and 2 are presented in Table 6.

Discussion

During the last three decades, laparoscopy has proven its indisputable advantages in many aspects over open surgery [14, 15]. Access to minimally invasive techniques had increased worldwide. In general, LA is considered a safe operation, although quite technically demanding and with potentially life-threatening morbidity [16–20]. Because of the complexity, advanced minimally-invasive techniques such as LA are still frequently thought to be somehow hazardous if performed by residents. However, there is no evidence supporting this opinion.

The problem of the safety of LA performed by residents in training supervised by an experienced surgeon was addressed. In our study, the course of the LA operation itself did not differ greatly when comparing residents and attending surgeons. The blood loss, conversion rate, and rate of adverse events were similar. Seib and Venkat showed that there was no difference in need of transfusion between the two groups [21, 22]. The risk of complication, readmission or reoperation related to the procedure was also no different. Similar findings have been reported by other authors. Goldfarb and Horesh showed that there were no significant differences between numbers of major complications when comparing residents and surgeons [23, 24]. Notably, Seib showed that resident participation was even associated with decreased odds of serious complications [21]. We noticed a lower incidence of serious perioperative complications than other authors [21, 22].

According to our results, the safety of these procedures performed by residents, regarding the surgery itself and its postoperative course, did not differ from operations performed by attending surgeons. This can likely be explained by our training program, which included liberal active proctoring. The key point into safe LA is training. Most authors agree that the LA learning curve stabilizes between the 20th and 40th surgery [16, 17, 25]. The steepness of a learning curve is related to several factors, including proper theoretical knowledge followed by practical training, the complexity of a procedure, previous experience with other procedures, proctorship and mentoring [21, 22]. According to the literature, the typical learning curve in LA is evaluated in the group of surgeons who already have some experience in advanced laparoscopic techniques, but not in the group of beginners [16, 18]. Another aspect related to the learning curve is the volume of procedures performed in a surgical unit, which should be substantial. Low volume is related to the poor quality of the learning curve [19]. Our department is a referral center for general surgery that specializes in minimally invasive techniques and a teaching hospital with experience in endocrine surgery and advanced laparoscopic procedures. We included several structured training step comprising theoretical background, training on simulators, and assistance in laparoscopic procedures. This is followed by an active participation in basic and advanced operations. We believe that the key point for safe and effective training is active tutoring. We understand this as active participation of a more experienced surgeon who proceeds instead of the prior operator in the most difficult

Table 4 Intraoperative difficulties requiring conversion of an operator

Parameter	Group 1(residents)	Group 2 (specialists)	p –value
Total	7 (12.96%)	18 (7.32%)	0.1741
Difficulty to achieve good and sufficient working space	2 (3.70%)	3 (1.22%)	
Intra-abdominal adhesions obstructing performance of the surgery	0 (0.00%)	3 (1.22%)	
Difficulty in preparation	2 (3.70%)	7 (2.85%)	
Difficulty in recognizing the anatomy, the layers	2 (3.70%)	2 (0.81%)	
Difficulty to achieve sufficient hemostasis	1 (1.85%)	3 (1.22%)	

Table 5 Perioperative complications

Clavien-Dindo Classification	Parameter	Group 1 (residents)	Group 2 (specialists)	*p*-value
	Total	3 (5.56%)	12 (4.88%)	0.6442
1	Fever of unknown origin	0 (0.00%)	2 (0.81%)	–
1	Surgical site infection	2 (3.70%)	3 (1.22%)	0.4812
2	Bleeding requiring transfusion	1 (1.85%)	3 (1.22%)	0.7732
2	Postoperative pneumonia	0 (0.00%)	2 (0.81%)	–
3	Other organ injury requiring reoperation	0 (0.00%)	1 (0.41%)	–
3	Bleeding requiring reoperation	0 (0.00%)	1 (0.41%)	–

steps of the operation. The incidence of intraoperative difficulties, which was based on the operator's subjective opinion, was higher in the residents' than the specialists' group. More than half of these difficulties enforced an active tutoring and a change of the operator. This parameter was never explored in the field of LA. Notably, the difference in operator conversion between the two groups was not statistically significant and was not related to a higher complication rate. This means that operator conversion was an effective tactic to prevent complications. However, it shows that LA can still be challenging even for specialists.

Another interesting finding is the similar operative time for residents and attending surgeons. Longer operative time seems somewhat natural in the course of a learning curve and for the sake of safety, no time pressure should be put on learning residents. A similar operative time for residents and specialists can be natural when related to the tactic of choosing potentially easier cases for beginners and more difficult (that is, longer-lasting surgeries) for more experienced surgeons. In our department, the tactic of choosing potentially easier cases for residents was not observed. The results were similar to those of Horesh but differ from these of Goldfarb, Seib, and Venkat, who showed that residents operate for longer. We think that this phenomenon could be due to "learning from the experience of the more experienced." This was described by Geubbels et al., who wrote that some surgeons benefit directly from the experience already gained by more experienced colleagues and then "learn to operate faster." Furthermore, institutional experience grows parallel to individual experience over time [26]. They confirmed surgical experience as the primary explanation for a decrease in surgical time but he emphasized that as decrease in operating time in case of bariatric procedures after every 50 patients is indeed well explained by an increase in experience, the differences among the surgeons are not [26]. Most attending surgeons at the beginning of our study were specialists just for 2–3 years, so were probably close to their learning curve stabilization point then. The mean operation time in our study was shorter than that in other reports [21–24].

Another interesting finding was that patients operated by residents had shorter LOS. Similarly to our findings, Seib [21] noted that residents participation as an operator has a positive effect on LOS. It is not clear why patients operated by specialists had a statistically significant longer hospital stay. It could be explained, again, by the selection bias resulting in more easy cases operated by residents as shown previously.

Recent surveys showed that surgical residents, even in highly developed countries, are concerned about their training in minimally invasive techniques and conclude

Table 6 End points of the study

Parameter	All	Group 1 (residents)	Group 2 (specialists)	*p* value
Mean operative time (min, ± SD))	103.5 (30–350, SD ±43.5)	106.5 (45–220, SD ± 33.35)	102.8 (30–350, SD ± 45.40	0.5761
Median blood loss (ml, IQR)	50 (20–100) ml	50 (30–100) ml	50 (20–100) ml	0.4325
Intraoperative adverse events, n (%)	26 (8.67%)	5 (9.26%)	21 (8.54%)	0.8643
Complications, n (%)	15 (5.00%)	3 (5.56%)	12 (4.88%)	0.6442
Intraoperative difficulties, n (%)	40 (13.33%)	13 (24.07%)	27 (10.98%)	0.0104
Conversion of the operator, n (%)	25 (8.33%)	7 (12.96%)	18 (7.32%)	0.1741
Conversion to open surgery, n (%)	2 (0.67%)	0 (0.00%)	2 (0.81%)	–
Reoperation, n (%)	2 (0.67%)	0 (0.00%)	2 (0.81%)	–
Readmission, n (%)	5 (1.67%)	0 (0.00%)	5 (2.03%)	–
Mean length of hospital stay (days, ± SD)	1.93 (1–2, SD ±1.11)	1.69 (1–2, SD ±0.97)	1.98 (1–2, SD ±1.14)	0.0422
30-day mortality rate, n (%)	0 (0.00%)	0 (0.00%)	0 (0.00%)	–

that most are unprepared for autonomous laparoscopic operations [27, 28]. Modifications of the residency program are required to fulfill both the needs of residents and expectations of the patients to get a laparoscopic approach to most of the abdominal pathologies. Residents should also be encouraged to use any sort of laparoscopic trainer to further improve their laparoscopic skills. However, safe minimally invasive techniques training should generally be limited to high volume centers.

This study has several limitations. Our institution is a referral center for general surgery specialized in minimally invasive techniques and a teaching hospital. It was impossible to include several variabilities such as the influence of previous experience of residents in minimally invasive techniques. Moreover, it was impossible to include individual skills and natural predispositions in surgical performance. Another limitation is the retrospective nature of the study, which was performed without randomization. Quite naturally for those settings, the group of patients was quite heterogenous and selection bias could impact the results. Therefore, a prospective study should be designed to confirm these findings.

Conclusions

The results of our study have shown that laparoscopic transperitoneal adrenalectomy performed by a supervised resident is a safe procedure. There is no difference in operating time between residents and specialists as operating surgeons. Patients operated on by residents have shorter LOS in hospital. Liberal use of "operator conversions" from resident to attending surgeon and from a surgeon to a senior surgeon provides reasonable safety and prevents complications.

In the setting of high volume centers of minimally invasive techniques, closed supervision allows residents to safely perform LA.

Abbreviations

BMI: body mass index; CI: confidence interval; CT: computed tomography; LA: laparoscopic adrenalectomy; LOS: length of hospital stay; MRI: magnetic resonance imaging; OR: odds ratio; PET: positron emission computed tomography; SD: standard deviation

Acknowledgements

Not applicable

Authors' contributions

JD – made substantial contributions to conception and design, analysis and interpretation of data, was involved in drafting the manuscript or revising it critically for important intellectual content. MW – made substantial contributions to acquisition of data, analysis and interpretation of data. AR – made substantial contributions to acquisition of data. MN - made substantial contributions to acquisition of data, analysis and interpretation of data. MP – made substantial contributions to analysis and interpretation of data. AB – was involved in drafting the manuscript or revising it critically for important intellectual content. PM – made substantial contributions to conception and design, was involved in drafting the manuscript or revising it critically for important intellectual content. All authors read and approved the final manuscript, agreed to be accountable for all aspects of the work in ensuring that questions related to the accuracy or integrity of any part of the work are appropriately investigated and resolved.

References

1. Gagner M, Lacroix A, Bolte E. Laparoscopic adrenalectomy in Cushing's syndrome and pheochromocytoma. N Engl J Med. 1992;327:1003.
2. Maccabee DL, Jones A, Domreis J, et al. Transition from open to laparoscopic adrenalectomy: the need for advanced training. Surg Endosc. 2003;17:1566–9.
3. Natkaniec M, Pedziwiatr M, Wierdak M, et al. Laparoscopic adrenalectomy for pheochromocytoma is more difficult compared to other adrenal tumors. Wideochir Inne Tech Maloinwazyjne. 2015;10(3):466–71.
4. Pędziwiatr M, Wierdak M, Ostachowski M, et al. Single center outcomes of laparoscopic transperitoneal lateral adrenalectomy - Lessons learned after 500 cases: A retrospective cohort study. Int Surg. 2015;20:88–94.
5. Zhang X, Wang B, Ma X, et al. Laparoscopic adrenalectomy for beginners without open counterpart experience: initial results under staged training. Urology. 2009;73:1061–5.
6. Sefr R, Penka I, Olivero R, et al. The impact of laparoendoscopic surgery on the training of surgical residents. Int Surg. 1995;80(4):358–60.
7. Itani KM, DePalma RG, Schifftner T, Sanders KM, Chang BK, et al. Surgical resident supervision in the operating room and outcomes of care in veterans affairs hospitals. Am J Surg. 2005;190:725.
8. Khuri SF, Henderson WG, Daley J, Jonasson O, Jones RS, et al. Successful implementation of the Department of Veterans Affairs' National Surgical Quality Improvement Program in the private sector: the patient safety in surgery study. Ann Surg. 2008;248:329.
9 Fischer CP, Hong JC. Early perioperative outcomes and pancreaticoduodenectomy in a general surgery residency training program. J Gastrointest Surg: official J Soc Surg Aliment Tract. 2006;10:478.
10. Zacharias M, Haese A, Jurczok A, Stolzenburg JU, Fornara P. Transperitoneal Laparoscopic Adrenalectomy: Outline of the Preoperative Management, Surgical Approach, and Outcome. *Eur Urol.* 2006; 49 (2006) 448–459.
11. Major P, Matlok M, Pedziwiatr M, et al. Do we really need routine drainage after laparoscopic adrenalectomy and splenectomy? Wideochir Inne Tech Maloinwazyjne. 2012;7(1):33–9.
12. Dindo D, Demartines N, Clavien PA. Classification of surgical complications: a new proposal with evaluation in a cohort of 6336 patients and results of a survey. Ann Surg. 2004;240(2):205–13. https://doi.org/10.1097/01.sla.0000133083.54934.ae.
13. World Medical Association. World medical association declaration of Helsinki: ethical principles for medical research involving human subjects. JAMA. 2013;310:2191–4.
14. Agha R, Muir G. Does laparoscopic surgery spell the end of the open surgeon? J Royal Society of Med. 2003;96(11):544–6.
15. Pędziwiatr M, Natkaniec M, Kisialeuski M, et al. Adrenal incidentalomas: should we operate on small tumors in the era of laparoscopy? Int J Endocrinol. 2014;2014:658483. https://doi.org/10.1155/2014/658483.
16. Fiszer P, Toutounchi S, Pogorzelski R, Krajewska E, Ciesla W, Skórski M. Laparoscopic adrenalectomy – assessing the learning curve. Pol Przegl Chir. 2012;84:293–7.
17. Guerrieri M, Campagnacci R, De Sanctis A, Baldarelli M, Coletta M, Perretta S. The learning curve in laparoscopic adrenalectomy. J Endocrinol Investig. 2008;31:531–6.
18. Goitein D, Mintz Y, Gross D, Reissman P. Laparoscopic adrenalectomy: ascending the learning curve. Surg Endosc. 2004;18:771–3.
19. Treter S, Perrier N, Sosa JA, Roman S. Telementoring: a multi-institutional experience with the introduction of a novel surgical approach for adrenalectomy. Ann Surg Oncol. 2013;20:2754–8.
20. Pędziwiatr M, Matłok M, Kulawik J, et al. Laparoscopic adrenalectomy by the lateral transperitoneal approach in patients with a history of previous abdominal surgery. Wideochir Inne Tech Maloinwazyjne. 2013;8(2):146–51. https://doi.org/10.5114/wiitm.2011.32942.
21. Seib CD, Greenblatt DY, Campbell MJ, et al. Adrenalectomy outcomes are superior with the participation of residents and fellows. J Am Coll Surg. 2014;219(1):53–60. https://doi.org/10.1016/j.jamcollsurg.2014.02.020.
22. Venkat R, Valdivia PL, Guerrero MA. Resident participation and postoperative outcomes in adrenal surgery. J Surg Res. 2014;190(2):559–64. https://doi.org/10.1016/j.jss.2014.05.025 Epub 2014 May 20.

23. Horesh N, Jacoby H, Dreznik Y, Nadler R, Amiel I, Dotan ZA et al. Teaching Laparoscopic Adrenalectomy to Surgical Residents. *J of Laparoendoscopic & Advanced surgical Techniques* 2016 Volume 26, Number 6, doi: https://doi.org/10.1089/lap.2015.0625.
24. Goldfarb M, Gondek S, Hodin R, Parangi S. Resident/fellow assistance in the operating room for endocrine surgery in the era of fellowships. Surgery. 2010;148(6):1065–71; discussion 1071-2. https://doi.org/10.1016/j.surg.2010.09.010.
25. Stefanidis D, Goldfarb M, Kercher KW, Hope WW, Richardson W, Fanelli RD. SAGES guidelines for minimally invasive treatment of adrenal pathology. Surg Endosc. 2013;27:3960–80.
26. Geubbels N, de Brauw LM, Acherman YI, van de Laar AW, Wouters MW, Bruin SC. The preceding surgeon factor in bariatric surgery:a positive influence on the learning curve of subsequent surgeons. Obes Surg. 2015; 25(8):1417–24. https://doi.org/10.1007/s11695-014-1538-x.
27. De Win G, Everaerts W, De Ridder D, et al. Laparoscopy training in Belgium: results from a nationwide survey, in urology, gynecology, and general surgery residents. Adv Med Educ Pract. 2015;6:55–63.
28. Qureshi A, Vergis A, Jimenez C, et al. MIS training in Canada: a national survey of general surgery residents. Surg Endosc. 2011;25(9):3057–65.

28

Outcome of buccal mucosa graft urethroplasty: A detailed analysis of success, morbidity and quality of life in a contemporary patient cohort at a referral center

Armin Soave†, Luis Kluth†, Roland Dahlem, Amelie Rohwer, Michael Rink, Philipp Reiss, Margit Fisch and Oliver Engel*

Abstract

Background: To evaluate outcome of buccal mucosa graft urethroplasty (BMGU) for the treatment of urethral stricture disease, including a detailed analysis of success, morbidity and quality of life (QoL).

Methods: Between 12/05/2008 and 07/21/2010, 187 patients with urethral stricture disease, who were treated with BMGU at our University Medical Center, received a standardized questionnaire, evaluating postoperative success, morbidity and QoL. The primary endpoint was the success, i.e., stricture recurrence-free survival plus patients' satisfaction with surgery. Secondary endpoints included erectile function, voiding symptoms, pain and health-related QoL, which were assessed with a modified Urethral Stricture Surgery Patient Reported Outcome Measure (USS PROM), including the Erectile Function domain of the International Index of Erectile Function (IIEF-EF), Incontinence Questionnaire Male Lower Urinary Tract Symptoms Module (ICIQ-MLUTS) and EuroQol-5 dimensions (EQ-5D).

Results: In total, 83 patients (51.9%) completed the questionnaire. Bulbar, penile and panurethral strictures were found in 69 patients (83.1%), 13 patients (15.7%) and one patient (1.2%), respectively. The median length of the stricture was 5 cm (range: 1–16). At a median follow-up of 46 months (range: 36–54), 65 patients (78.3%) had no stricture recurrence and were satisfied with BMGU. Median scores for ICIQ-MLUTS, IIEF-EF and EQ-5D visual analogue scale were 6, 22 and 80, respectively. Based on USS PROM, postoperative improvement of QoL and satisfaction with BMGU was found in 67 patients (80.7%) and 68 patients (81.9%), respectively.

Conclusions: In patients with urethral stricture disease, BMGU offers excellent success, morbidity and QoL.

Keywords: Urethra, Urethral stricture, Buccal mucosa, Reconstructive surgical procedure, Treatment outcome

Background

Substitution urethroplasty is the gold standard treatment for long primary urethral strictures and recurrent urethral stricture disease [1]. Depending on the stricture's length, location and etiology, various single-stage and two-stage techniques for substitution urethroplasty have been successfully established in daily clinical practice [2], including ventral onlay [3], dorsal inlay [4] or modified procedures [5]. Due to its favorable availability, simple processing and durable integration in the urethra [6], autologous buccal mucosa currently remains the most commonly used transplant for substitution urethroplasty [1, 7].

Several studies confirmed excellent stricture recurrence-free survival of buccal mucosa graft urethroplasty (BMGU) for the treatment of USD [5, 8]. In contrast, outcome comprising morbidity and health-related quality of life (QoL) has been poorly investigated thus far. In addition, previous studies included heterogeneous patient

* Correspondence: o.engel@uke.de
†Armin Soave and Luis Kluth contributed equally to this work.
Department of Urology, University Medical Center Hamburg-Eppendorf, Martinistraße 52, 20246 Hamburg, Germany

cohorts, various urethroplasty procedures and mainly lack of standardized validated instruments such as patient-reported outcome measures (PROM) [9–11], which might complicate the comparability of results. In 2011, Jackson et al. introduced Urethral Stricture Surgery (USS) PROM, facilitating a standardized outcome evaluation of voiding symptoms, health related QoL (HRQoL) and satisfaction with treatment [12]. A German language version of USS PROM with additional assessment of erectile function and urinary incontinence has recently been validated [13].

The aim of the present study was to evaluate in detail success, morbidity and HRQoL of BMGU for the treatment of urethral stricture disease in a contemporary, homogeneous patient cohort, using USS PROM.

Methods

Patient cohort

Data on 187 patients with urethral stricture disease, who were treated with BMGU at the University Medical Center Hamburg-Eppendorf between 12/05/2008 and 07/21/2010, were prospectively collected in the local urethroplasty database and retrospectively reviewed following Institutional Review Board approval (local ethics committee approval number PV4123). Patients were included following written consent from each patient. Inclusion criteria were patients with urethral stricture disease, who were treated with BMGU at our institution. Patients' refusal to participate in the study was an exclusion criteria.

Surgical procedure

BMGU has previously been described extensively [8, 13]. In brief, based on the location and length of the urethral stricture, single-stage or two-stage BMGU was performed [3, 5, 14, 15].

Questionnaire

All patients received the validated German language version of the USS-PROM [13], addressing voiding symptoms, patients' satisfaction and HRQoL including the following questionnaires: The International Consultation on Incontinence Questionnaire Male Lower Urinary Tract Symptoms (ICIQ-MLUTS) with an additional LUTS-specific QoL question from the ICIQ-MLUTSqol [16, 17]; The Peeling's voiding picture; The EuroQuol 5D including pain evaluation and a visual analogue scale (VAS) [18]. In order to assess erectile function, the Erectile Function domain of the International Index of Erectile Function (IIEF-EF) [19] was added. On July 25th 2013, the questionnaire was sent to 187 patients in paper form by post. Patients received the questionnaire at home.

Statistical analysis

The primary endpoint was the success rate following BMGU. Success was defined as stricture recurrence-free survival plus patients' satisfaction with BMGU. Stricture recurrence was defined as any re-intervention and/or instrumentation following BMGU, including catheterization of the bladder or dilatation of the urethra. Patients' satisfaction with BMGU was assessed with the question "Are you satisfied with the outcome of BMGU?" with the following answering possibilities: "very satisfied", "satisfied", "undecided", "dissatisfied" and "very dissatisfied". Only patients answering "very satisfied" or "satisfied" were classified as satisfied with BMGU. Erectile function, voiding symptoms, pain and health-related QoL were secondary endpoints of the present study. Stricture recurrence-free survival and success probabilities were assessed with the Kaplan-Meier method. Differences between groups were measured using the Logrank statistic. Univariable Cox regression was used to assess time to stricture recurrence. Associations between categorical variables were evaluated with the Fisher exact and χ^2-tests. Differences in continuous variables were evaluated with the Mann-Whitney-U test (two categories) and the Kruskal-Wallis test (three or more categories). All tests are two-sided. A p-value of < 0.05 was defined to be statistically significant. All analyses were made with SPSS 23 (SPSS Inc., IBM Corp., Armonk, NY).

Results

Patients' characteristics

In total, 187 patients underwent BMGU for urethral stricture disease between 12/05/2008 and 07/21/2010 at our center. Of these, 83 patients (44.4%) completed the questionnaire and were included in analyses. Table 1 presents clinical characteristics of the study cohort. In total, 69 patients (83.1%) had a stricture of the bulbar urethra. Single-stage BMGU was performed in 75 patients (90.4%). Prior surgical urethral interventions included direct visual internal urethrotomy, urethroplasty and dilatation in 59 patients (71.1%), 17 patients (20.5%) and 40 patients (48.2%), respectively.

Outcome

At a median follow-up of 46 months (range: 36–54 months), success was found in 65 patients (78.3%), and 73 patients (88.0%) had no stricture recurrence (Fig. 1). There was no difference in the probability of success and stricture recurrence-free survival among patients with and without previous surgical urethral interventions, according the stricture length stratified by ≤5 cm and > 5 cm, as well as according patients' age stratified by ≤60 years and > 60 years (Fig. 2).

Following BMGU, post-micturition dribbling and streaking the urethra was observed in 45 patients

Table 1 Clinical characteristics of 83 patients with urethral stricture disease treated with buccal mucosa graft urethroplasty

Age years [median (range)]	61 (16; 77)
Follow-up months [median (range)]	46 (36; 54)
Location of the stricture patients (%)	
Bulbar urethra	69 (83.1)
Penile urethra	13 (15.7)
Panurethral	1 (1.2)
Length of the stricture cm [median (range)]	5 (1; 16)
Procedure patients (%)	
Single-stage	75 (90.4)
Two-stage	8 (9.6)
Previous surgical urethral interventions patients (%)	63 (75.9)
Number of direct visual internal urethrotomies	
1	12 (14.5)
2–5	38 (45.8)
> 5	9 (10.8)
Number of urethroplasties	
1	14 (16.9)
> 1	3 (3.6)
Number of dilatations	
≥ 1	40 (48.2)

(54.2%) and 39 patients (46.1%), respectively. Severe penile shortening, penile curvature and hypoesthesia of the glans or scrotum was reported by 2 patients (2.4%), respectively. Fifty patients (60.3%) had erections with normal or slightly reduced rigidity. Forty-three patients (51.8%) had a normal or slightly reduced ejaculate volume and 9 patients (10.8%) had painful sensations during ejaculation. In total, 7 patients (8.4%) described a strong impairment of sexuality.

Table 2 displays data on erectile function, voiding symptoms, pain and QoL. Based on USS PROM, 67 patients (80.7%) and 68 patients (81.9%) reported improvement of HRQoL and satisfaction with the surgical procedure, respectively. There was no difference in ICIQ-MLUTS, Peeling's voiding picture, IIEF-EF, ICIQ-MLUTSqol and EQ-5D among patients with and without previous surgical urethral interventions as well as according the stricture length stratified by ≤5 cm and > 5 cm (data not shown). There was no difference in ICIQ-MLUTS, Peeling's voiding picture, ICIQ-MLUTSqol and EQ-5D among patients with an age ≤ 60 years and > 60 years (data not shown). Patients ≤60 years of age had elevated IIEF-EF scores compared to patients > 60 years of age (median IIEF-EF in patients ≤60 years vs. > 60 years: 29 vs. 3; *p*-value≤0.001).

Risk factor analysis for reduced success and stricture recurrence

In univariable Cox regression analysis, neither previous surgical urethral interventions, nor stricture length, nor patients' age were associated with a reduced success or increased stricture recurrence following BMGU (data not shown).

Discussion

We found that BMGU offers excellent outcome in a contemporary patient cohort with urethral stricture disease. Nearly 90% of patients did not require any form of re-intervention or instrumentation at a maximum follow-up exceeding 4 years, which is in line to results of earlier studies with 66 to 100% stricture recurrence-free survival at 15 to 83 months follow-up [7]. Based on strict success criteria, we found that the success rate of 78% was lower than the stricture recurrence-free survival. A reason for this discrepancy may certainly be the fact that outcome measure comprising the factor patients' satisfaction may facilitate a more patient-oriented evaluation of the success of BMGU. Thus, our findings emphasize the importance of the inclusion of PROM in the evaluation of BMGU outcome. Indeed, although PROM does not allow an objective assessment of surgical complications, it adds crucial information on patients' subjective morbidity, including voiding symptoms, erectile function, pain and health-related QoL following BMGU.

We found favorable Peeling's voiding picture and ICIQ-MLUTS scores following BMGU, which corresponds to earlier reports [8, 13, 20]. Conversely, voiding symptoms including post-micturition dribbling and streaking the urethra were quite frequently reported in the present study. This discrepancy may indicate that patients do not consider these symptoms to be bothering. Indeed, based on ICIQ-MLUTSqol, more than 80% of patients reported that urinary symptoms did not interfere with life, which is comparable to the results of earlier studies [20]. The median IIEF-EF score showed mild erectile dysfunction, and a relevant proportion of patients reported erections with reduced rigidity. Other impairments of sexual function comprised reduced ejaculate volume, painful ejaculation, penile shortening and curvature as well as hypoesthesia of the glans or scrotum, which corresponds to previously reported findings [8, 21, 22]. However, more than 90% of patients did not report a strong deterioration of their sexuality. Other authors have previously shown variable impairment of sexual function and IIEF scores following BMGU [8, 13, 23–25]. Heterogeneity across different studies may be due to variable evaluation methods of sexual and erectile function, including inconsistent implementation of IIEF [21, 22, 26]. Importantly, our findings emphasize again the need of a standardized

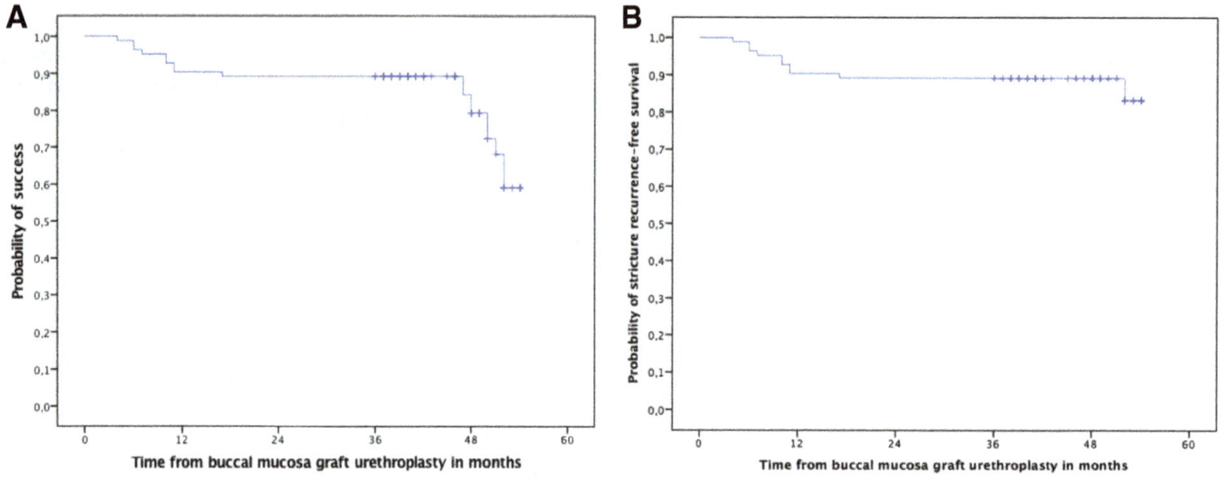

Patients at risk for success

Months				
0	**12**	**24**	**36**	**48**
83	75	74	55	21

Patients at risk for stricture recurrence

Months				
0	**12**	**24**	**36**	**48**
83	75	74	54	18

Fig. 1 Kaplan-Meier plots of success (**a**) and stricture recurrence-free survival (**b**) in 83 patients with urethral stricture disease treated with buccal mucosa graft urethroplasty

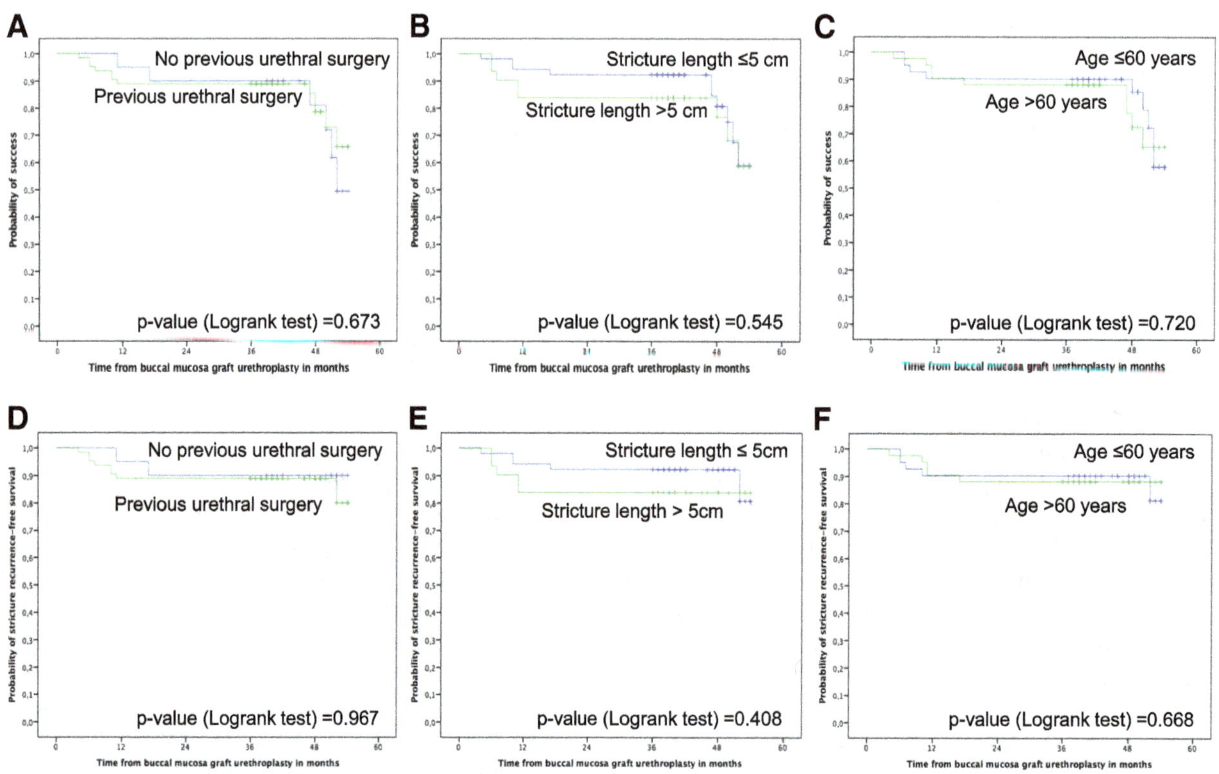

Fig. 2 Kaplan-Meier plots of success (**a**, **b**, **c**) and stricture recurrence-free survival (**d**, **e**, **f**) in 83 patients with urethral stricture disease treated with buccal mucosa graft urethroplasty stratified by previous urethral surgery status (**a**, **d**), stricture length (**b**, **e**) and age (**c**, **f**)

Table 2 Erectile function, voiding symptoms, pain and health related quality of life of 83 patients with urethral stricture disease treated with buccal mucosa graft urethroplasty

Voiding symptoms	
ICIQ-MLUTS score [median (range)]	6 (0; 17)
Peeling's voiding picture [median (range)]	2 (1; 4)
Erectile function	
IIEF-EF score [median (range)]	22 (1; 30)
Health related quality of life	
ICIQ-MLUTSqol	
Urinary symptoms interfere with life – a little or not at all [patients (%)]	68 (81.9)
EQ-5D: severe pain postoperatively [patients (%)]	1 (1.2)
EQ-5D VAS [median (range)]	80 (20; 100)
Surgical outcome	
USS PROM: improvement of quality of life [patients (%)]	67 (80.7)
USS PROM: satisfaction with surgical procedure [patients (%)]	68 (81.9)

assessment of sexual and erectile function following BMGU. We found that the majority of patients did not experience strong pain postoperatively, which is reflected by low EQ-5D VAS scores and corresponds to earlier findings [8, 13, 20]. In accordance to a favorable postoperative morbidity, more than 80% of patients described an improvement of HRQoL and satisfaction with BMGU.

We did not find differences in success and morbidity among patients with and without previous urethral interventions as well as according to stricture length and patients' age. Not surprisingly, these factors were not associated with an increased risk for failure and stricture recurrence in univariable analysis. In contrast, other authors have previously identified prior urethral interventions, stricture length and age as potential independent predictors for stricture recurrence and failure [27–29]. Variable findings across studies may be due to differences in cohort sizes, surgical urethroplasty techniques, follow-up and the definition of success. For example, patients with posterior urethral stricture were excluded from analyses [28] and stricture recurrence-free survival was assessed by urethrocystoscopy and symptom inquiry [29]. In fact, further studies are needed to clearly define risk factors for stricture recurrence and failure following BMGU.

The present study has relevant limitations. First and foremost are limitations inherent to the retrospective study design including a limited follow-up. Patients did not receive USS PROM preoperatively. Thus, baseline data on ICIQ-MLUTS, Peeling's voiding picture, IIEF-EF, ICIQ-MLUTSqol, EQ-5D and VAS was not available. This represents an important limitation of the present study, since a comparison of preoperative and postoperative voiding, erectile function, urinary continence and quality of life was not possible. Thus, there remains a risk of bias regarding the impact of urethroplasty on patient reported outcomes. In addition, the response rate is limited and to draw conclusion regarding the patients who did not answer the questionnaire is not possible, which might represent a source of bias. The specific reasons for the limited response rate remain unknown. Patients received the questionnaire at variable time points following BMGU, which might have influenced the results, since the length of follow-up seems to be a predictor for stricture recurrence [27]. Data on buccal mucosa donor site complications were not available, although donor site morbidity may certainly have a detrimental impact on patients' satisfaction and QoL [30]. Moreover, the present study did not comprise instrument-based outcome measure, i,e. urethral calibration, uroflowmetry, urethrography and urethrocystoscopy. These techniques may allow a more surgery-oriented outcome evaluation. In addition, instrument-based outcome measure and comparison to baseline values allows objective evaluation of surgical results. Missing data on urethral calibration, uroflowmetry, urethrography and urethrocystocopy following BMGU represents a limitation of the present study. Urethral calibration can identify narrowing of the urethral diameter and may detect stricture recurrence early following urethroplasty. However, stricture recurrences have to narrow the urethra to a caliber <10F to result in a relevant decrease of urinary flow rates [7]. In addition, urethrography implicates the use of radiation, and urethrocystoscopy is an invasive procedure, which may be problematic for monitoring patients with USD. Finally, urethral calibration, uroflowmetry, urethrography and urethrocystoscopy may not allow assessing adequately the morbidity of BMGU, which was a secondary endpoint of the present study. The present study did focus on success, morbidity and HRQoL of urethroplasty. Therefore, the utilization of USS-PROM is appropriate, since it represents a validated instrument allowing standardized patient-orientated outcome evaluation of success, voiding symptoms, quality of life and satisfaction.

Conclusions

In patients with urethral stricture disease, BMGU offers excellent outcome, success, morbidity and QoL, independently of previous urethral interventions, patients' age and stricture length. Prior surgery, patients should be counseled on morbidity of BMGU, including voiding symptoms, pain and impairment of sexual and erectile function. USS PROM allows a detailed and standardized analysis of success, morbidity and HRQoL, and should therefore be consistently utilized in outcome reporting of BMGU.

Abbreviations

EQ-5D VAS: Euro QoL 5D Visual Analogue Scale; EQ-5D: Euro QoL 5D; ICIQ-MLUTS: Incontinence Questionnaire Male Lower Urinary Tract Symptoms Module; ICIQ-MLUTSqol: LUTS-specific QoL Question of Incontinence Questionnaire Male Lower Urinary Tract Symptoms Module; IIEF-EF: Erectile Function domain of the International Index of Erectile Function; PROM: Patient Reported Outcome Measure; QoL: Quality of life

Acknowledgements

None.

Authors' contributions

AS, conception and design, analysis and interpretation of data, paper writing. LK, acquisition of data and analysis of data, paper writing. RD, drafting the manuscript and revising it critically. AR, conception and design, acquisition of data, analysis and interpretation of data. MR, involved in drafting the manuscript and revising it critically. PR, analysis and interpretation of data. MF, conception and design, drafting the manuscript and revising it critically. OE, conception and design, analysis and interpretation of data, paper writing and drafting the manuscript. All authors have read and approved of the final version and the publication of the manuscript.

References

1. Chapple C, Andrich D, Atala A, et al. SIU/ICUD consultation on urethral strictures: the Management of Anterior Urethral Stricture Disease Using Substitution Urethroplasty. Urology. 2014;83:S31–47.
2. Mundy AR, Andrich DE. Urethral strictures. BJU Int. 2011;107:6–26.
3. Ahyai SA, Schmid M, Kuhl M, et al. Outcomes of ventral Onlay buccal mucosa graft Urethroplasty in patients after radiotherapy. J Urol. 2015;194: 441–6.
4. Marshall SD, Raup VT, Brandes SB. Dorsal inlay buccal mucosal graft (Asopa) urethroplasty for anterior urethral stricture. Transl Androl Urol. 2015;4:10–5.
5. Pfalzgraf D, Kluth L, Isbarn H, et al. The Barbagli technique: 3-year experience with a modified approach. BJU Int. 2013;111:E132–6.
6. Soave A, Steurer S, Dahlem R, et al. Histopathological characteristics of buccal mucosa transplants in humans after engraftment to the urethra: a prospective study. J Urol. 2014;192:1725–9.
7. Mangera A, Patterson JM, Chapple CR. A systematic review of graft augmentation Urethroplasty techniques for the treatment of anterior urethral strictures. Eur Urol. 2011;59:797–814.
8. Kluth LA, Dahlem R, Reiss P, et al. Short-term outcome and morbidity of different contemporary Urethroplasty techniques—a preliminary comparison. J Endourol. 2013;27:925–9.
9. Barbagli G, Kulkarni SB, Fossati N, et al. Long-term Followup and deterioration rate of anterior substitution Urethroplasty. J Urol. 2014;192:808–13.
10. Elliott SP, Metro MJ, McAninch JW. Long-term Followup of the ventrally placed buccal mucosa Onlay graft in bulbar urethral reconstruction. J Urol. 2003;169:1754–7.
11. Kellner DS, Fracchia JA, Armenakas NA. Ventral onlay buccal mucosal grafts for anterior urethral strictures: long-term followup. J Urol. 2004;171:726–9.
12. Jackson MJ, Sciberras J, Mangera A, et al. Defining a patient-reported outcome measure for urethral stricture surgery. Eur Urol. 2011;60:60–8.
13. Kluth LA, Dahlem R, Becker A, et al. Psychometric validation of a German language version of a PROM for urethral stricture surgery and preliminary testing of supplementary ED and UI constructs. World J Urol. 2015;34:369–75.
14. Riechardt S, Fisch M. Two-stage urethroplasty with buccal mucosa. BJU Int. 2012;109:150–62.
15. Riechardt S, Pfalzgraf D, Dahlem R, et al. Dorsal buccal mucosal inlay for penile urethroplasty. BJU Int. 2009;103:1444–7.
16. Donovan JL, Abrams P, Peters TJ, et al. The ICS-'BPH' study: the psychometric validity and reliability of the ICSmale questionnaire. Br J Urol. 1996;77:554–62.
17. Donovan JL, Peters T, Abrams P, et al. Scoring the short form ICSmaleSF questionnaire. International continence society. J Urol. 2000;164:1948–55.
18. EurQoL Group. EuroQol--a new facility for the measurement of health-related quality of life. Health Policy. 1990;16:199–208.
19. Rosen RC, Riley A, Wagner G, et al. The international index of erectile function (IIEF): a multidimensional scale for assessment of erectile dysfunction. Urology. 1997;49:822–30.
20. Jackson MJ, Chaudhury I, Mangera A, et al. A prospective patient-centred evaluation of Urethroplasty for anterior urethral stricture using a validated patient-reported outcome measure. Eur Urol. 2013;64:777–82.
21. Erickson BA, Wysock JS, McVary KT, et al. Erectile function, sexual drive, and ejaculatory function after reconstructive surgery for anterior urethral stricture disease. BJU Int. 2007;99:607–11.
22. Sharma V, Kumar S, Mandal AK, et al. A study on sexual function of men with anterior urethral stricture before and after treatment. Urol Int. 2011;87: 341–5.
23. Erickson BA, Granieri MA, Meeks JJ, et al. Prospective analysis of erectile dysfunction after anterior Urethroplasty: incidence and recovery of function. J Urol. 2010;183:657–61.
24. Dogra PN, Saini AK, Seth A. Erectile dysfunction after anterior Urethroplasty: a prospective analysis of incidence and probability of recovery—single-center experience. Urology. 2011;78:78–81.
25. Blaschko SD, Sanford MT, Cinman NM, et al. De novo erectile dysfunction after anterior urethroplasty: a systematic review and meta-analysis. BJU Int. 2013;112:655–63.
26. Levine MA, Kinnaird AS, Rourke KF. Revision Urethroplasty success is comparable to primary Urethroplasty: a comparative analysis. Urology. 2014; 84:928–32.
27. Han JS, Liu J, Hofer MD, et al. Risk of urethral stricture recurrence increases over time after urethroplasty. Int J Urol. 2015;22:695–9.
28. Breyer BN, McAninch JW, Whitson JM, et al. Multivariate analysis of risk factors for long-term Urethroplasty outcome. J Urol. 2010;183:613–7.
29. Hoy NY, Kinnaird A, Rourke KF. Expanded use of a dorsal onlay augmented anastomotic Urethroplasty with buccal mucosa for long segment bulbar urethral strictures: analysis of outcomes and complications. Urology. 2013; 81:1357–61.
30. Rourke K, McKinny S, St. Martin B. Effect of wound closure on buccal mucosal graft harvest site morbidity: results of a randomized prospective trial. Urology. 2012;79:443–7.

Permissions

All chapters in this book were first published by BioMed Central; hereby published with permission under the Creative Commons Attribution License or equivalent. Every chapter published in this book has been scrutinized by our experts. Their significance has been extensively debated. The topics covered herein carry significant findings which will fuel the growth of the discipline. They may even be implemented as practical applications or may be referred to as a beginning point for another development.

The contributors of this book come from diverse backgrounds, making this book a truly international effort. This book will bring forth new frontiers with its revolutionizing research information and detailed analysis of the nascent developments around the world.

We would like to thank all the contributing authors for lending their expertise to make the book truly unique. They have played a crucial role in the development of this book. Without their invaluable contributions this book wouldn't have been possible. They have made vital efforts to compile up to date information on the varied aspects of this subject to make this book a valuable addition to the collection of many professionals and students.

This book was conceptualized with the vision of imparting up-to-date information and advanced data in this field. To ensure the same, a matchless editorial board was set up. Every individual on the board went through rigorous rounds of assessment to prove their worth. After which they invested a large part of their time researching and compiling the most relevant data for our readers.

The editorial board has been involved in producing this book since its inception. They have spent rigorous hours researching and exploring the diverse topics which have resulted in the successful publishing of this book. They have passed on their knowledge of decades through this book. To expedite this challenging task, the publisher supported the team at every step. A small team of assistant editors was also appointed to further simplify the editing procedure and attain best results for the readers.

Apart from the editorial board, the designing team has also invested a significant amount of their time in understanding the subject and creating the most relevant covers. They scrutinized every image to scout for the most suitable representation of the subject and create an appropriate cover for the book.

The publishing team has been an ardent support to the editorial, designing and production team. Their endless efforts to recruit the best for this project, has resulted in the accomplishment of this book. They are a veteran in the field of academics and their pool of knowledge is as vast as their experience in printing. Their expertise and guidance has proved useful at every step. Their uncompromising quality standards have made this book an exceptional effort. Their encouragement from time to time has been an inspiration for everyone.

The publisher and the editorial board hope that this book will prove to be a valuable piece of knowledge for researchers, students, practitioners and scholars across the globe.

List of Contributors

Min Seok Kim, Won Sik Jang, Doo Yong Chung, Dong Hoon Koh, Jong Soo Lee and Hyeok Jun Goh
Department of Urology and Urological Science Institute, Yonsei University College of Medicine, 50-1, Yonsei-ro, Seodaemun-gu, Seoul 03722, Republic of Korea

Young Deuk Choi
Department of Urology, Severance Hospital, Urological Science Institute, Yonsei University College of Medicine, 50-1, Yonsei-ro, Seodaemun-gu, Seoul 03722, Republic of Korea

Yoann Koskas, François Lannes, Nicolas Branger, Dominique Rossi and Cyrille Bastide
Department of Urology, Hopital Nord, Chemin des Bourrely, 13015 Marseille, France

Sophie Giusiano
Department of Anatomic Pathology, Hôpital nord, Chemin des Bourrely, 13015 Marseille, France

Géraldine Pignot and Jochen Walz
Departement of urology, Institut Paoli-Calmettes, 13008 Marseille, France

Nicolas Guibert
Centre hospitalier universitaire de Lyon, Lyon, France
Hopital Edouard Herriot, 69003 Lyon, France

Tyler Overholt
School of Medicine, West Virginia University, Morgantown, USA

Morris Jessop, John Barnard and Osama Al-Omar
Department of Urology, West Virginia University, Morgantown, USA

Mehdi Shirazi
Department of Urology, Shiraz University of Medical Sciences, Shiraz, Iran
Histomorphometry and Stereology Research Center, Shiraz University of Medical Sciences, Zand Ave., Shiraz 71348-45794, Iran

Mohammad-Bagher Rajabalian, Zahra Jahanabadi and Faisal Ahmed
Department of Urology, Shiraz University of Medical Sciences, Shiraz, Iran

Ali Noorafshan and Saied Karbalay-Doust
Histomorphometry and Stereology Research Center, Shiraz University of Medical Sciences, Zand Ave., Shiraz 71348-45794, Iran
Anatomy Department, School of Medicine, Shiraz University of Medical Sciences, Shiraz, Iran

Anna Pallisera-Lloveras, Laura Mora-López, Sheila Serra-Pla, Salvador Navarro-Soto and Xavier Serra-Aracil
Coloproctology Unit, General and Digestive Surgery Department, Parc Taulí University Hospital, Sabadell, UniversitatAutònoma de Barcelona, Parc Taulí s/n. 08208 Sabadell, Barcelona, Spain

Paula Planelles-Soler, Naim Hannaoui, Jesús Muñoz-Rodriguez, Arturo Dominguez-Garcia and Joan Prats-López
Urology Department, Parc Taulí University Hospital, Sabadell, Universitat Autònoma de Barcelona, Parc Taulí s/n 08208, Sabadell, Barcelona, Spain

Howard Kynaston and Nicholas Bullock
Division of Cancer and Genetics, Cardiff University School of Medicine, Cardiff, UK
Department of Urology, Cardiff and Vale University Health Board, University Hospital of Wales, Cardiff, UK

Krishna Narahari
Department of Urology, Cardiff and Vale University Health Board, University Hospital of Wales, Cardiff, UK

Andrew Simpkin
School of Mathematics, Statistics and Applied Mathematics, National University of Ireland, Galway, Ireland

Sarah Fowler
British Association of Urological Surgeons, London, UK

Murali Varma
Department of Cellular Pathology, Cardiff and Vale University Health Board, University Hospital of Wales, Cardiff, UK

Annemarie Uhlig, Lutz Trojan and Arne Strauss
Department of Urology, University Medical Center Goettingen, Goettingen, Germany

Johannes Uhlig
Department of Diagnostic and Interventional Radiology, University Medical Center Goettingen, Goettingen, Germany
Division of Interventional Radiology, Department of Radiology and Biomedical Imaging, Yale School of Medicine, New Haven, CT, USA

Marc Hinterthaner and Alexander von Hammerstein-Equord
Department of Thoracic and Cardiovascular Surgery, University Medical Center Goettingen, Goettingen, Germany

Hasan Suat Arslantas
Faculty of Medicine, Department of Radiation Oncology, Cukurova University, Adana, Turkey

Yildirim Bayazit, Mustafa Zuhtu Tansug and Volkan Izol
Faculty of Medicine, Department of Urology, Cukurova University, Adana, Turkey

Serkan Gokcay
Department of Medical Oncology, Mehmet Akif Inan Training and Research Hospital, Sanliurfa, Turkey

Hatice Coskun
Faculty of Medicine, Department of Radiation Oncology, Gaziantep University, Gaziantep, Turkey

Yasar Sertdemir
Faculty of Medicine, Department of Biostatistics, Cukurova University, Adana, Turkey

Fundagul Andic
Faculty of Medicine, Department of Radiation Oncology, Cukurova University, Adana, Turkey
Balcali Hastanesi, Radyasyon Onkolojisi AD, Cukurova Universitesi, 01330 Sarıcam, Adana, Turkey

Christoph Oehler, Michel Zimmermann, Lukas Adam and Daniel R. Zwahlen
Department of Radiation Oncology, Kantonsspital Graubünden, Loëstrasse 170, 7000, Chur, Switzerland

Juergen Curschmann, Marcin Sumila and Uwe Schneider
Center for Radiation Oncology, Hirslanden Klinik, Zürich, Switzerland

Räto T. Strebel
Department of Urology, Kantonsspital Graubünden, Chur, Switzerland

Richard Cathomas
Division of Medical Oncology, Kantonsspital Graubünden, Chur, Switzerland

Qiyu Li
Statistics Unit, SAKK Coordinating Center, Bern, Switzerland

Alessio Tognarelli, Francesca Manassero and Cesare Selli
Department of Translational Research and New Technologies in Medicine and Surgery, Sections of Urology, University of Pisa, via Paradisa 2, 56126 Pisa, Italy

Lorenzo Faggioni
Diagnostic and Interventional Radiology, University of Pisa, Pisa, Italy

Angiolo Gadducci
Department of Clinical and Experimental Medicine, Section of Gynecologic Oncology, University of Pisa, Pisa, Italy

Yukari Bando, Koji Chiba, Junya Furukawa, Kenichi Harada, Takeshi Ishimura, Yuzo Nakano and Masato Fujisawa
Department of Urology, Kobe University Graduate School of Medicine, 7-5-1 Kusunoki-cho Chuo-ku, Kobe 650-0017, Japan

Nobuyuki Hinata
Department of Urology, Kobe University Graduate School of Medicine, 7-5-1 Kusunoki-cho Chuo-ku, Kobe 650-0017, Japan
Training Center for Advanced Surgery and Endoscopy, Kobe University School of Medicine, Kobe, Japan

David Bock
Department of Surgery, Institute of Clinical Sciences, Sahlgrenska Academy, University of Gothenburg, SSORG (Scandinavian Surgical Outcomes Research Group), Sahlgrenska University Hospital/Östra, 416 85 Gothenburg, Sweden
Health Metrics Unit, Sahlgrenska Academy, University of Gothenburg, Gothenburg, Sweden

Eva Angenete, Sofie Walming and Eva Haglind
Department of Surgery, Institute of Clinical Sciences, Sahlgrenska Academy, University of Gothenburg, SSORG (Scandinavian Surgical Outcomes Research Group), Sahlgrenska University Hospital/Östra, 416 85 Gothenburg, Sweden

Anders Bjartell
Department of Urology, Skåne University Hospital, Malmö, Sweden

Jonas Hugosson
Department of Urology, Institute of Clinical Sciences, Sahlgrenska Academy, University of Gothenburg, Sahlgrenska University Hospital, Gothenburg, Sweden

Gunnar Steineck
Division of Clinical Cancer Epidemiology, Department of Oncology, Institute of Clinical Sciences, Sahlgrenska Academy, Gothenburg, Sweden

Peter Wiklund
Department of Molecular Medicine and Surgery, Section of Urology, Karolinska Institutet, Stockholm, Sweden

Hong Koo Ha
Department of Urology, Pusan National University Hospital, Busan, South Korea
Pusan National University School of Medicine, Busan, South Korea
Biomedical Research Institute, Pusan National University Hospital, Busan, South Korea

Henk B. Luiting
The Clinical Research Institute, Sydney, Australia
Faculty of Medical Sciences, University of Groningen, Groningen, The Netherlands

Petra L. Graham
Centre for Economic Impacts of Genomic Medicine (GenIMPACT), Macquarie University, Sydney, Australia

Manish I. Patel
Department of Urology, Westmead Hospital, Sydney, Australia
Discipline of Surgery, Sydney Medical School, The University of Sydney, Sydney, Australia

Jaspreet S. Sandhu
Urology Service, Department of Surgery, Memorial Sloan- Kettering Cancer Center, New York, USA

Oguz Akin
Department of Radiology, Memorial Sloan- Kettering Cancer Center, New York, USA

Sean F. Mungovan
The Clinical Research Institute, Sydney, Australia
Westmead Private Physiotherapy Services, Westmead Private Hospital, Suite 6, 16-18 Mons Road, Westmead, NSW 2145, Australia
Department of Health Professions, Faculty of Health, Arts and Design, Swinburne University of Technology, Melbourne, Australia

Xiao Wang, Yiqi Wu, Jia Guo, Hui Chen, Xiaodong Weng and Xiuheng Liu
Department of Urology, Renmin Hospital of Wuhan University, 238Jiefang Road, Wuhan 430060, People's Republic of China

Sigrun Holze, Karl V. Healy and Jens-Uwe Stolzenburg
Department of Urology, University of Leipzig, Liebigstr. 20, 04103 Leipzig, Germany

Meinhard Mende
Coordination Centre for Clinical Trials, University of Leipzig, Härtelstr. 16-18, 04107 Leipzig, Germany

Norbert Koehler and Lutz Gansera
Department of Medical Psychology and Medical Sociology, University of Leipzig, Philipp-Rosenthal-Str. 55, 04103 Leipzig, Germany

Michael C. Truss
Department of Urology, Klinikum Dortmund, Beurhausstr. 40, 44137 Dortmund, Germany

Udo Rebmann
Department of Urology, Diakonissenkrankenhaus Dessau, Gropiusallee 3, 06846 Dessau, Germany

Stephan Degener
Department of Urology, Helios Klinikum Wuppertal, Heusnerstr. 40, 42283 Wuppertal, Germany

Jeffrey Albaugh, Cecilia Chang and Nicholas Kirwen
Northshore University HealthSystem, Evanston, IL, USA

Brittany Adamic and Joshua Aizen
University of Chicago Medical Center, Chicago, USA

Akihiro Nakane, Hiroki Kubota, Yusuke Noda, Tomoki Takeda and Yasuhiko Hirose
Department of Urology, The Aichi Prefectural Federation of Agricultural Cooperatives for Health and Welfare Kainan Hospital, Yatomi, Japan
Department of Nephro-urology, Nagoya City University Graduate School of Medical Sciences, 1 Kawasumi, Mizuho-cho, Mizuho-ku, Nagoya 467-8601, Japan

Atsushi Okada, Noriyasu Kawai, Keiichi Tozawa and Takahiro Yasui
Department of Nephro-urology, Nagoya City University Graduate School of Medical Sciences, 1 Kawasumi, Mizuho-cho, Mizuho-ku, Nagoya 467-8601, Japan

Kentaro Mizuno and Yutaro Hayashi
Department of Pediatric Urology, Nagoya City University Graduate School of Medical Sciences, Nagoya, Japan

Timothy R. Ackland and Daniel J. Green
School of Human Sciences (Exercise and Sport Science), The University of Western Australia, Crawley, Western Australia 6009, Australia

Joanne E. Milios
School of Human Sciences (Exercise and Sport Science), The University of Western Australia, Crawley, Western Australia 6009, Australia
Faculty of Science, School of Human Services (Sport Science, Exercise and Health), University of Western Australia, Parkway Rd, Crawley, Western Australia 6009, Australia

Joanne Nyaboe Nyarangi-Dix, Magdalena Görtz, Luisa Hofer, Viktoria Schütz, Claudia Gasch, Jan Philipp Radtke and Markus Hohenfellner
Department of Urology, University Hospital Heidelberg, Im Neuenheimer Feld 110, 69120 Heidelberg, Germany

Georgi Gradinarov
Ruprecht-Karls University of Heidelberg, Medical Faculty, Heidelberg, Germany

Da-chao Zheng, Min-kai Xie, Shi-bo Fu, Jian-hua Guo, Wen-ji Li, Hai-jun Yao and Zhong Wang
Department of Urology, Shanghai 9th People's Hospital, Shanghai JiaoTong University School of Medicine, NO.369, ZhiZaoJu Road, HuangPu District, Shanghai 200011, China

Hualiang Yu, Yongliang Lu, Yi Xiao, Jiaxiang Guo, Xiaotao Yin, Yu Yang and Jiangping Gao
Department of Urology, The Fourth Medical Center of Chinese PLA General Hospital, 51th Fucheng Street, Haidian District, Beijing 100048, China

Hongwei Wang
Department of Pathology, The Fourth Medical Center of Chinese PLA General Hospital, 51th Fucheng Street, Haidian District, Beijing 100048, China

Asaf Shvero, Dorit Zilberman, Yoram Mor, Harry Winkler and Nir Kleinmann
Department of Urology, The "Chaim Sheba" Medical Center, Ramat-Gan, Israel. Affiliated to Sackler School of Medicine, Tel-Aviv University, Tel-Aviv, Israel

Haim Herzberg
Department Of Urology, Sourasky Medical Center, Tel-Aviv, Israel

Fan Zhang and Shengkun Sun
Department of Urology, The First Medical Center of Chinese PLA General Hospital, Beijing, China
Department of Urology, Hainan Hospital of Chinese PLA General Hospital, Sanya, China

Xu Zhang, Hongzhao Li, Xin Ma and Gang Guo
Department of Urology, The First Medical Center of Chinese PLA General Hospital, Beijing, China

Lisong Shan, Jiahui Yin, Luyang Liu, Pengchao Wang and Qiming Liu
Department of Urology, Hainan Hospital of Chinese PLA General Hospital, Sanya, China

Mohamed Selim, Shady Salem, Eid Elsherif, Atef Badawy and Mohamed Elshazely
Department of Urology, Faculty of Medicine, Menoufia University, Governorate, Menoufia, Egypt

Maher Gawish
Department of Urology, Faculty of Medicine, Alazhar University, Governorate, Assiut, Egypt

Jinghai Hu
Department of Urology, First Hospital of Jilin University, Changchun 130021, People's Republic of China

Shengxian Li
Department of Urology, First Hospital of Jilin University, Changchun 130021, People's Republic of China
Key Laboratory of Polymer Ecomaterials, Changchun Institute of Apllied Chemistry, Chinese Academy of Sciences, Changchun 130022, People's Republic of China

Yuchen Pan
Department of Clinical Epidemiology, First Hospital of Jilin University, Changchun 130021, People's Republic of China

Mmatsie Manentsa, Hilary Mukudu, Nthabiseng Koloane, Ashley Ringane, Eleanor Matta, Neil A. Martinson and Limakatso Lebina
Perinatal HIV Research Unit (PHRU), SA MRC Soweto Matlosana Collaborating Centre for HIV/AIDS and TB, University of the Witwatersrand, Johannesburg, South Africa

Jadwiga Dworak, Michał Wysocki, Anna Rzepa, Michał Natkaniec, Michał Pędziwiatr, Andrzej Budzyński and Piotr Major
2nd Department of General Surgery, Jagiellonian University Medical College, Kopernika 21 St., 31-501 Kraków, Poland

Armin Soave, Luis Kluth, Roland Dahlem, Amelie Rohwer, Michael Rink, Philipp Reiss, Margit Fisch and Oliver Engel
Department of Urology, University Medical Center Hamburg-Eppendorf, Martinistraße 52, 20246 Hamburg, Germany

Index